Nancy Beth Massaro, M.Sc., RN

WORKBOOK FOR

PEARSON'S NURSING ASSISTANT TODAY

First Edition

Francie Wolgin, MSN, RN
Julie French, DNP, RN, CNE
Kate Smith, RN

PEARSON

Boston Columbus Indianapolis New York San Francisco Upper Saddle River
Amsterdam Cape Town Dubai London Madrid Milan Munich Paris Montreal Toronto
Delhi Mexico City Sao Paulo Sydney Hong Kong Seoul Singapore Taipei Tokyo

10 9 8 7 6

PEARSON

ISBN 10: 0-13-510177-8
ISBN 13: 978-0-13-510177-3

Contents

Introduction

This workbook has been written to motivate interest, to instruct, to evaluate, and to involve you, the student, actively in the learning process. We ask you to

- Locate, recall, and recognize information
- Change information into different forms, such as from pictures to words
- Discover relationships, facts, definitions, rules, procedures, and skills
- Find solutions to lifelike situations
- Learn by doing

A variety of exercises have been included in an effort to meet your individual learning needs and to provide an effective learning experience that is compatible with your learning style. The knowledge and skill you gain will help you face the new experiences on the job as a nursing assistant. Question and exercise formats include

- Key Terms Review
- Multiple Choice Questions
- True or False Questions
- Fill-in-the-Blank
- Labeling Exercises
- Matching Exercises
- Completion Exercises
- The Nursing Assistant in Action
- Learning Activities

This workbook is not intended to be used alone. It is totally dependent and coordinated with the textbook *Pearson's Nursing Assistant Today.* It is planned to guide you through the textbook, and it is absolutely essential that you read the textbook as you do each assignment. If you read something that puzzles you, ask your instructor to explain it.

This is not a book of tests, and it is recommended that you keep your textbook open as you complete each assignment. The questions in this workbook were written to help you learn to do the nursing tasks and procedures you will be reading about and studying in your textbook. In addition, procedure checklists appear at the end of the workbook chapters.

You can also use the workbook to review your classroom and clinical learning experiences. By completing these assignments, you can fix the procedures and key ideas firmly in your mind. If you are willing to be an active participant in the learning experiences, this workbook can help you with key terms and can be an effective learning tool.

The more you read, review, and practice, the easier it will be for you to take the step from being a student to being a nursing assistant.

ACKNOWLEDGMENTS

The publisher would like to thank the following individuals for their contributions to, and review of, this workbook:

Teresa K. Novy, MSN, RN-BC
Assistant Professor of Nursing
Heartland Community College

Patricia Graham, MSN, RN, CNE
Nurse Aide Program Director
Front Range Community College, CO

The Health Care System

1

Key Terms Review

Match the key terms in the right column with the definitions in the left column by placing the letter of each correct answer in the space provided.

____ 1. Physician's determination of a patient's disease or condition.

____ 2. Diagnostically related groups of patients.

____ 3. A method of organizing the health care team in which the head nurse assigns and directs all patient care responsibilities for the nursing staff.

____ 4. Hospital, hospice, nursing home, convalescent home, or clinic where health care services are provided on both an inpatient and outpatient basis.

____ 5. An extended, or long-term, care facility that provides health care services to terminally ill patients and their families.

____ 6. A short-term, or emergency, care facility that provides health care services to patients.

____ 7. An individual responsible for providing direction, critiquing performance, and giving feedback related to that performance.

____ 8. A team of professionals and nonprofessionals from different disciplines that plans and implements patient-focused care.

Terms

A. Nurse

B. Hospice

C. Diagnosis

D. DRGs

E. Multidisciplinary team

F. Functional nursing or direct assignment

G. Health care institution

H. Immediate supervisor

I. Hospital

J. Managed Care or Managed Lives Contract

K. Team nursing

L. Team leader

M. Task oriented

N. Nurse manager

O. Primary nursing

P. Nursing assistant

Q. Patient-focused care

____ 9. A person educated and trained to provide health care for people, working with physicians and other health care team members; licensed as RNs and LPNs.

____ 10. A person who helps the registered nurse care for patients.

____ 11. The RN leader responsible for the care delivery, personnel supervision, and operating budget of a unit, area, or facility.

____ 12. A care delivery model in which multidisciplinary teams plan and implement care based on the patient's individual needs.

____ 13. A patient-oriented method of organizing the health care team in which the professional RNs are responsible and accountable for the entire nursing care of the patient.

____ 14. Care provided under a wide variety of prepayment agreements, negotiated contracts and discounts, agreements for prior service authorization or approval, and performance audits.

____ 15. Nursing care arranged according to what must be done.

____ 16. The nurse responsible for one area of a nursing unit, including patient care assignments.

____ 17. A task-oriented method of organizing the health care team in which the team leader gives patient care assignments to each team member.

____ 18. A company that provides health care and physician services to members for a discounted price as long as they use services within the plan.

____ 19. A person who has more than one disease or chronic illness.

____ 20. Nursing care arranged according to what must be done.

____ 21. A team made up of either a nurse or primary care nurse and a nursing assistant who work as partners to deliver patient care.

____ 22. A federal U.S. government program funded by Social Security and available to all individuals over age 65, regardless of income.

____ 23. A U.S. federal public assistance program paid out of general taxes. Each state manages the money received from this program to pay for the medical and health care needs of low-income individuals or families.

____ 24. Federal law that sets minimum training and competency evaluation requirements for nursing assistants.

R. Preferred Provider Organization

S. Comorbities

T. HIPAA

U. Manager

V. Task oriented

W. OBRA

X. Medicare

Y. Partners in practice

Z. Medicaid

_____ **25.** Federal regulation that governs the privacy of medical records.

_____ **26.** The RN leader responsible for the care delivery, personnel supervision, and operating budget of a unit, area, or facility.

MULTIPLE-CHOICE QUESTIONS

Circle the letter next to the word or statement that best completes the sentence or answers the question.

1. Many societal and financial factors affect the health care system directly. Which factor affects how health care is delivered in America?
   a. Government legislation
   b. Nursing assistants
   c. Children
   d. Floral deliveries

2. The nursing assistant in his role is able to contribute directly to the health care system if he can effectively participate in
   a. culturally sensitive care.
   b. the team approach.
   c. cost-effective quality care.
   d. all of the above.

3. It is important to understand the organizational structure in the facility you work because
   a. knowing about this hierarchy helps you be more successful in your role.
   b. this information might be asked on a test.
   c. you will get paid more for knowing this.
   d. you want to impress your friends.

4. At the center of the multidisciplinary team approach is the
   a. nurse.
   b. nursing assistant.
   c. doctor.
   d. patient.

5. What is one of the goals of OBRA?
   a. To allow nursing assistants to do what they think is best for the resident.
   b. To take away the rights of the resident.
   c. To govern hospitals.
   d. To set important guidelines as to how people living in nursing homes are cared for.

6. Preventing disease is an important aspect of the _______ system.
   a. postal
   b. digestive
   c. infective
   d. health care

7. Because the health care system is continually changing, the successful nursing assistant will be looking for opportunities to
   a. work fewer hours.
   b. learn new skills to keep up with these changes.
   c. remain the same, because it always worked in the past.
   d. do her best to resist change.

8. Which of the following is a type of insurance?
   a. DRG
   b. Blue Cross
   c. OBRA
   d. HIPAA

9. DRG stands for
   a. divisional regulated growth.
   b. diagnostic rules and groups.
   c. diagnosis-related groups.
   d. diagonally related growth.

10. HIPAA was created to
  a. allow anyone working in health care access to a patient's health information.
  b. create a universal medical record that could be accessed from anywhere in the country to obtain information about a person's health status and health history.
  c. create safeguards and restrictions regarding disclosure of patient health records.
  d. create rules and methods to lock up health records so a patient could never gain access to his own health information.

11. CPT–4 stands for
  a. *Cost-Preventive Treatment,* 4th edition.
  b. *Currently Posted Trials,* 4th edition.
  c. *Collective Procedural Terminology,* 4th edition.
  d. *Current Procedural Terminology,* 4th edition.

12. *Health care delivery* refers to ______, who provide health care services to patients.
  a. nursing assistants, doctors, nurses, and therapists
  b. hospitals, clinics, and surgical centers
  c. rehabilitation centers, hospices, and home care agencies
  d. all of the above

13. There are several different kinds of nursing care team structures, but a common element is
  a. a nurse accountable for the patient's nursing care.
  b. a nursing assistant as part of the team.
  c. fee-for-service payment.
  d. a doctor performing nursing tasks.

14. Which of the following is a responsibility of the nursing assistant?
  a. Maintaining confidentiality about the patient's health issues
  b. Diagnosing a patient's condition
  c. Withholding care because of a patient's religious beliefs
  d. Offering financial advice

15. No matter what team the nursing assistant works on, the most important element of his success is
  a. to discuss his assignments with the patient.
  b. to discuss his assignment and any questions he may have with his immediate supervisor.
  c. to discuss everything with the team.
  d. to discuss the patients he cares for with his friends.

16. Based on the ______, nursing assistants must complete an approved training program before working in skilled nursing facilities and nursing homes.
  a. Omnibus Budget Reconciliation Act (OBRA) of 1987
  b. direction of the Skilled Nursing Act
  c. American Nursing Home Authority
  d. TEFRA of 1982

17. Which is true about the Medicare program?
  a. All low income persons can receive help from this program.
  b. It is a federally funded program.
  c. Most people who are 35 years or older can apply to receive these benefits.
  d. It is a state funded program.

18. Which is an example of a community-based outreach service that provides assessment or screening?
  a. Having a tooth filled at the dentist's office.
  b. Having a broken bone fixed in the emergency room of a hospital.
  c. A high blood pressure test done by a nurse at the hospital.
  d. A high blood pressure screening done by a nurse at a senior citizen organization.

19. What type of health care facility would a person diagnosed with cancer and who had only a few weeks to live use?

a. Hospice
b. Hospital
c. Long term care (nursing home)
d. Clinic

20. Which type of care model is believed to provide more direct patient care in the form of a team who is cross-trained?

a. Partners in practice
b. Patient-focused care team
c. Primary nursing
d. Functional nursing

21. Which is part of the nurse's responsibility?

a. Diagnose the problem
b. Assess the patient
c. Assign CPT codes
d. Manage the schedule of laboratory technicians

22. Which model of care allows for a nursing assistant and a nurse to work closely together and share in the care taking responsibilities of a group of patients assigned to them?

a. Partners in practice
b. Patient-focused care
c. Functional nursing
d. Team nursing

23. What should be taken into account when offering age-specific care?

a. Recognizing that no matter how old a patient is, everyone should get the same exact care.
b. An older person needs more care because he has the greatest health care needs.
c. The same equipment is used with everyone, no matter what their age.
d. Recognizing that there are different needs a patient may have based on how old they are and their maturity level.

24. The nursing assistant will

a. never be asked to take a competency test.
b. always work alone providing safe and efficient care.
c. never be included in the multidisciplinary team meetings.
d. report any problems with the patient to the nurse supervisor.

25. Which professional name can be used to distinguish a nursing assistant depending on where he or she works?

a. PCT
b. DRG
c. RN
d. EMT

TRUE OR FALSE QUESTIONS

Determine whether each question is true or false. In the space provided, write "T" for true and "F" for false. If the statement is false, rewrite it on the line provided to make it a true statement.

____ **1.** *Patient-focused care* means that the patient's needs are considered first when planning individualized care.

____

____ **2.** To be effective, health care must go beyond the care provided in the hospital to consider the health needs of the community.

____

____ **3.** Most cataract surgery can be done in an outpatient or ambulatory setting.

____

____ **4.** A facility that is separate from a hospital and offers chest x-rays and blood work is a good example of an outpatient facility.

____

____ 5. Providing compassionate care is very important to offering quality customer service.

____

____ 6. Housekeeping staff should be included in the multidisciplinary team.

____

____ 7. A family member is not a customer.

____

____ 8. It is important for a nursing assistant to attend in-services and workshops provided by a facility to update skills and learn about new ways to offer health care to patients.

____

____ 9. A nursing assistant who does not have the same cultural or religious background of a patient can refuse to take care of that patient.

____

____ 10. If a nursing assistant is asked to do something they have not been taught, it is alright to perform this skill or task.

____

FILL-IN-THE-BLANK QUESTIONS

Provide the meaning of the following abbreviations:

1. DRGs ______________________________
2. HIPAA ______________________________
3. RN ______________________________
4. OBRA ______________________________
5. LPN or LVN ______________________________
6. PPO ______________________________
7. HMO ______________________________
8. HHS ______________________________
9. CPT ______________________________
10. AMA ______________________________
11. NA ______________________________
12. NAII ______________________________
13. PCA ______________________________
14. PCT ______________________________

EXERCISE 1-1

Objective: To apply what you have learned about organizational structures and the nursing assistant's "chain of command."

Directions: Label the blank spaces on the organizational chart in Figure 1-1. Place the words from the following word list in the proper order on the diagram.

Word List

Board of Directors	Staff Nurses	Director of Nurses
VP of Operations	LPNs	Nursing Assistants
Nurse Managers	President	

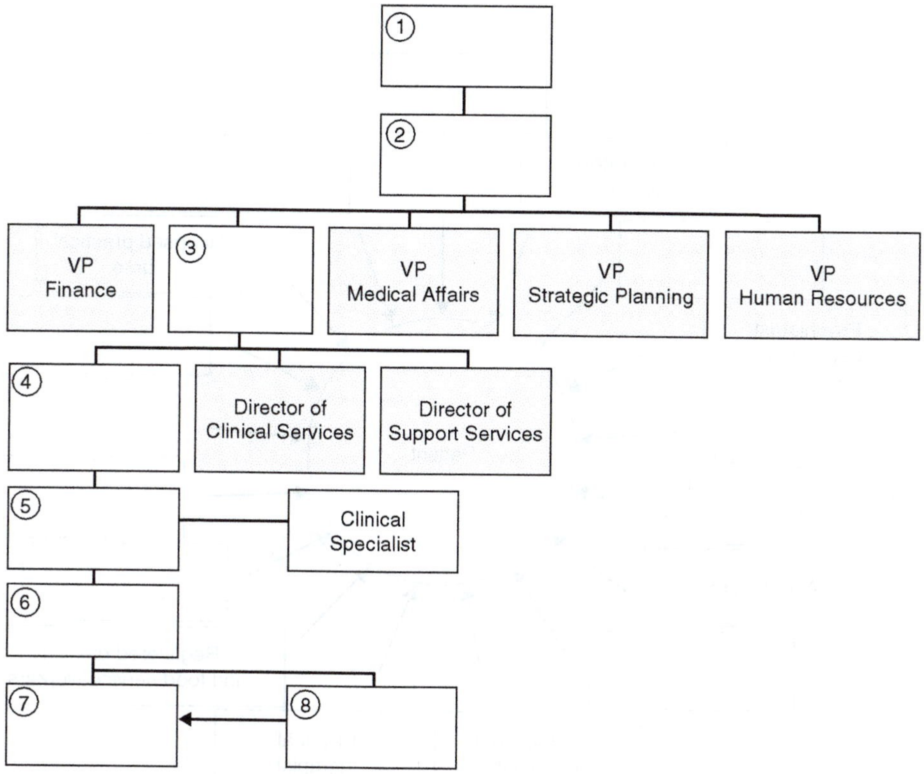

FIGURE 1-1

EXERCISE 1-2

Objective: To apply what you have learned about the multidisciplinary patient care team.

Directions: Label the multidisciplinary patient care team diagram in Figure 1-2 with the correct words from the following word list. Choose from the list only those who are part of this team.

Word List

Clergy	Pharmacist	Beautician	Nursing Assistant
Patient	Veterinarian	Physician	Speech Therapist
Manicurist	Family	Social Worker	Coach
Dentist	Engineer	Pilot	Registered Nurse
			Patient Care Technician

FIGURE 1-2

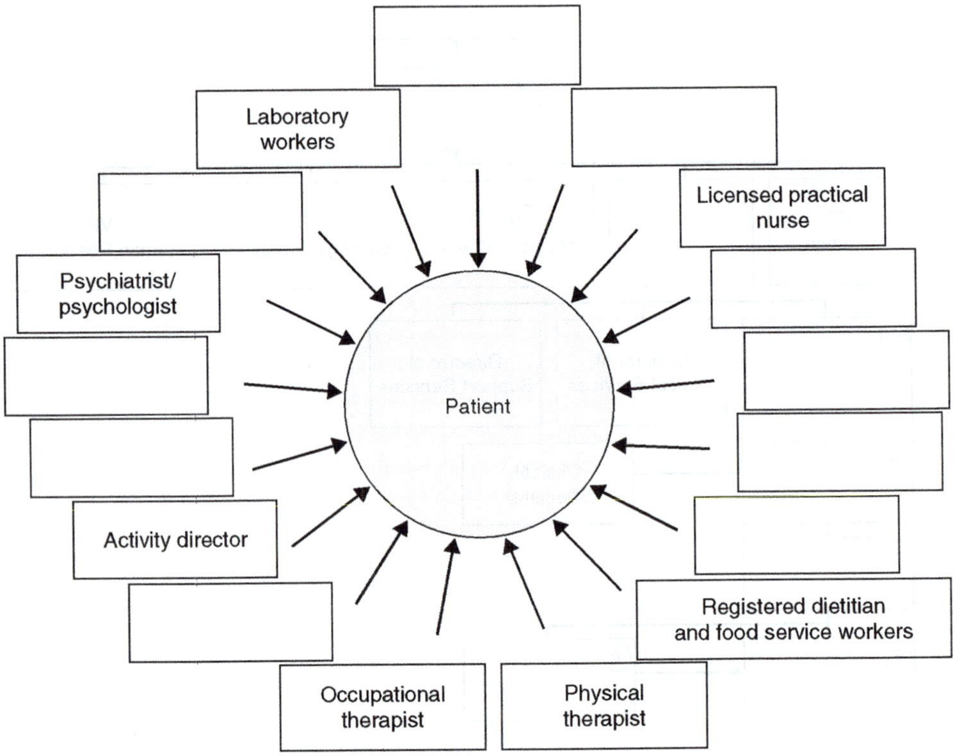

EXERCISE 1-3

Objective: To recognize and correctly spell words related to the health care system.

Directions: Unscramble the words in the following word list and write the correct answer on the line provided.

1. RDG ____________________
2. AANMDGE RAEC ____________________

3. AETM ______________________________

4. IMRPRYA ______________________________

5. AKST ______________________________

6. SPRUEVRIOS ______________________________

7. TAIPNET OCFSDUE ______________________________

8. SRGIETEEDR ESRUN ______________________________

9. AIPHA ______________________________

EXERCISE 1-4

Select from the "Models of Care" the letter of the procedure that best answers each question. Write the correct letter(s) on the blank line next to the question.

A. Functional nursing

B. Team nursing

C. Primary nursing

D. Partners in practice

E. Patient-focused care

____ 1. Which care model(s) could both the nursing assistant and the nurse work closely together and offer their assigned patients the best care?

____ 2. In which care model(s) are small, cross-trained teams used to provide more personalized care to the patient?

____ 3. In which care model(s) does the team leader become teacher, advisor, and helper?

____ 4. The charge nurse or nurse manager assigns nursing staff patient care responsibilities in which care model(s)?

____ 5. The nurse acts as a resource and divides staff into teams offering an assigned group of patients care in which model(s)?

THE NURSING ASSISTANT IN ACTION

1. Your patient is an Orthodox Jew and refuses to eat any food on his tray because he claims it is not kosher. What should you do?

____

____

____

____

2. You are a male nursing assistant and are assigned to give a bath to a Muslim woman. She tells you she cannot have a man see her naked or touch her body because of her culture and religion. What should you do?

3. A patient complains about the care he is being given. Knowing what you know about chain of command, who should you tell on the health care team?

4. A family member calls into the facility via the phone and demands to know what his mother is being treated for and the results of her blood tests. What should you do?

5. A colleague from another floor stops by to visit her aunt, who is one of your patients. A few minutes later, you find this colleague going through this patient's medical records. You know this is a HIPAA violation. What should you do?

LEARNING ACTIVITIES

1. On a piece of paper, list as many outpatient care facilities you can think of that exist in your community. Use the telephone book or Internet if needed. Then compare your list with a friend in class. Pick three outpatient care facilities you are not familiar with and either call to speak with staff or visit the facility. Identify what services are provided. This information will help you gain a broader understanding of healthcare offered in your community and help you decide where you may want to work in the future.

2. Using Figure 1-1 in this workbook as a guide, create your own organizational chart in the facility you plan to work or are already working. Discuss your answer with a friend in class, your instructor, or your current employer to understand the chain of command in a facility.

2

The Role of the Nursing Assistant, Workplace Ethics, and Legal Aspects of Patient Care

Key Terms Review

Match the key terms in the right column with the definitions in the left column by placing the letter of each correct answer in the space provided.

____ **1.** To be answerable for one's behavior; legally or ethically responsible for the care of another.

____ **2.** The quality of being exact or correct; exact conformity to truth and rules; free from errors or flaws.

____ **3.** A skill or ability that may be demonstrated.

____ **4.** Working or acting together; uniting to produce an effect or to share an activity that benefits both parties.

____ **5.** A polite or considerate helpful act or comment.

____ **6.** To authorize, entrust, or assign responsibility to another person to perform nursing tasks within their scope of practice in a given situation.

____ **7.** Being reliable; for example, coming to work every day on time, or doing what is asked at the proper time and in the proper manner.

____ **8.** A physical, mental, or emotional tension or strain triggered by a stimulus that requires some response or type of adjustment.

____ **9.** Planning, prioritizing, and organizing your work and tasks to be completed in a certain period of time.

____ **10.** Identifying a target or desired end and making an action plan to meet it.

Terms

A. Accountable
B. Accuracy
C. Dependability
D. Delegate
E. Courtesy
F. Competency
G. Cooperation
H. Hazard
I. Incident
J. Time management
K. Goal setting
L. Ethical behavior
M. Ethics
N. Libel
O. Defamation of character
P. Malpractice
Q. False imprisonment
R. Patient abandonment
S. Criminal law

____ **11.** Source of danger; possible cause of an accident.

____ **12.** An unforeseen event that occurs without intent.

____ **13.** The science that deals with the preservation of health. When used to describe an object or a person, it means clean and sanitary.

____ **14.** Skills used in interacting with other persons, such as courtesy. Good interpersonal skills help people to interact or work together in a productive and satisfying manner.

____ **15.** The obligation or duty to perform some act, assignment, or function—responsibility.

____ **16.** Actions limited to those that the law allows for specific education and experience, and specific demonstrated competency.

____ **17.** A spoken untrue statement (gossip).

____ **18.** *Carelessness;* a legal term that means either acting or not acting in a way that should have been done. By either acting or not acting, the person fails to behave in the way a reasonably prudent or sensible person would have in the same or similar conditions.

____ **19.** A false statement made in writing, print, or through a picture, cartoon, or drawing.

____ **20.** Negligence when applied to the performance of a professional person.

____ **21.** Unlawful restriction or restraint against the will of an individual's personal liberty or freedom of movement.

____ **22.** The act of leaving, walking off the premises, deserting, or neglecting a patient.

____ **23.** Laws concerned with offenses against the public or society.

____ **24.** Making written or spoken false or damaging statements or misrepresentations about another that harms that person's reputation.

____ **25.** A voluntary act by which a person gives permission for someone else to do something for him. The person must be conscious and mentally competent when giving permission.

____ **26.** To keep promises and do what you should; to follow the rules or standards for right conduct or practice.

____ **27.** The rules or standards that govern right conduct or practice.

T. Informed consent
U. Slander
V. Negligence
W. Responsibility
X. Scope of practice
Y. Hygiene
Z. Interpersonal skills
AA. Stress

MULTIPLE-CHOICE QUESTIONS

Circle the letter next to the word or statement that best completes the sentence or answers the question.

1. Making false or damaging statements about another person is
  a. known as defamation of character.
  b. known as a good standard of care.
  c. a breach of duty.
  d. a way to strengthen a relationship.

2. Working well with others to allow for safe and efficient care is known as
  a. goal setting.
  b. cooperation.
  c. courtesy.
  d. time management.

3. Leaving your patients without permission or without notifying the immediate supervisor is
  a. acceptable if you are sick.
  b. acceptable at the end of your shift, even if no other caregiver has arrived to take your place.
  c. known as abandonment.
  d. important to you.

4. If a nursing assistant leaves a weak, unstable patient alone in the bathroom and the patient is seriously injured,
  a. the nursing assistant is guilty of malpractice.
  b. there is no breach of duty.
  c. the nursing assistant is protected under the Good Samaritan Act.
  d. the nursing assistant may be charged with negligence.

5. Putting a patient in a restraining device without a written doctor's order is known as
  a. invasion of privacy.
  b. liability.
  c. false imprisonment.
  d. a prudent practice.

6. Planning, organizing, and prioritizing tasks allows for tasks to be completed in a certain length of time and is known as
  a. time management.
  b. responsibility.
  c. cooperation.
  d. accuracy.

7. A patient falls out of a bed that was left in the highest position with the rails down. A nursing assistant
  a. does not have to report the fall because the patient does not complain of pain.
  b. must write an incident report and place it in the patient's chart immediately.
  c. must report the incident to the nurse supervisor immediately and write an incident report.
  d. will immediately be fired because of this accident.

8. A quality shown by coming to work every day on time and doing what is asked at the proper time and in the proper way is known as
  a. good hygiene.
  b. malpractice.
  c. liability.
  d. dependability.

9. When professionals, such as registered nurses, are negligent, they can be charged with
  a. the patient's hospital bill.
  b. an advance directive.
  c. impersonating a Good Samaritan.
  d. malpractice.

10. The document from the American Hospital Association describing the basic rights of how the patient and family will be treated is known as
  a. the Good Samaritan Act.
  b. the Hospital Bill of Rights.
  c. a living will.
  d. the Patient Care Partnership.

11. Stress that comes from what a person thinks or does is called
  a. external stress.
  b. internal stress.

c. threat.

d. frustration.

12. Planning family events, balancing work demands, and living up to the expectations of others can increase

a. external stress.

b. internal stress.

c. flexibility.

d. interpersonal skills.

13. The nursing assistant may share a patient's health information with

a. the patient's doctor.

b. housekeeping staff.

c. another healthcare provider.

d. the staff who directly work with the patient.

14. A nursing assistant who is a devote church-goer is assigned to care for a patient who does not believe in God. The nursing assistant should

a. scold the patient for not believing in a higher order.

b. pray for his soul.

c. respect the patient's beliefs.

d. offer minimal care to this non-believer.

15. A patient receives a care package left by his granddaughter. The nursing assistant should

a. open the package for the patient while he is in testing to surprise him when he returns to his room.

b. open the package and help herself to the cookies the granddaughter sent.

c. share the contents of the package with the patient's roommate.

d. keep the package in a safe place and then give the patient the unopened package when he returns from testing.

16. Which is an example of neglect?

a. Leaving a patient in soiled clothing for the shift

b. Withholding water when the patient is NPO

c. Assisting the patient with toileting

d. Initiating measures to prevent a patient from falling

17. A nursing assistant will

a. be rigid in her approach to offering care.

b. cover up any accident that occurs so she does not get in trouble.

c. provide privacy when bathing a patient.

d. share information about the patient with any of his family members.

18. *Ethics* is defined as

a. an action plan that is made to meet a desired goal.

b. rules that govern the correct conduct and practice.

c. obligations a health care worker must perform.

d. giving permission to another person to offer care in a safe manner.

19. The nursing assistant accidentally drops a patient's hearing aid and now it does not work correctly. The nursing assistant should

a. return the hearing aid to the patient and act like nothing happened.

b. tell the patient's wife the hearing aid is broken.

c. tell the audiologist.

d. check to see if it works and tell the nurse in charge.

20. When a new patient is admitted to the unit, the nursing assistant should

a. tell the roommate about the common health conditions both he and the new patient have in common so they have something to talk about.

b. place all money and jewelry the patient arrived with in the patient's dresser for safekeeping.

c. greet them by the name they want to be called and orient them to the room and facility.

d. let the patient figure out how to order meals and work the television and bed controls for himself.

21. A nursing assistant should remember
a. that patients are entitled to respectful care.
b. she does not have to work under the same high standards as other colleagues.
c. she can do exactly what a registered nurse can do.
d. that laws concerning patients and workers in health care facilities protect only the patient.

22. A colleague is frustrated by a patient who has soiled herself many times during the shift. This nursing assistant goes into patient's room, stating, "I have had it with you." The nursing assistant grabs the patient's arm, twists it and the patient's bone breaks. This is an example of
a. assault.
b. battery.
c. slander.
d. libel.

23. You confront a colleague about the tone he uses with patients. He threatens you by stating, "If you tell on me, I will beat you up after work." This is an example of
a. assault.
b. battery.
c. slander.
d. libel.

24. A nursing assistant can maintain safety in the workplace by
a. greeting families with a smile and a welcoming comment.
b. keeping wheelchairs in the proper storage area to reduce clutter in the hallways.
c. avoiding conflict with colleagues.
d. calling off from work when she feels like she needs a break.

25. What is an example of how a nursing assistant can maintain confidentiality?
a. Discuss the patient's diagnosis with his family in a private room.
b. Discuss the patient's condition with other colleagues and ask for advice about this patient's care.
c. Discuss the patient's condition during shift report in a closed room.
d. Allow a colleague from another floor to see the patient's chart while in a locked medication room.

TRUE OR FALSE QUESTIONS

Determine whether each question is true or false. In the space provided, write "T" for true and "F" for false. If the statement is false, rewrite it on the line provided to make it a true statement.

____ **1.** Patients have the right to refuse care, even if they are not conscious.

____

____ **2.** Good Samaritan laws have been developed to protect individuals who try to help people who need emergency care.

____

____ **3.** Escorting patients for a blood test is not a nursing assistant's job.

____

____ **4.** Only housekeeping should disinfect tubs after a patient uses the whirlpool tub.

____

____ **5.** Voluntary acts by which a conscious and mentally competent person gives permission for someone else to do something for him is known as a civil law.

____

____ **6.** It is acceptable to wear the same uniform to work two days in a row and then wash it.

____

____ **7.** A nursing assistant should document all vital signs and any Intake and Output results noted only in the last 5 minutes of her shift.

____

____ **8.** An acceptable and reliable method to reduce stress is to engage in binge drinking.

____

____ **9.** A nursing assistant witnesses a colleague slap a patient. She does not have to report this behavior because the patient did not get hurt or cry.

____

____ **10.** A person can give written instructions in advance that life-support systems shall not be used in the event that they are sick.

____

FILL-IN-THE-BLANK QUESTIONS

Provide the meaning of the following abbreviations.

1. IV ______________________________
2. D/C ______________________________
3. I&O's ______________________________
4. CVC ______________________________
5. HS ______________________________
6. ROM ______________________________

EXERCISE 2-1

Objective: To apply what you have learned about personal hygiene and appearance.

Directions: Look carefully at the pictures in Figure 2-1. Choose the number of the sentence on the Personal Hygiene List that indicates the correct personal grooming rule you must practice on a daily basis. Label the item in Figure 2-1 with the matching number.

Personal Hygiene List

1. Dress properly and neatly. Follow the dress code of the health care institution where you work.
2. Use good personal hygiene, bathing or showering daily.
3. Keep your mouth and teeth clean and in good condition.
4. Keep your hair clean and neatly combed. Long hair should be braided, pulled back, or pinned up.

5. Keep your nails short and clean. Wear only clear nail polish, if any.
6. Wear no or very little makeup.
7. Try to be completely free of odor. Do not use heavy perfume, scented sprays, or heavy shaving lotion. Use an unscented deodorant.
8. Get plenty of sleep. Be alert when you come to work.
9. Keep your body fit; do daily exercises.
10. Wear your nametag where patients can see it.
11. Wear comfortable, low-heeled, enclosed shoes with nonskid soles and heels.
12. Keep your shoes polished and the laces clean.
13. Repair rips and hems and replace missing buttons on your clothing.
14. Eat a well-balanced diet every day.
15. Always wear your nametag and institutional badge.
16. Always wear a wristwatch with a second hand.
17. Always carry a pen and a pad of paper.

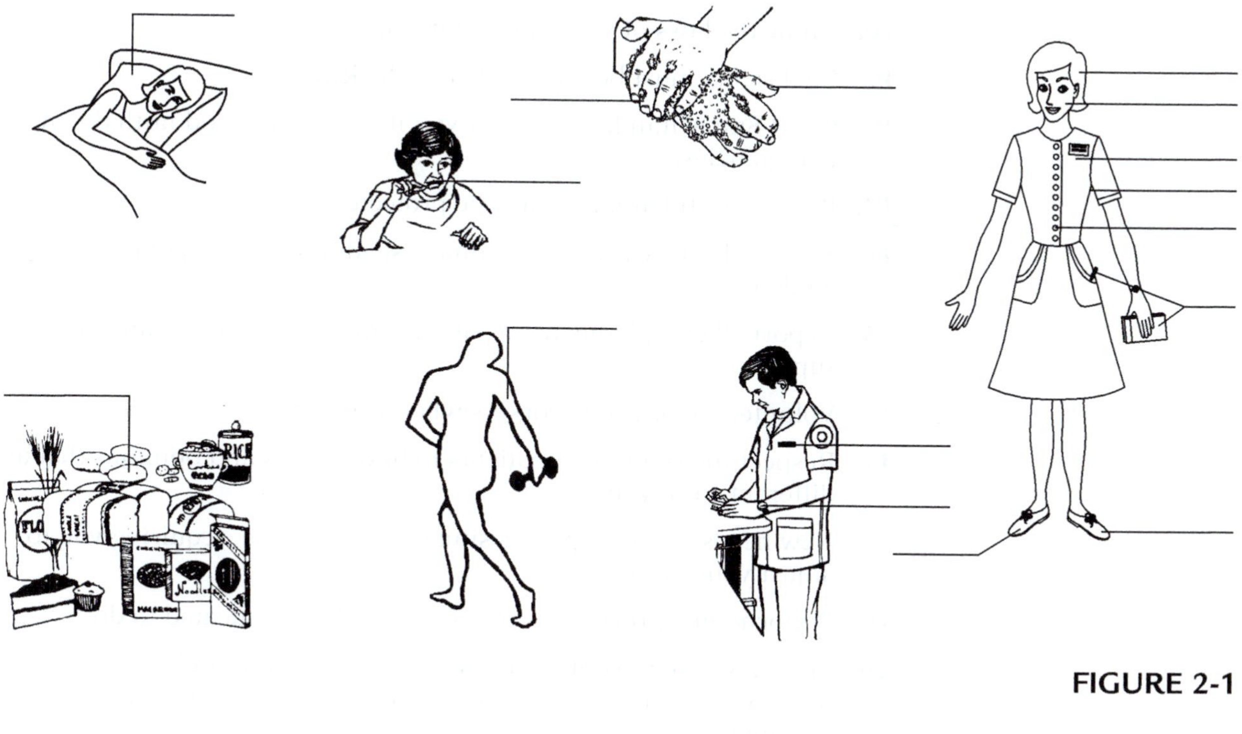

FIGURE 2-1

EXERCISE 2-2

Objective: To be able to recognize important concepts of work organization, ethics, work rules, staff relationships, and the legal requirements of patient care.

Directions: Place the correct letters next to the closest matching phrase. There may be more than one correct answer.

WO—Work Organization
WR—Work Rules
LR—Legal Requirements
SR—Staff Relationships
E—Ethics

____ **1.** The Patient's Bill of Rights or Patient Care Partnership.

____ **2.** Never discuss your personal problems with patients.

____ **3.** Do not waste or destroy supplies or equipment.

____ **4.** Check the patient's ID bracelet for accuracy.

____ **5.** Prioritize your work.

____ **6.** Understand how the law affects you and your patient.

____ **7.** Dependability means more than coming to work on time every day.

____ **8.** Work to be a good team member.

____ **9.** Be ready to adjust quickly to new situations.

____ **10.** Know the laws of your particular state.

____ **11.** Civil rights must be guaranteed to all citizens.

____ **12.** Good Samaritan laws protect you if you act in good faith during emergencies.

____ **13.** Patient confidentiality must be protected.

____ **14.** Standards of care are based on laws, administrative policy, and guidelines.

____ **15.** Report all complaints from patients and visitors to the immediate supervisor.

____ **16.** Volunteer to assist coworkers when you can.

____ **17.** Respect the right of all patients to have beliefs and opinions that are different from yours.

____ **18.** New needs and unexpected situations may arise, requiring you to adjust your priorities.

____ **19.** Perform only procedures that you have been educated to do.

____ **20.** Make a written list of your assignments. Review or change the list as you prioritize your work, and check off each item as it is completed.

EXERCISE 2-3

Objective: To apply principles of ethical behavior to challenging situations in which you may be involved.

Directions: Next to each Practice Description, write the letter of the correct response.

Practice Description

_____ **1.** A patient offers you a tip.

_____ **2.** A patient inquires about another patient across the hall.

_____ **3.** The patient's ID bracelet is on the bedside stand.

_____ **4.** You discover that Mrs. Chang, who is on a low-salt diet, has eaten all of her lunch from a regular diet tray, which you gave her earlier by mistake.

_____ **5.** You have a headache, and nothing seems to be going the way it should today.

Response

A. Refrain from sharing your personal problems as you provide care for others.

B. You notify your immediate supervisor at once.

C. You say, "No, thank you," and pleasantly explain that it is against written policy to accept.

D. You follow the policy of your institution to place the ID bracelet on the patient's wrist for safety.

E. You give no information about the patient, but you do explain the institution's policy on confidentiality.

THE NURSING ASSISTANT IN ACTION

1. You are working the night shift and check on your patients a little after midnight. You find the room dark and hear moaning. You see your patient lying on the floor next to his bed. The bed is in the locked position. The height of the bed is in the highest position. What should you do?

____

____

____

____

2. You are ready to leave for the day and stop in to say goodbye to your patient. She tells you that she soiled herself. You realize that the colleague assigned to this patient is doing a complete bath at this time. What should you do?

____

____

____

____

LEARNING ACTIVITIES

1. Turn to a peer and practice interviewing each other for a potential job for a nursing assistant position. Include questions about qualities and characteristics they need to improve on and what qualities would make them a strong part of the team. Offer each other feedback about the answers offered.

2. Find music that is soothing. Lie down somewhere quiet. Practice one method to help reduce stress called *progressive muscle relaxation.* Listen to the music. Take long, deep breaths, filling your lungs as much as possible. Then let the air out slowly, allowing all air to be expelled. Close your eyes. Continue to breathe. Focus on your toes. Tighten muscles by clenching your toes hard. Hold for 5 seconds. Release and let the tension flow out of your body. Next, move to the muscles in the back of your lower legs. Tighten, hold, and release. Then move to the muscles in your upper legs. Tighten, hold, and release. Slowly, move up your body, focusing on muscles in your back, stomach, chest, hands, arms, and then finally the face, always tightening, holding, and then relaxing while breathing. When finished, be sure to rest for a few minutes—slow your breathing and enjoy your relaxed body. Incorporate new methods to reduce stress so you can stay a healthy and productive health care worker.

Communication Skills: Interpersonal, Written, and Electronic

3

Key Terms Review

Match the key terms in the right column with the definitions in the left column by placing the letter of each correct answer in the space provided.

____ **1.** Nonverbal communication sent through hand movements (gestures), facial expressions, body movements, and touch.

____ **2.** To start up the computer.

____ **3.** The "computer brain," where information is stored or directed to appropriate pathways.

____ **4.** Flashing bar or symbol on the computer screen that shows where the next character is to be placed.

____ **5.** The actual physical equipment used by a computer to process data.

____ **6.** A device similar to a typewriter keyboard; it allows the user to enter, or input, information into the computer. It also has additional keys that allow the user to make selections to direct computer activity.

____ **7.** Computer monitor that allows the computer operator to see input and output on a screen.

____ **8.** Medical records kept electronically on a computer.

____ **9.** A handheld device shaped like a pen that has an electronic sensor for entering information or making selections on a computer screen.

Terms

A. Subjective reporting

B. Subjective observation

C. Empathy

D. Courtesy

E. Tact

F. Body language

G. Feedback

H. Communication

I. Emotional control

J. Constructive criticism

K. Objective observation

L. Objective reporting

M. Observation

N. Pediatric patient

O. Boot up

P. Central processing unit (CPU)

Q. Confidential

R. Prompt

____10. To sign on to the computer using a password or personal identification number (PIN).

____11. A type of computer program designed to provide privacy and prevent phosphor burn-in on plasma computer monitors. It works by blanking the screen or filling it with moving images or patterns when the computer is not in use.

____12. Set or sets of instructions that direct computer operations; computer programs.

____13. Information that a user enters into a computer.

____14. The capacity of the computer to store data.

____15. Several computers connected together, having access to central computer programs; can interface to obtain information; located at different workstations.

____16. A screen, similar to a television screen that allows the user to see input and output.

____17. A pointing and selecting device to input data; a small, tabletop electronic pointing device used to make selections on a computer screen.

____18. A word or phrase that identifies a person and allows access to or entry to a program or record.

____19. A unique combination of letters and numbers used to gain access to your computer system or software programs; your security.

____20. To recall data stored in computer memory.

____21. A portion of data displayed at one time within the confined area of the computer monitor.

____22. An output device for creating a hard copy.

____23. A reminder that the user must take some action so further processing of the data can continue.

____24. Personal or private data, information or knowledge that is not shared with others.

____25. Any patient who is younger than 16 years of age.

____26. Doing or saying the right things at the right time.

____27. The exchange of thoughts, messages, or ideas by speech, signals, gestures, or writing between two or more people.

____28. Response of the receiver to the sender's message; it lets the sender know if the message is acknowledged and clearly understood.

____29. Feedback or advice meant to improve, correct, or help the receiver.

S. Electronic medical record (EMR)

T. Cursor

U. Retrieval

V. Printer

W. Hardware

X. Keyboard

Y. Password

Z. Screen

AA. Mouse

BB. Personal identification number (PIN)

CC. Screensaver

DD. Memory

EE. Software

FF. Data

GG. Network

HH. Terminal

II. Light pen

JJ. Log on

KK. Monitor

_____ **30.** Remaining calm and maintaining self-control in the presence of another individual who may upset you.

_____ **31.** Being polite and considerate.

_____ **32.** The ability to put yourself in another's place and to see things as they see them.

_____ **33.** Gathering information about the patient by noticing any changes.

_____ **34.** Sign that can be observed and reported exactly as it is seen.

_____ **35.** Reporting exactly what you observe.

_____ **36.** Any symptom that can be felt and described only by the patient.

_____ **37.** Giving your opinion about what you have observed.

MULTIPLE-CHOICE QUESTIONS

Circle the letter next to the word or statement that best completes the sentence or answers the question.

1. A patient rings his call bell at mealtime. The nursing assistant answers the signal and the patient says angrily, "What's wrong with this place? I have no fork and my coffee is cold!" The nursing assistant should respond by saying,

a. "I'll do something about it later."

b. "I'll get you a fork and hot coffee right now."

c. "The dietary department must have a lot of new help."

d. "Well, that's the way it is around here."

2. A patient signals by ringing the call bell every 15 to 20 minutes. The nursing assistant responds and notices that the patient is making a lot of small requests, such as, "Please raise the window shade," "Please lower the window shade," "Please turn on the radio," or "Please turn my pillow." The nursing assistant should respond by

a. telling the patient politely not to ring so often.

b. deliberately delaying in answering the call signal or neglecting to answer it at all.

c. explaining to the patient that she has other work to do.

d. reporting to the immediate supervisor, asking what to do and how to handle the situation, and asking the nurse to visit the patient; something is obviously wrong.

3. Mrs. White, a nursing assistant, finished her assignment and is walking down the hall toward the nurses' lounge when another nursing assistant approaches her and says, "Please get Mrs. Smalling in 203-B back to bed for me now. Her doctor is on the nursing unit in another room and wants to examine her. Thank you, Mrs. White. I have to go and get the dressing cart for the nurse so the doctor can change my patient's bandages." The nursing assistant on her way to the lounge should respond by saying,

a. "That's not my job, because it is not my patient."

b. "I will do this right away. By the time you get to Mrs. Smalling's room, she will be in bed."

c. "I am going to complain to the nurse that you are always asking me to do your work."
d. "I am tired from my own assignment, and if this hospital wants me to do two jobs, let them pay me two salaries."

4. The nursing assistant has just been told by the nurse that walking to the linen closet five times during one patient's bed bath is bad technique, time consuming, and not acceptable. One trip should be made, and all the linen needed for one patient must be brought into the room at one time. The nursing assistant should respond by saying,
a. "Thank you for taking the time to teach me. I will try your suggestion now that I understand that what I have been doing is not acceptable."
b. "How dare you criticize me!"
c. "I went to school to learn how to be a nursing assistant, and you have no right to tell me how to do anything."
d. "You always manage to think of something else I do that you do not like; this is the fourth time this morning that you have told me that I am doing something wrong."

5. Miss Smith, a nursing assistant, is told to go to bed 201-A to give the patient, Mrs. Joseph, a message from her family. Miss Smith has never met this patient, and even though other staff members refer to all of the patients by room and bed number, she does not feel this is right. What would be the right way for Miss Smith to greet the patient?
a. "Are you 201-A bed? Your husband called, . . ."
b. "How do you do, Mrs. Joseph. I am Miss Smith, a nursing assistant. May I check your identification bracelet? Thank you. The nurse asked me to give you this message, . . ."
c. "Hi, your husband called, . . ."
d. "Hi, are you the diabetic patient? Well, I have a message for you, . . ."

6. Both verbal and nonverbal communication involves which three important elements?
a. A criticizer, a moderator, and an evaluator
b. A host, an audience, and a sponsor
c. A stretcher, a toner, and an exerciser
d. A sender, a receiver, and a message

7. An example of good body language to use when providing care to a patient is to
a. pause briefly to ask, "How are you?" and then leave quickly before the reply is completed.
b. back slowly out of the room as you are talking.
c. glance out the window often while speaking to the patient about his level of pain.
d. look directly at the arm the patient is describing as painful.

8. A key to good communication is to be ___________when you listen.
a. talking
b. nonjudgmental
c. ready to reply
d. opinionated

9. To distract the child when he is unhappy or fearful means to
a. discipline him for crying.
b. turn his attention to other things, such as a toy or book.
c. tell him to be happy.
d. contact the parents immediately.

10. Being sensitive to times when a patient may not want to talk means
a. you sing happy songs so he won't feel he has to talk to you.
b. you convey your support with positive body language instead of carrying on a conversation with him.
c. you encourage him to "talk things over" with you so he will feel better.
d. you should be offended that he does not talk to you.

11. Pediatric patients are sometimes grouped according to age because
   a. children of different ages play well together.
   b. children of different ages need different kinds of care.
   c. children age differently.
   d. children do better if grouped.

12. What is the most accurate statement about pediatric patients?
   a. Family members need to be with their children.
   b. Most children first learn about the world from their friends.
   c. Family members are usually concerned about the child.
   d. The less serious the illness, the less the child needs his/her family.

13. If you suspect the child has been abused by the family,
   a. ask them if they have stopped beating the child.
   b. report your suspicions and any objective observations to your immediate supervisor at once.
   c. call 911.
   d. take the child away from them immediately.

14. When visitors bring food for the patient,
   a. you must taste the food before the patient eats it.
   b. ask if you may have some.
   c. tell them it is not allowed.
   d. find out if the nurse or doctor has approved this practice.

15. If your patient has a visual impairment, make sure you
   a. have him demonstrate to you that he can use the call light.
   b. leave the call light on the bedside table.
   c. remind him to shut off the light.
   d. all of the above.

16. A(n) __________ has pictures of the patient's equipment and is a tool to help you communicate with the patient.
   a. bulletin board
   b. story board
   c. communication board
   d. notice board

17. Incidents, such as a patient fall, should be reported to your immediate supervisor as soon as you
   a. have time to do so after your break.
   b. observe it or it is reported to you.
   c. can after completing your daily assignment.
   d. can after discussing it with the patient's family.

18. As a nursing assistant, you should be aware of the ________________ in your institution so that you can follow it when you or others have a complaint that must be resolved by your employer.
   a. grievance procedure
   b. complaint process
   c. professional boundary setting
   d. Right to Privacy Act

19. Computers are tools to assist in ______________________ information and getting work done.
   a. entering
   b. storing
   c. retrieving
   d. all of the above

20. Because all patient computer information deals with the private and personal care of the patient, it must be treated in a _______________ manner.
   a. public
   b. confidential
   c. humorous
   d. all of the above

21. Communication is basic to the mutual exchanges of messages that make a connection between the nursing assistant and the patient. What types of things would you do to show good communication skills?
   a. Show an interest in what the patient is saying.
   b. Speak in a pleasant tone.

c. Use good manners, courtesy, emotional control, sympathy, empathy, and tact.
d. All of the above.

22. Your patient appears to be very irritable. What would you do?
a. Try to calm him down.
b. Try to be an attentive and a sympathetic listener.
c. Report this excessive irritability to the nurse or immediate supervisor.
d. Answer the patient in the same irritable manner.

23. Your objective is to report your observations. Which of the following best describes this process?
a. Tell the nurse or immediate supervisor what you think is wrong with the patient.
b. Tell the nurse or immediate supervisor to give the patient some pills.
c. Tell the nurse or immediate supervisor exactly what you saw, smelled, or felt, or what the patient said.
d. Tell the nurse or immediate supervisor to observe the patient.

24. The nurse or immediate supervisor has given you instructions to report exactly what the patient eats at mealtime and not to give the patient anything between meals. However, during visiting hours, you notice that the patient is eating a hot dog that was brought in by a visitor. What would you do?
a. Speak to the patient and take the food away immediately.
b. Call the visitors outside the room and send them home.
c. Tell the doctor.
d. Report this to the nurse or immediate supervisor right away.

25. Which is the correct way to document in military time 8:05 AM?
a. 0805
b. 2005
c. 1805
d. 8005

TRUE OR FALSE QUESTIONS

Determine whether each question is true or false. In the space provided, write "T" for true and "F" for false. If the statement is false, rewrite it on the line provided to make it a true statement.

____ **1.** The sender must send a clear message.

____

____ **2.** The receiver should ask for clarification if necessary.

____

____ **3.** When working with patients, the message should be unclear, complex, disorganized, and complicated in order to challenge the listening skills of the receiver.

____

____ **4.** A smile can communicate many positive things to a child.

____

____ **5.** Addressing adults in the manner they prefer, such as "Mrs. Smith" rather than "Grandma," shows that you respect them as people.

____

____ **6.** Communicating with patients who have hearing or speaking impairments is helped by the use of a pad of paper and a pencil to communicate in writing.

____

____ **7.** If your patient speaks a different language or needs sign language, your employer or institution must address that need.

____

_____ 8. Giving your password and PIN number to another colleague promotes good communication and teamwork.

____

_____ 9. If a mistake is made in documenting, you should take a black marker and color the mistake so no one can see what was written in the chart.

____

_____ 10. Stating, "I am going to take your vital signs now" is the correct way to tell a two-year-old you will obtain his temperature, pulse, respirations, and blood pressure.

____

FILL-IN-THE-BLANK QUESTIONS

Provide the meaning of the following abbreviations.

1. EMR _______________________________
2. CPU _______________________________
3. PIN _______________________________
4. CBT _______________________________
5. ID _______________________________
6. IS _______________________________

EXERCISE 3-1

Label the correct parts of the computer using the following word list.

1. Monitor
2. Mouse
3. Screen
4. Terminal
5. Cursor
6. Bar code
7. Scanner or bar code reader
8. Keypad
9. Light pen
10. Keyboard
11. Printer

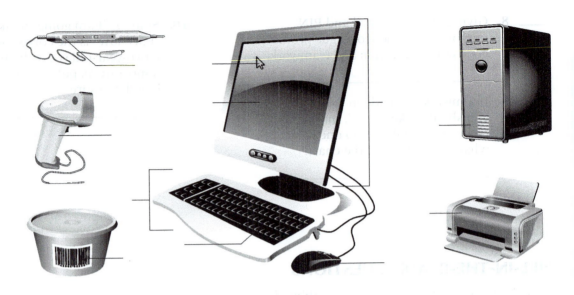

EXERCISE 3-2

Place the military time on the clocks shown next.

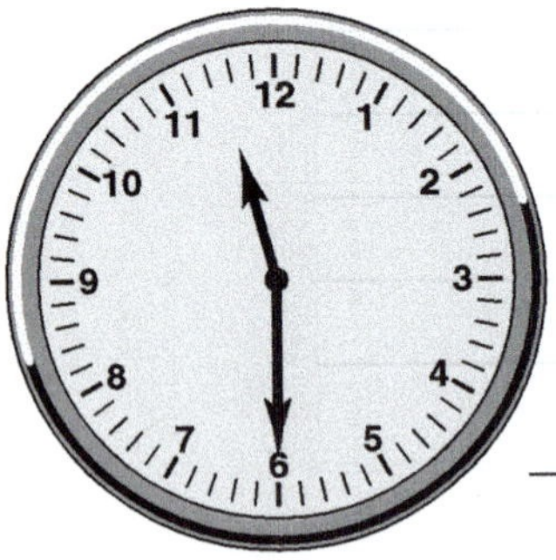

______________ (Morning)

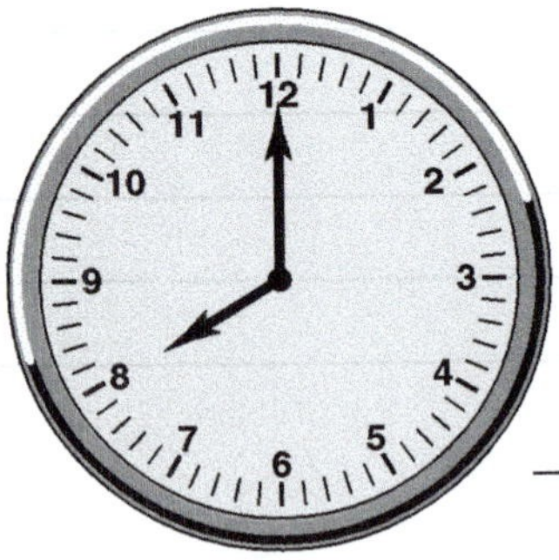

______________ (Morning)

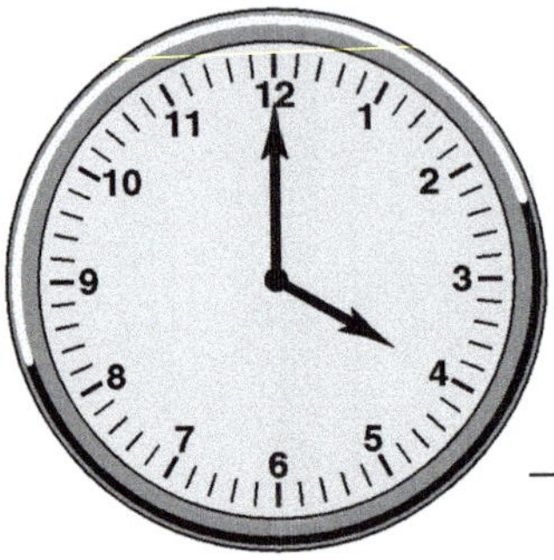

______________ (Afternoon)

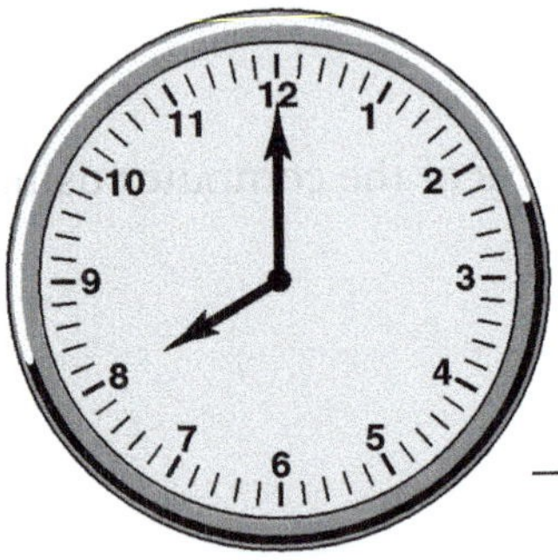

______________ (Night)

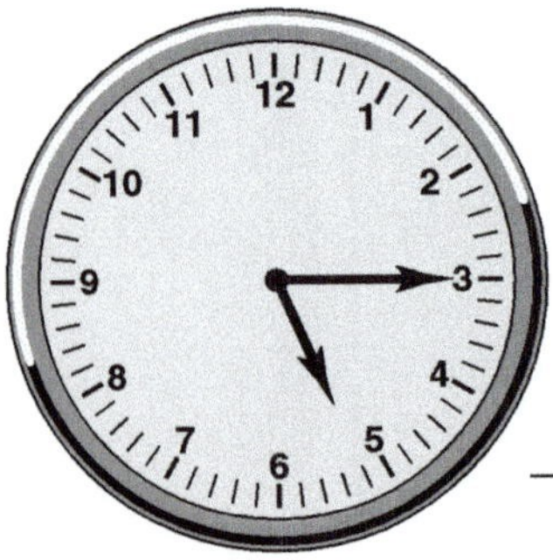

______________ (Morning)

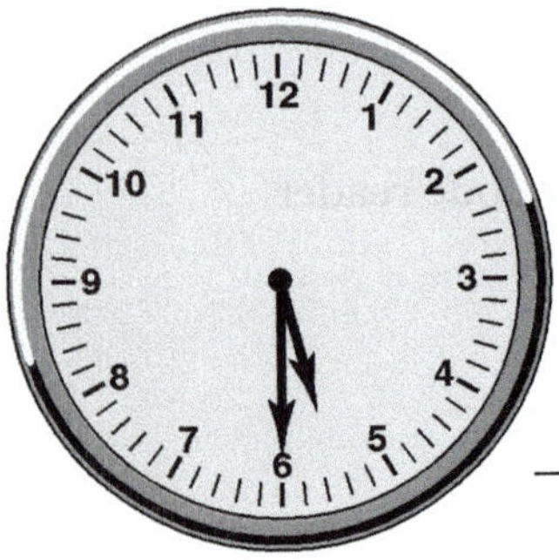

______________ (Evening)

EXERCISE 3-3

Read each statement below. Write "S" for subjective or "O" for objective where it applies.

_____ **1.** The father of a pediatric patient tells you, "My son had his appendix removed last year."

_____ **2.** The infant you are taking care of has been crying for 1 hour.

_____ **3.** A postsurgical patient is holding his stomach tightly and is bent over in bed.

_____ **4.** A teenage patient whimpers and cries out when you touch his arm.

_____ **5.** A frail older patient states, "I have not gone to the bathroom or had a bowel movement in a week."

_____ **6.** You set a patient up for a bed bath and notice she is sweating profusely.

_____ **7.** You smell alcohol on the patient's breath.

_____ **8.** You put a patient back to bed and see his feet are purple and very swollen.

_____ **9.** The patient screams out, "This medicine in my IV feels like it is burning my veins!"

_____ **10.** A 90-year-old patient tells you, "King Henry VIII came to visit me last night."

THE NURSING ASSISTANT IN ACTION

1. Mrs. Hernandez is receiving a blood transfusion that has been running for the past hour. As you are making her bed, you notice that the color of the patient's face has changed. She now has very red cheeks. Mrs. Hernandez cannot speak English and communicating with her is difficult. You then notice that Mrs. Hernandez is scratching her arms and legs and seems very agitated. What should you do?

____

____

____

____

2. A patient complains to you that his IV hurts. You look at the area on the patient's arm around the needle. It appears red and swollen. What should you do?

____

____

____

____

3. You have been taking care of Mrs. Jones for the past 2 days. Mrs. Jones has been able to get out of bed and brush her teeth in the bathroom; however, today she says to you, "I will brush my teeth later. I don't feel so good today. I am going to stay in bed. Don't bring me any breakfast." What should you do?

4. Your patient was fine this morning and was able to get out of bed and walk around his room. However, after lunch, you notice that the patient is lying very quietly in his bed, does not answer when you talk to him, and his face is very red. What should you do?

5. Mr. Murray had four bowel movements in the past 2 hours. The last time he wasn't able to wait for the bedpan and soiled the bed. Yesterday, he had one bowel movement the entire day. What should you do?

LEARNING ACTIVITIES

1. Pair with a classmate or friend. One of the pair should be blindfolded and pretend to be a patient with a visual impairment. The other partner should pretend to be a nursing assistant. Make believe the patient who is living with a visual impairment is new to the unit. Take 5 minutes to figure out how you will orient the patient to the layout of the room she is assigned, the equipment in the room, and make the necessary introductions with the roommate and the staff. Take into consideration any safety issues and customer service measures that will assure smooth transition to the unit. Allow for some time to discuss how it felt to be the patient. Allow for discussion about what things were done well by the nursing assistant and what things could have been added to insure optimal care and safety of a visually impaired patient were initiated.

2. Have a classmate or a friend get a piece of blank paper. Do not show them the following picture, and do not look at what they are drawing. Using good communication skills, have them draw what you describe on the blank piece of paper. Allow 5 minutes or less. When the time is up, compare the following drawing to the drawing your partner produced. Discuss the strong and weak points made when communication occurred.

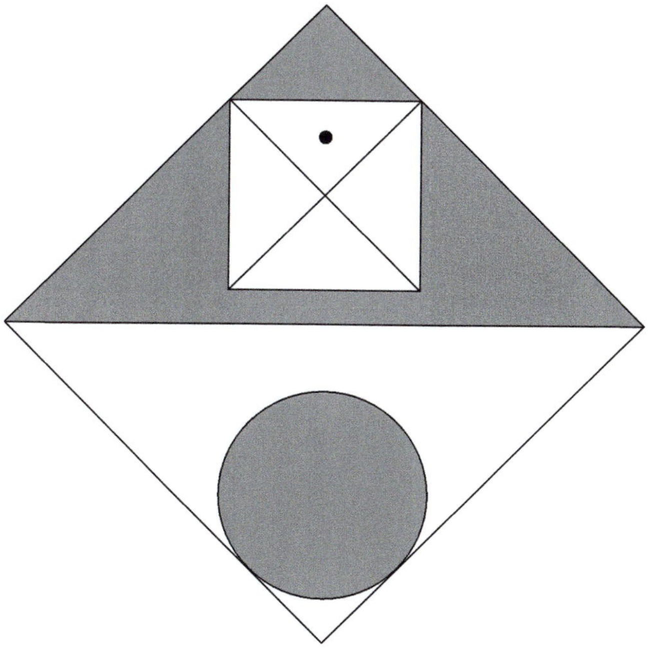

Now think of a situation in your life when miscommunication occurred. Identify some things that could improve on how the message was sent and how the message was received.

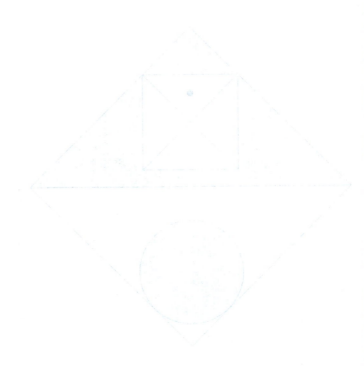

4

Medical Terminology, Abbreviations, and Specialties

Key Terms Review

Match the key terms in the right column with the definitions in the left column by placing the letter of each correct answer in the space provided.

____ **1.** The word root plus the combining vowel, which is always written with a backward slash (/) between the root word and combining vowel.

____ **2.** A vowel (usually *o*) placed between word parts that makes it possible to pronounce medical terms.

____ **3.** A shortened form of a word commonly recognized as representing that word.

____ **4.** The study of medical words and their uses.

____ **5.** A word part added in front of the word root. It often gives information about the location of an organ, the number of parts, or the time.

____ **6.** A word part attached to the end of a word. It often indicates a condition, disease, or procedure.

____ **7.** The part of a medical term that gives a word its essential meaning.

Terms

A. Root word

B. Suffix

C. Prefix

D. Abbreviation

E. Combining form

F. Medical terminology

G. Combining vowel

MULTIPLE-CHOICE QUESTIONS

Circle the letter next to the word or statement that best completes the sentence or answers the question.

1. A *prefix* is
- a. placed at the end of a word.
- b. the main part of the word.
- c. placed at the beginning of the word.
- d. a shortened form of a word.

2. Which medical term means *small*?
- a. Macro
- b. Grande
- c. Micro
- d. Megaly

3. The suffix *–ectomy* means
- a. surgical removal.
- b. surgical incision.
- c. cutting into and leaving an open wound.
- d. surgical repair.

4. How would you abbreviate *electrocardiogram*?
- a. EEC
- b. EKG
- c. ECG
- d. Both b and c are accepted abbreviations

5. DX means
- a. discontinue.
- b. discharge.
- c. disregard the chart.
- d. diagnosis.

6. Which is the correct way to spell the medical term meaning heart attack?
- a. Myocardial infarction
- b. Myocardial infartion
- c. Mycardiac infarction
- d. MI

7. A patient who has *dysuria*
- a. may have a difficult time or pain when urinating.
- b. may have difficulty swallowing.
- c. may have a difficult time seeing.
- d. may have pain when having a period (menses).

8. *Postsurgical* means
- a. during surgery.
- b. before surgery.
- c. stop surgery.
- d. after surgery.

9. A medication that is ordered *STAT* means
- a. the medication should be given immediately.
- b. the medication should be stopped immediately.
- c. the nurse should start the antibiotic today.
- d. give the medication when needed.

10. An order that reads "Perform ROM QID" means
- a. range of motion should be given every day.
- b. range of motion should be given every other day.
- c. range of motion should be offered as needed.
- d. range of motion should be given four times a day.

11. The abbreviation *NKA* means
- a. no known antibodies.
- b. no known allergies.
- c. nothing kept away.
- d. None of the above

12. Because the Joint Commission discourages the use of abbreviations, you should
- a. never abbreviate medical terms.
- b. check with your facility about their policy when abbreviating.
- c. use only those terms the Joint Commission approves.
- d. use only those abbreviations you remember when documenting.

13. Fluid intake can be documented using a metric unit of measurement known as
a. mL.
b. I&O.
c. kg.
d. oz.

14. Which abbreviation is used when documenting the patient cannot have anything to drink?
a. NKA
b. PO
c. NPO
d. mL

15. Which physician is the best one to use if urinary problems occur?
a. Obstetrician
b. Gastroenterologist
c. Internist
d. Urologist

16. Corrective lenses can be ordered by a(n)
a. ophthalmologist.
b. otolaryngologist.
c. nurse.
d. general practitioner.

17. Your patient had a CVA. She may need
a. help with performing ADLs.
b. help getting on and off the BSC.
c. extra ROM.
d. all of the above.

18. Which is the correct abbreviation for *every two hours*?
a. QD
b. QOD
c. Q2h
d. BID

19. The correct spelling of the medical term that means removal of the appendix is
a. appendectomy.
b. appendicitis.
c. appendoma.
d. appendices.

20. A patient has been diagnosed with *pericarditis*. This means he has
a. a heart transplant.
b. inflammation surrounding the heart.
c. pain in the heart.
d. a cut in the heart that has become inflamed.

21. Prefixes and suffixes combined with ______ make a medical term.
a. root words
b. abbreviations
c. plurals
d. specialists

22. When adding an *a-* to the beginning of a word, it changes the meaning of the root to mean
a. first.
b. without.
c. against.
d. pertaining to.

23. When adding *-ic* as a suffix, it means
a. pertaining to.
b. against.
c. without.
d. last.

24. The suffix *-ology* means
a. specialist.
b. study of.
c. science.
d. disease.

25. Which two medical prefixes can be used to note the size of something?
a. Macro- and micro-
b. Large and small
c. Kg and mL
d. anti- and a-

TRUE OR FALSE QUESTIONS

Determine whether each question is true or false. In the space provided, write "T" for true and "F" for false. If the statement is false, rewrite it on the line provided to make it a true statement.

____ **1.** A shortened word or phrase used to represent the complete form is a(n) abbreviation.

____

____ **2.** The special vocabulary used in health care professions is referred to as *medical terminology*.

____

____ **3.** The word element that is always added to the end of a root to change or add meaning is the prefix.

____

____ **4.** The body or the main part of a word is the root.

____

____ **5.** A physical therapist (PT) can work with patients who are rehabilitating from disabilities caused by a stroke.

____

____ **6.** The abbreviation *"HOH"* means hard of hearing.

____

____ **7.** Specialists usually continue their schooling in order to treat illnesses that affect a particular body system.

____

____ **8.** An oncologist treats patients living with tumors that are either cancerous or non-cancerous.

____

____ **9.** An ENT doctor is an otolaryngologist.

____

____ **10.** It is easy to understand a new medical term by breaking the word into three parts to decipher its meaning: the prefix, the root, and the suffix.

____

EXERCISE 4-1

Use the following words to fill in the blanks correctly in the following sentences.

Word List

abbreviation
medical terminology
prefix
root
suffix

1. A shortened word or phrase used to represent the complete form is a(n) __________.

2. The special vocabulary used in the health care profession is referred to as __________.

3. The word element always added to the end of a root to change or add meaning is the __________.

4. The body or main part of a word is the __________.

5. A(n) __________ is a word element added to the beginning of a root.

EXERCISE 4-2

Recognize and label correctly abbreviations of terms using the lines provided.

1. Nothing by mouth ____________________
2. Oxygen ____________________
3. Intravenous ____________________
4. Before surgery ____________________
5. Head of bed ____________________

EXERCISE 4-3

Write the meaning of the abbreviation using the lines provided.

1. RN ____________________
2. ADL ____________________
3. H&P ____________________
4. HOH ____________________
5. BSC ____________________
6. CVA ____________________
7. HTN ____________________
8. OOB ____________________
9. LPN ____________________

EXERCISE 4-4

Draw a line from the first column, which identifies the type of physician, with the correct answer in the second column, which defines what kind of care this physician provides.

Physician	Description
Allergist	Treats patients with diseases of the heart and circulatory system.
Cardiologist	Treats diseases and disorders of the muscular and skeletal systems.
Gynecologist	Treats patients with allergies.
Orthopedist	Treats patients with mental disorders.
Psychiatrist	Treats patients with diseases of the female reproductive organs.

THE NURSING ASSISTANT IN ACTION

1. You review the patient care plan and find the following is ordered for your patient:

   OOB with assist X 1 QID

   What does this mean?

   ____
   ____
   ____
   ____

2. You are getting report during shift change and your supervisor explains that a new patient will be admitted shortly.

   He is HOH and needs a BSC.

   What does this mean, and what equipment must you get?

   ____
   ____
   ____
   ____

3. A patient living with a CVA arrives on your unit. Her orders read:

   ROM to left arm TID; reposition Q2h; OOB to w/c with assist X 2 PRN

   What does this mean?

   ____
   ____
   ____
   ____

4. You are assigned to care for the patient who has a DX of DM. Her orders read:

   Obtain a FBS via fingerstick ac and call MD STAT if FBS > 240 mg/dL

   What does this mean and what must you do?

   ____
   ____
   ____
   ____

5. A patient is getting prepared for open-heart surgery. His H&P states:

   Past HX: MI in 2011

   Primary DX: HTN, DM

   NKA

The orders read:

NPO after midnight

Obtain a UA via Foley catheter STAT

Obtain CBC STAT

Obtain EKG STAT

BP X Q4h

OOB PRN

Interpret what this means and what you must do.

____

____

____

____

LEARNING ACTIVITIES

1. **Objective:** To learn the list of abbreviations and their meanings. This is a long list, and there is a lot of important information to learn. It will be easier to remember what all the different abbreviations are if you try to learn them one at a time. One way to learn the list is to study from flashcards. You can create your own set of flashcards by using 3" × 5" index cards. Write the abbreviation on one side and the meaning on the other side. Now you can test yourself.
   1. Arrange all the cards so the name of the abbreviations is facing up and the meaning is facing down.
   2. Read the name of the first abbreviation in your stack.
   3. Try to remember the meaning from studying your textbook.
   4. Say the meaning out loud.
   5. Turn the card over and read the meaning to see if you were right.
   6. If you were correct, put the card in a pile on the left. You are finished studying this card.
   7. If you were wrong, put the card in a pile on the right, so you can study it later.
   8. Repeat this for all the cards.
   9. Now go back to the pile of cards on the right and study these.
   10. Read each card, front and back, five times.
   11. Close your eyes and try to say the name of the abbreviation and its meaning.
   12. Open your eyes and see if you were correct.
   13. Repeat this for all the cards that you originally put on the right side.
   14. When you believe that you have learned them all, test yourself again.
   15. Ask someone to test you by holding the first card up to you can see the abbreviation. Read the abbreviation and recite the meaning.
   16. Your friend can read the meaning to determine if you are correct.
   17. Repeat for all the cards.

18. Turn the stack upside down.
19. Now go through the cards, read the meanings, and tell the name of the abbreviations.
20. Repeat this until you have learned all the abbreviations and their meanings.

2. Using the flashcards that you made from the previous learning activity, try to combine words. For instance, take a flashcard for a prefix, add a root, then add the suffix and see if you can drop the combining vowel correctly and spell a new medical term. Check if this actually is a medical term, if you spelled it correctly, and define the new meaning of the word by using one of the resources mentioned in your textbook, such as one of the following:
   - *Taber's Cyclopedic Medical Dictionary*
   - *Merriam-Webster's Medical Dictionary*
   - Rice, Jane. *Medical Terminology: A Word-Building Approach,* 7th Edition. Pearson/Prentice Hall. 2012. ISBN: 0132148021
   - Turley, Susan. *Medical Language: Immerse Yourself,* 2nd Edition. Pearson/Prentice Hall, 2011. ISBN: 0135055784
   - www.online-medical-dictionary.org

5

Patients, Residents, and Clients

Key Terms Review

Match the key terms in the right column with the definitions in the left column by placing the letter of each correct answer in the space provided.

____ **1.** The variety of races, religions, and cultures in the world.

____ **2.** The thoughts, beliefs, and values of a social group.

____ **3.** Factors such as attentiveness, quality of food, and cleanliness of environment that affect the care and comfort of the individual receiving health care.

____ **4.** A requirement for survival.

____ **5.** Care designed to meet the needs of patients, residents, and clients (customers).

____ **6.** An individual cared for in a nursing home or other long-term/extended care facility.

____ **7.** An individual cared for by a home health agency or provider.

____ **8.** An individual admitted to an inpatient or outpatient hospital, physician's office, or clinic.

____ **9.** Ways for dealing with a dangerous situation involving a patient, resident, or client.

Terms

A. Service

B. Ethnic diversity

C. Culture

D. Patient

E. Client

F. Resident

G. Physical crisis management

H. Customer-focused care

I. Need

MULTIPLE-CHOICE QUESTIONS

Circle the letter next to the word or statement that best completes the sentence or answers the question.

1. Patients, families, and visitors judge the care given to their loved one based on
   a. the helpfulness of the staff.
   b. employee behavior.
   c. personal attentiveness and interaction of the staff.
   d. all of the above.

2. Dissatisfied customers may complain about the care they receive to an average of _______ other relatives, friends, or acquaintances.
   a. 4
   b. 7
   c. 200
   d. 20

3. Currently, _______ make up the largest growing minority population in America.
   a. Latinos
   b. Chinese
   c. African Americans
   d. Pacific Islanders

4. Which level of need is the most basic, according to Maslow?
   a. Esteem needs
   b. Belonging needs
   c. Security needs
   d. Physiological needs

5. To be respectful of a patient's cultural differences, the nursing assistant should _______ rather than evaluate his behavior.
   a. listen
   b. observe
   c. describe
   d. all of the above

6. _______ are not easily translated into other languages, cultures, or value systems and are usually misunderstood.
   a. Directions
   b. Songs
   c. Poems
   d. Jokes

7. Part of the job of the nursing assistant is to try to show the patient that the health care institution is a friendly place and that the major concern is for the patient's
   a. discharge.
   b. well-being.
   c. cure.
   d. cultural diversity.

8. If a patient appears upset because of difficulty communicating, the nursing assistant should
   a. explain to him that the care team is friendly.
   b. report this to your immediate supervisor and reassure the patient.
   c. speak louder.
   d. write the directions on a flash card.

9. Because of cultural differences regarding modesty, it is a good idea to
   a. drape the patient's entire body at all times to be safe.
   b. ask your supervisor for suggestions to protect the patient's modesty.
   c. ask the patient to stop being so different.
   d. keep the privacy curtain closed at all times.

10. In Maslow's hierarchy, _______ needs must be met before higher-level needs.
   a. lower-level
   b. middle-level
   c. end-level
   d. beginning-level

11. An example of a lower-level need is
   a. food.
   b. music.
   c. love.
   d. self-esteem.

12. Unmet needs can cause people to show physical reactions, such as
   a. anger.
   b. depression.

c. weakness.
d. all of the above.

13. It is during sleep that
a. muscles contract.
b. brain activity is at its highest.
c. tissues heal.
d. body temperature is highest.

14. People need to spend enough time in ______ sleep each night to feel rested.
a. ROM
b. REM
c. NREM
d. PROM

15. The nursing assistant must make ______ a priority when dealing with disruptive patients or families.
a. safety
b. humor
c. speed
d. sleep

16. Remember that many people want their *say,* not their
a. *pay.*
b. *way.*
c. *day.*
d. *play.*

17. A patient is angry. The nursing assistant should
a. remain calm.
b. frown and explain you disapprove of their behavior.
c. speak loudly and tell them to calm down.
d. turn your back on them and stand as far away as you can.

18. A patient appears very stressed and anxious. The nursing assistant should
a. be supportive.
b. ignore them and let them have time to work things out.
c. stare at them until they talk about their concerns.
d. suggest they exercise.

19. A patient is crying, moaning, and pacing back and forth in her room. The patient tells you she is not in any pain. The nursing assistant should
a. increase the volume of music in her room to help calm her.
b. suggest she walk around the floor so she has some time to think about her problems.
c. tell the nurse what the patient said and what was observed.
d. suggest she sleep.

20. When patients hallucinate, the nursing assistant should
a. immediately bring them to their rooms.
b. restrain them at all times.
c. keep other patients away from them.
d. protect them from hurting others and themselves.

21. A patient speaks very little English, but his family tells you he understands English well. You should
a. first touch his arm to make sure you have his attention and then speak softly.
b. speak slowly and calmly, and then ask the patient to explain to you what was said.
c. shout to the patient so you are sure he can hear everything you have to say.
d. give the patient a pad of paper and pencil to take notes.

22. Usually for Americans and Canadians, personal space where comfortable communication can occur in is usually within
a. 1½ feet.
b. 5–50 inches.
c. 6 feet.
d. 2 inches.

23. A newborn baby may require ______ hours of sleep a day.
a. 6–8
b. 20
c. 2
d. 12

24. What is the best statement to consider before touching a patient?

a. When caring for most Americans and Canadians, stay approximately 5 feet away so this patient feels comfortable.

b. Consider the patient's cultural background and assess body language before touching a patient.

c. All patients should be all right with receiving help with personal hygiene regardless of their culture.

d. If any patient is crying, it is your duty to hold their hand or hug them to make them feel comforted.

25. *Culture* is defined as

a. the variety of races, religions, and cultures in the world.

b. the behavior of the patient.

c. the thoughts, beliefs, and values of a social group.

d. the intellectual development of a person.

TRUE OR FALSE QUESTIONS

Determine whether each question is true or false. In the space provided, write "T" for true and "F" for false. If the statement is false, rewrite it on the line provided to make it a true statement.

____ **1.** Dissatisfied customers may not complain, but they may often return to the same institution.

____

____ **2.** There are 17 goals of customer service.

____

____ **3.** Ethnic diversity is decreasing in the United States.

____

____ **4.** *Different* means the wrong way of doing things.

____

____ **5.** It is a good idea to use culturally diverse gestures when communicating.

____

____ **6.** Whenever possible, plan care to accommodate the patient's sleep preferences.

____

____ **7.** In some cultures, you should not handle the body until certain religious authorities arrive.

____

____ **8.** Some vegetarians will not eat anything that is produced by an animal, such as butter, eggs, and meat.

____

____ **9.** Avoid asking questions where the response may be "yes" or "no." This ensures better communication.

____

____ **10.** Transcultural care means that a nursing assistant must deliver care to many people with different backgrounds and many different beliefs.

____

FILL-IN-THE-BLANK QUESTIONS

Provide the meaning of the following abbreviations.

1. REM ____
2. NREM ____

EXERCISE 5-1

Label Maslow's Hierarchy of Needs by placing the correct need from the list provided into the correct section of the pyramid.

Word List

Physiology
Self-actualization
Love and belonging
Esteem
Safety

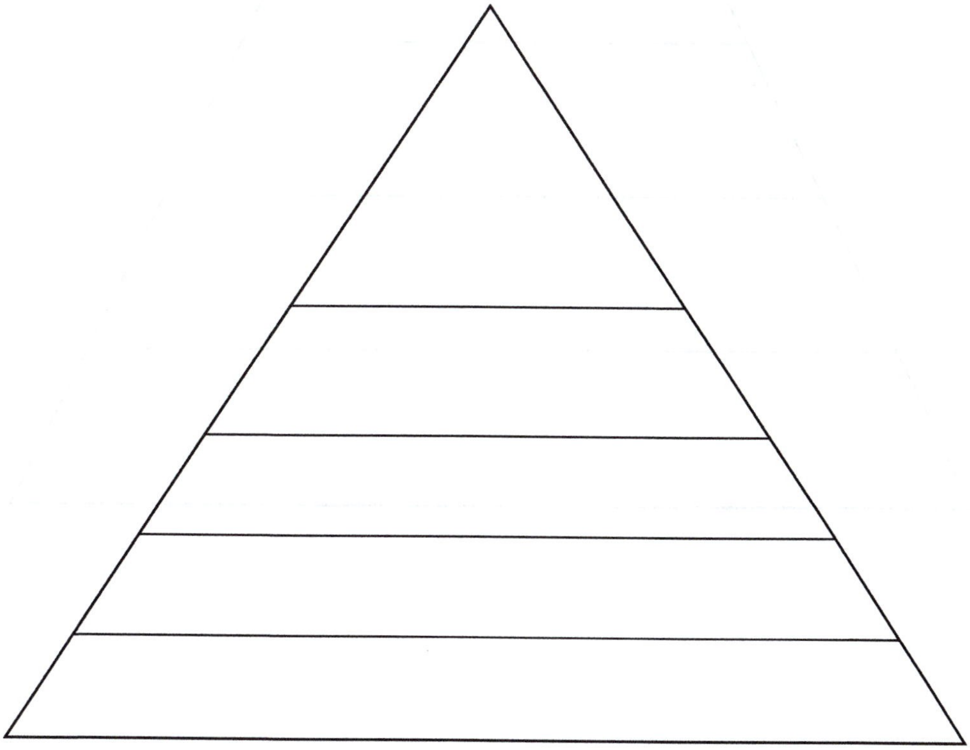

EXERCISE 5-2

Using the previous labeling exercise, write an example of one thing that would be important to the patient in each level of the pyramid.

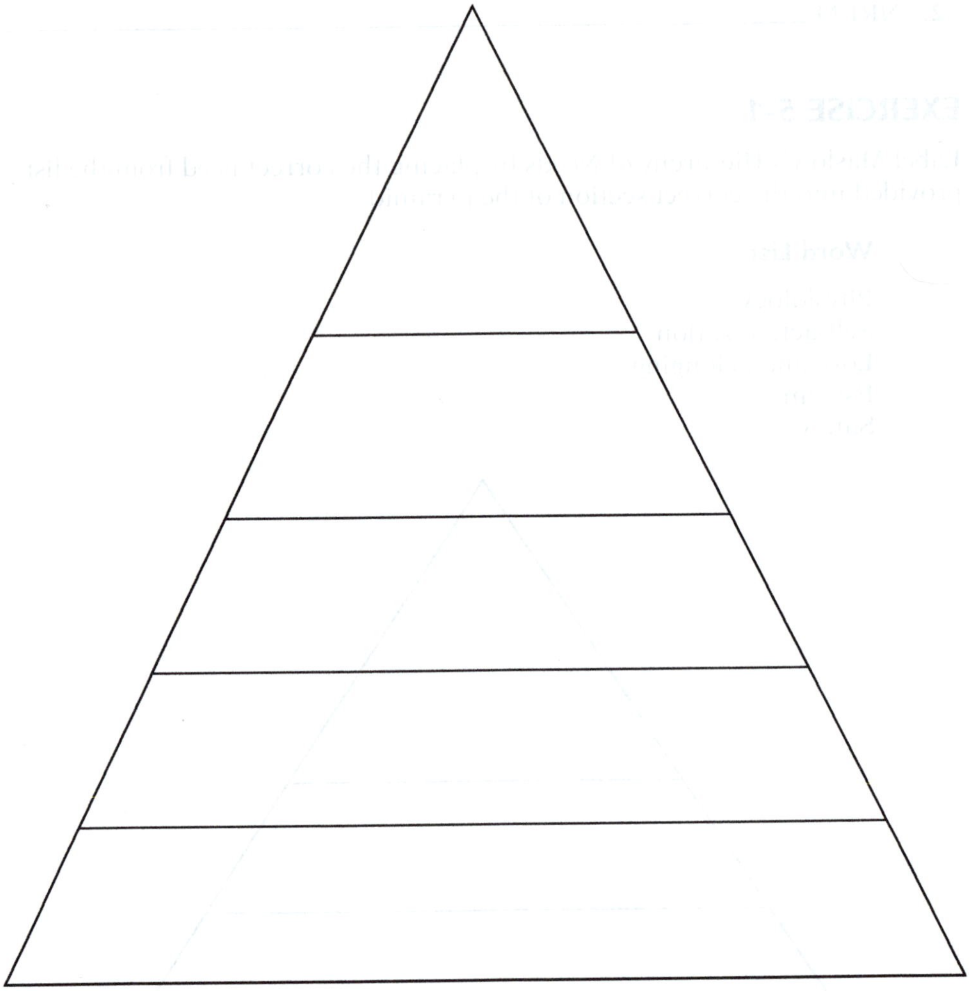

EXERCISE 5-3

Sleep is very important to help tissues heal; restore the body to optimal performance; increase mental alertness; and decrease stress, tension, and anxiety. Factors that can affect sleep have been placed in the top half of the boxes that follow. Write an example of your own or offered from the reading as to how a nursing assistant can help promote sleep for patients.

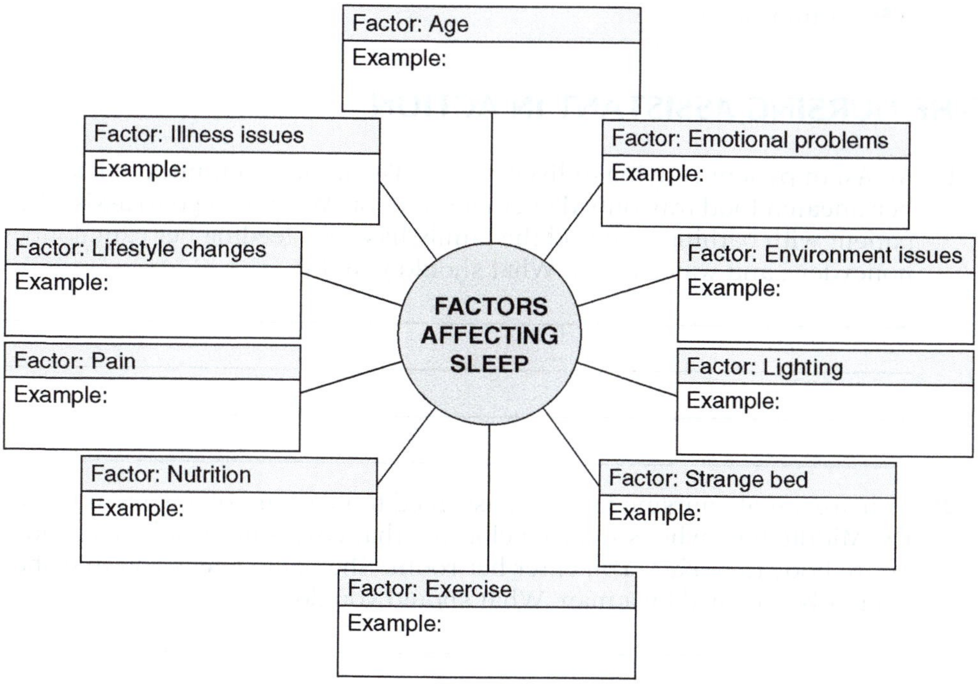

EXERCISE 5-4

Place the correct letters next to the matching phrase. More than one answer may apply.

CF—customer-focused care goal
FAS—factors affecting sleep
SS—sleep stages

____ 1. Keep door closed at night to reduce noise.

____ 2. Information is communicated to patients or to staff.

____ 3. Body rests and restores

____ 4. Patient may not be comfortable with her roommate, so a change may be needed.

____ 5. Muscles completely relax.

____ 6. Care provided reflects respect for the individual.

____ 7. Avoid exertion less than 2 hours prior to sleeping time.

____ 8. Family and friends are involved.

____ 9. Vivid dreaming.

____ **10.** The patient is relieved of fear when possible.

____ **11.** Easily aroused.

____ **12.** May be allowed to have pillow from home.

____ **13.** Lower vital signs.

____ **14.** Caregivers work together in a planned way.

____ **15.** Sound sleep.

THE NURSING ASSISTANT IN ACTION

1. An Asian patient is dying of liver failure. The family continues to leave her uneaten food tray outside her closed door. When you go to assist the patient with bathing, you find the family has been feeding her cantaloupe, honeydew, and watermelon. What should you do?

____

____

____

____

2. You are a male nursing assistant assigned to take care of a woman from the Middle East who is wearing clothing that covers her head, face, and entire body (a *burka*). You enter her room. She politely tells you that she cannot be touched by a man. What should you do?

____

____

____

____

3. Your patient is a strict vegetarian who does not eat anything that originally came from an animal. A food tray arrives that contains mashed potatoes with butter, cream of broccoli soup, and gelatin. He tells you he cannot eat anything on this food tray. What should you do?

____

____

____

____

4. You enter a patient's room to find him naked, standing on top of his bed and screaming that there are bugs biting him. He has scratched his arms and legs and they are bleeding. What should you do?

____

____

____

____

5. A patient tells you he is exhausted and being in the hospital has left him even more tired and fatigued. He cannot sleep because there is so much noise throughout the day and the staff keeps waking him up throughout the night. What should you do?

____

____

____

____

LEARNING ACTIVITIES

1. Identify a culture that fascinates you. Using the Internet, find information about the health care beliefs of this culture. For example, research their religious beliefs about death and dying, organ donation, food practices, birthing rituals, and ideas surrounding touch and eye contact. Share your findings with your classmates and use this new knowledge when caring for someone from this culture.
2. Create a small booklet or a ring with flashcards that contain some key health care phrases in another language. Alternatively, add some pictures of common items that can be found on the unit to help promote better communication between you and a person who has a different language than yours. Some examples of phrases are "Are you hungry?" "Do you have to use the bathroom?" or "Are you in pain?"

Infection Control

6

Key Terms Review

Match the key terms in the right column with the definitions in the left column by placing the letter of each correct answer in the space provided.

____ **1.** A living thing that is so small it cannot be seen with the naked eye, but only through a microscope.

____ **2.** Microorganisms necessary for health and usually live and grow in specific locations; they are nonpathogenic when in or on a natural reservoir.

____ **3.** Disease-producing microorganism.

____ **4.** A type of microorganism, much smaller than bacteria, that can survive only in other living cells.

____ **5.** Blood-borne disease affecting the liver; easily transmitted within the health care setting following parenteral exposure.

____ **6.** Prior to 1988, this was known as *non-A non-B hepatitis;* transmitted best through needlesticks and may result in chronic liver disease.

____ **7.** Viral respiratory illness spread by close person-to-person contact.

____ **8.** A type of bacteria called *Enterococci* that is difficult to treat because of its resistance to many antibiotics, including vancomycin.

____ **9.** A condition in humans in which the immune system begins to fail, leading to the development of life-threatening opportunistic infections.

Terms

A. Universal precautions
B. Standard precautions
C. Transmission-based precautions
D. Transmission
E. Microorganism
F. Pathogen
G. Virus
H. Normal flora
I. Bacteria
J. Spores
K. Infection
L. Local infection
M. Health care–associated infection (HAI)
N. Nosocomial infection
O. Iatrogenic infection
P. Systemic infection
Q. Infection control
R. *Clostridium difficile* (*C. diff*)

_____ **10.** A retrovirus that causes acquired immunodeficiency syndrome.

_____ **11.** Unicellular microorganism.

_____ **12.** Bacteria that have formed hard shells around themselves as a defense.

_____ **13.** A bacterium that causes diarrhea and more serious intestinal infections that is primarily associated with health care settings.

_____ **14.** A bacterial infection that is highly resistant to some antibiotics.

_____ **15.** A common bacterium that can cause disease in particular susceptible individuals; it is resistant to many antibiotics.

_____ **16.** An example of bacteria found in the tissues of fleas, lice, ticks, and other insects; Rickettsiae are transmitted to humans by insect bites.

_____ **17.** Results from a pathogen producing a reaction that may cause soreness, tenderness, redness, pus, fever, change in drainage, and other symptoms.

_____ **18.** An infection contained in a specific area of the body.

_____ **19.** An infection that is in the blood stream and spread throughout the body.

_____ **20.** An infection acquired in a health care setting.

_____ **21.** An infection caused by medical treatment.

_____ **22.** Hospital-acquired infection.

_____ **23.** The effort to prevent the spread of pathogens.

_____ **24.** The process of rubbing two surfaces together, such as skin.

_____ **25.** General term that applies to handwashing, antiseptic handwash, antiseptic hand rub, or surgical hand antisepsis.

_____ **26.** The absence of microorganisms (germs).

_____ **27.** Germ-free; without disease-producing organisms.

_____ **28.** Device used to make an item sterile through heat, pressure, and steam.

_____ **29.** The process of killing all microorganisms, including spores.

_____ **30.** An organic compound, also called *phenol,* used to kill germs.

_____ **31.** The process of destroying as many harmful organisms as possible.

S. *Psuedomonas aeruginosa*

T. Methicillin-resistant *Staphylococcus aureus* (MRSA)

U. Rickettsiae

V. Surgical conscience

W. Sterile field

X. Asepsis

Y. Aseptic

Z. Mucous membranes

AA. Sharps

BB. Parenteral

CC. Perinatal

DD. Friction

EE. Hand hygiene

FF. Autoclave

GG. Disinfection

HH. Isolation

II. Carbolic acid

JJ. Sterilization

KK. Hepatitis C

LL. Hepatitis B

MM. Acquired Immunodeficiency Syndrome (AIDS)

NN. Human Immunodeficiency Virus (HIV)

OO. Vancomycin-resistant Enterococci (VRE)

PP. Severe Acute Respiratory Syndrome (SARS)

_____ 32. To separate or set apart.

_____ 33. A membrane that lines body cavities and canals that lead to the outside; these include structures of the mouth, eyes, and nose.

_____ 34. Direct inoculation of blood on a needle through the skin.

_____ 35. The period immediately before and after birth.

_____ 36. Any sharp device or equipment used in health care, such as hypodermic needles, scalpels, sutures, blood collection devices, and disposable razors.

_____ 37. An area created to work from when you are doing a sterile procedure.

_____ 38. Used to describe the way you must act and think when you are working with sterile technique.

_____ 39. The spread of microorganisms.

_____ 40. A set of precautions used in addition to standard precautions and designed for patients with suspected or confirmed highly transmissible pathogens for which additional precautions are needed to interrupt transmission.

_____ 41. A set of precautions used to prevent the spread of microorganisms and that assumes every person is potentially infected or colonized with an organism that could be transmitted in the health care setting.

_____ 42. A set of precautions designed to prevent the spread of microorganisms.

MULTIPLE-CHOICE QUESTIONS

Circle the letter next to the word or statement that best completes the sentence or answers the question.

1. The autoclave sterilizes or completely destroys microorganisms by combining
   a. soap with hot water under pressure.
   b. ammonia with steam under pressure.
   c. heath with steam under pressure.
   d. water and bleach under pressure.

2. Autoclaves are used to kill
   a. bad germs only.
   b. all bacteria and viruses, including spores.
   c. parasites.
   d. viruses only.

3. When an object is free of all __________, it is sterile.
   a. grease
   b. bacteria
   c. microorganisms
   d. dirt

4. The source of microorganisms
   a. can only be the patient and health care worker.
   b. is never really known.
   c. can be anyone, including objects in the environment.
   d. is a susceptible host only.

5. Standard Precautions are designed to provide safety to
   a. health care workers.
   b. patients.
   c. nursing assistants who are in training.
   d. all of the above.

6. To prevent or control the transmission of diseases, you
   a. must study very hard.
   b. must understand how a disease is spread.
   c. must protect yourself and your patient.
   d. both b and c.

7. The ability of a patient to resist infection depends on his
   a. personality.
   b. lifestyle.
   c. age.
   d. health status and exposure to pathogens.

8. Standard Precautions apply to
   a. blood, all body fluids, and non-intact skin and mucous membranes.
   b. saliva, semen, and blood.
   c. care of a burn victim.
   d. all of the above.

9. Which is important to consider when maintaining a sterile field?
   a. Keep a 2-inch border around the field.
   b. Place the field behind you.
   c. Keep the field below your waist.
   d. Once the field becomes wet, it is no longer sterile.

10. Cleanliness is important. Be sure that your fingernails are
   a. kept short and cleaned frequently.
   b. colorful and attractively painted at all times.
   c. kept long and in good repair to help open IV bags and perform personal care.
   d. extend more than ½" beyond the fleshy tip of your fingers.

11. The key to good handwashing is
   a. washing a long time to ensure all bacteria is removed.
   b. using friction and hand cream to protect against chapping.
   c. using bar soap instead of soap from a dispenser.
   d. using adequate soap with lots of tepid water and friction.

12. While washing your hands, if your hands touch the inside of the sink, you should
   a. start the procedure of handwashing all over again.
   b. rinse 30 seconds longer and then use a paper towel to wipe the edges of the sink.
   c. use adequate paper towels and friction to dry your hands to assure bacteria is removed.
   d. keep washing your hands because the leftover soap will help to kill the germs.

13. Which is a sign of infection?
   a. Redness noted at the site
   b. Swelling around the area
   c. Pus draining from the wound
   d. All of the above

14. A localized infection
   a. is confined to specific body area.
   b. cannot spread to the bloodstream.
   c. is always uncomplicated and easy to treat.
   d. can be treated with bleach.

15. Which type of microbe cannot be seen with a microscope?
   a. Virus
   b. Bacteria
   c. Fungi
   d. Protozoa

16. Most microbes need a moist, dark, and warm place to grow. Some even need __________ to thrive.
   a. oxygen
   b. carbolic acid
   c. pasteurization
   d. toxins

17. MRSA, VRE, and *C. diff*
  a. usually affect patients with a strong ability to fight infection.
  b. are easy to get rid of.
  c. may occur when persons are hospitalized for long periods of time.
  d. cannot affect the nursing assistant in any way.

18. A urinary tract infection may occur
  a. when *Escherichia coli* (*E. coli*) is introduced into the urinary tract.
  b. if a nursing assistant does not wash her hands correctly.
  c. when proper care of a catheter is not offered.
  d. all of the above.

19. Personal protective equipment
  a. includes gloves, gowns, and masks.
  b. must be provided by the employer per OSHA regulations.
  c. help provide a barrier between pathogens and the nursing assistant.
  d. all of the above.

20. Gloves do not need to be worn when providing care to a patient who
  a. is sweating.
  b. is vomiting.
  c. has a bloody dressing that needs to be changed.
  d. had diarrhea and needs help cleaning herself.

21. HBV and HIV can be spread through
  a. sharing needles with an IV drug user.
  b. having unprotected sex with an infected partner.
  c. birth, if the mother is positive for these diseases
  d. all of the above.

22. If a patient is diagnosed with the flu, usually __________ precautions are advised.
  a. contact
  b. airborne
  c. droplet
  d. isolation

23. __________ precautions are activated when a patient is diagnosed with tuberculosis (TB).
  a. Contact
  b. Airborne
  c. Droplet
  d. Reverse isolation

24. When a patient is placed in isolation, he
  a. should be given very little explanation about what he can and cannot do
  b. may need support coping with loneliness.
  c. will want to be alone and sleep.
  d. should have as many visitors as possible at one time to promote socialization.

25. A dry, non-sterile dressing
  a. increases further injury to the tissue.
  b. allows other microorganisms to get into the wound.
  c. promotes would healing.
  d. does not absorb drainage.

TRUE OR FALSE QUESTIONS

Determine whether each question is true or false. In the space provided, write "T" for true and "F" for false. If the statement is false, rewrite it on the line provided to make it a true statement.

____ **1.** To be *reinfected* means you or your patent have become infected a second time by the same microorganism.

____

____ **2.** *Cross contamination* means becoming infected from a different microorganism through equipment or from another patient or even from a staff member.

____

_____ 3. Gloves provide a complete barrier to contamination.

____

_____ 4. Hands must be washed after removing gloves.

____

_____ 5. A latex allergy can result in anaphylactic shock.

____

_____ 6. A minimum of 5 ounces of hand sanitizing gel should be used when washing one's hands.

____

_____ 7. The Centers for Disease Control and Prevention (CDC) recommends that handwashing using soap and water be performed for a minimum of 20 seconds.

____

_____ 8. If you sneeze in a respirator mask, you do not have to change the mask because it is suppose to catch 95% of all airborne pathogens.

____

_____ 9. Rubbing alcohol is an acceptable cleaning solution to use on scalpels.

____

_____ 10. A nursing assistant should remove gloves first when taking her gown off.

____

FILL-IN-THE-BLANK QUESTIONS

Provide the meaning of the following abbreviations.

1. CDC ______________________________
2. HCW ______________________________
3. HAI ______________________________
4. SARS ______________________________
5. VRE ______________________________
6. MRSA ______________________________
7. UTI ______________________________
8. AIDS ______________________________
9. HIV ______________________________
10. OSHA ______________________________
11. RSV ______________________________
12. VZIG ______________________________
13. TB ______________________________
14. HRS ______________________________
15. DI ______________________________
16. DH ______________________________
17. CN ______________________________
18. A ______________________________

19. C ______________________________

20. D ______________________________

21. S ______________________________

22. TB ______________________________

EXERCISE 6-1

Directions: Apply what you have learned about handwashing. Use numbers 1–7 (1 is first, 7 is last) and rank the sentences in an order that makes the most sense and maintains infection control measures.

____ Use a paper towel to dry hands and dispose of it in a wastebasket.

____ Use a paper towel to turn the faucet off and dispose of it in a wastebasket.

____ Use friction to scrub front and back of hands, wrists, and under fingernails by scratching the palms for 20 seconds or more.

____ Wet hands and adjust water flow and temperature.

____ Keep fingers pointed downward.

____ Get soap.

____ Rinse all surfaces of hands and wrists.

EXERCISE 6-2

Directions: Apply what you have learned about using a mask. Use numbers 1–7 (1 is first, 7 is last) and rank the sentences in an order that makes the most sense and maintains infection control measures.

____ Wash hands.

____ Tie lower strings behind neck.

____ Obtain mask.

____ Place mask on face.

____ Tie strings securely at crown of head.

____ Adjust pliable nosepiece until it fits securely.

____ Grasp bottom portion of mask and spread mask to cover below chin.

EXERCISE 6-3

Directions: Apply what you have learned about using a gown. Use numbers 1–9 (1 is first, 9 is last) and rank the sentences in an order that makes the most sense and maintains infection control measures.

____ Wash your hands. Roll up your sleeves.

____ Unfold the isolation gown so the opening is at the back

____ Put your arms into the sleeves of the isolation gown.

____ Don gloves, making sure they cover the wrist of the gown.

____ Tie the waist ties in a bow or fasten the adhesive strip.

____ Reach behind and tie the neck back with a simple shoelace bow or fasten an adhesive strip.

____ Grasp the edges of the gown and pull to the back.

____ Fit the gown at the neck, making sure your uniform is covered.

____ Overlap the edges of the gown, completely closing the opening and covering your uniform completely.

EXERCISE 6-4

Objective: To recognize and correctly spell words related to infection control.

Directions: Unscramble the words in the word list and place the answer on the line provided.

1. GNESHOPTA ____________________
2. THSO ____________________
3. SRECOU ____________________
4. RTSNAMSISION ____________________
5. IONTLASIO ____________________
6. DHWNASHAGNI ____________________
7. TCIFRNIO ____________________
8. TITPHEAIS ____________________
9. RELSIET ____________________

THE NURSING ASSISTANT IN ACTION

1. You check on Mr. Taylor, who complains of pain in his arm where his IV is located. What signs and symptoms of an infection should you check for and report?

   ____

   ____

   ____

   ____

2. You are assigned to empty a bedpan in a room where a patient is on droplet isolation. He had an episode of diarrhea and has soiled his bed linens. What should you do?

____

____

____

____

3. You are assigned to assist the nurse in setting up a sterile field to change a surgical dressing. What should you do to help facilitate this process?

____

____

____

____

4. You are asked to transport a patient on airborne precautions to another unit. What should you do?

____

____

____

____

5. You are asked to clean some medical equipment on the floor. What should you do?

____

____

____

____

LEARNING ACTIVITIES

1. Investigate the category-specific isolation precautions in your facility and report your findings to your classmates. Identify diseases that require using specific precautions. Become familiar with the types of personal protective equipment you should use when caring for a patient who is on any of these isolation precautions.
2. Participate in an in-service about OSHA regulations highlighting Standards for Occupational Exposure to Bloodborne Pathogens, or review your facility's policy manual.

PROCEDURE CHECKLISTS

PROCEDURE 6-1: HANDWASHING

Name : ______________________ Date: ______________________

STEPS	S	U	COMMENTS
1. Assemble your equipment. (soap, paper towels, warm running water, and wastepaper basket).			
2. Completely wet your hands and wrists under the running water. Keep your fingertips pointed downward.			
3. Apply soap.			
4. Hold your hands lower than your elbows while washing.			
5. Work up a good lather. Spread it over the entire area of your hands and wrists. Get soap under your nails and between your fingers.			
6. Clean under your nails by rubbing your nails across the palms of your hand.			
7. Use a rotating and rubbing (frictional) motion for 20 seconds. a. Rub vigorously. b. Rub one hand against the other hand and wrist. c. Rub between your fingers by interlacing them. d. Rub up and down to reach all skin surfaces on your hands, between your fingers, and 2" above your wrists. e. Rub the tips of your fingers against your palms to clean with friction around the nail beds.			
8. Rinse well. Rinse from 2" above your wrists to the hands. Hold your hands and fingertips down under running water.			
9. Dry thoroughly with paper towels and throw them away.			
10. Turn off the faucet, using a second new, clean, dry paper towel. Never touch the faucet with your hands after washing.			
11. Discard the paper towel into the wastepaper basket. Do not touch the basket.			

Charting:

____

____

____

____

Date of Satisfactory Completion ______________________

Instructor's Signature ______________________

PROCEDURE 6-2: WATERLESS HAND HYGIENE

Name : ____________________ Date: ____________________

STEPS	S	U	COMMENTS
1. Locate wall-mounted dispenser and push release lever with one hand while holding the other, open hand underneath the nozzle of the dispenser.			
2. One squirt of gel is delivered onto the open hand. Obtain another 1–2 mL if needed to have enough to cover the skin of both hands.			
3. Rub the gel into the skin of both hands.			
4. Allow hands to dry, usually about 30 seconds.			

Charting:

____

____

____

____

Date of Satisfactory Completion ____________________

Instructor's Signature ____________________

PROCEDURE 6-3: PUTTING ON DISPOSABLE GLOVES

Name : ______________ Date: ______________

STEPS	S	U	COMMENTS
1. Remove jewelry and wash hands. Remove two gloves from box or package.			
2. Slip your hands into the gloves, one hand at a time.			
3. Work the gloves down to the base of the fingers to make sure they fit comfortably.			
4. Gloves should be neither too tight nor too loose at the fingertips or wrists.			
5. Upon application, inspect gloves for integrity.			

Charting:

____

____

____

____

Date of Satisfactory Completion ______________

Instructor's Signature ______________

PROCEDURE 6-4: REMOVING GLOVES

Name : ____________________ Date: ____________________

STEPS	S	U	COMMENTS
1. With both hands gloved, with the gloved fingers of one hand grasp the glove of the other hand just below the cuff.			
2. Turn or peel one glove inside out, starting at the cuff. Hold it in the gloved hand, making sure to avoid contact with inside of other hand.			
3. Place your ungloved index and middle fingers inside the cuff of the remaining glove.			
4. With the ungloved hand, peel the second glove from the inside, tucking the first glove inside the second as you remove your hand.			
5. Upon removal of gloves, be sure to discard used gloves directly into the trash.			
6. Wash your hands.			

Charting:

____

____

____

____

Date of Satisfactory Completion ____________________

Instructor's Signature ____________________

PROCEDURE 6-5: PUTTING ON A MASK

Name : ____________________ Date: ____________________

STEPS	S	U	COMMENTS
1. Wash hands.			
2. Obtain mask.			
3. Place mask on face and adjust pliable nosepiece until it fits securely.			
4. Tie strings securely at crown of head.			
5. Tie lower strings behind neck.			

Charting:

____

____

____

____

Date of Satisfactory Completion______________

Instructor's Signature______________________

PROCEDURE 6-6: WEARING A MASK TO PREVENT CROSS-INFECTION

Name : ____________________ Date: ____________________

STEPS	S	U	COMMENTS
1. The mask should be handled only by the strings, thereby keeping the hands uncontaminated by a soiled mask. • Never lower mask to hang loosely around the neck or place it in a pocket. • Promptly discard mask into the proper receptacle on removal. • Change mask if it becomes wet or moist, or if you sneeze into the mask. • Change mask between procedures or cases in operating rooms or ambulatory surgery settings			
2. An N-95 respirator may be used for a shift when used by the same caregiver providing care to a patient on airborne precautions. Should the N-95 respirator become contaminated, it should be changed.			
3. If the mask is worn by a health care worker to provide an uncontaminated air environment for patient, and the health care worker has excessive facial hair, a hood must be worn to cover the neck area.			
4. Wash hands following discard.			

Charting:

____

____

____

____

Date of Satisfactory Completion ____________________

Instructor's Signature ____________________

PROCEDURE 6-7: APPLYING A GOWN

Name : ____________________ Date: ____________________

STEPS	S	U	COMMENTS
1. Wash your hands. If you are wearing a long-sleeve uniform, roll your sleeves above your elbows.			
2. Unfold the isolation gown so the opening is at the back.			
3. Put your arms into the sleeves of the isolation gown.			
4. Fit the gown at the neck, making sure your uniform is covered.			
5. Reach behind and tie the neck back with a simple shoelace bow or fasten an adhesive strip.			
6. Grasp the edges of the gown and pull to the back.			
7. Overlap the edges of the gown, completely closing the opening and covering your uniform completely.			
8. Tie the waist ties in a bow or fasten the adhesive strip.			
9. Don gloves, making sure they cover the wrist of the gown.			

Charting:

____

____

____

____

Date of Satisfactory Completion________________

Instructor's Signature____________________

PROCEDURE 6-8: REMOVING A GOWN

Name : ____________________ Date: ____________________

STEPS	S	U	COMMENTS
1. Keep gloves on, and then untie the waist belt or ties.			
2. Untie the neck ties, being cautious not to come in contact with neck, or have someone else untie the gown for you.			
3. Pull the sleeve off by grasping each shoulder at the neckline.			
4. Turn the sleeves inside out as you remove them from your arms.			
5. Holding the gown away from your body by the inside of the shoulder seams, fold it inside out, bringing the shoulders together.			
6. Roll the gown up with the inside out and discard.			
7. Remove gloves, being careful to not contaminate yourself. Be sure to discard used gloves directly into the trash. Wash your hands.			
8. Remove mask, touching only the strings, and discard.			
9. Wash hands.			

Charting:

____

____

____

____

Date of Satisfactory Completion ____________________

Instructor's Signature ____________________

PROCEDURE 6-9: PUTTING ON STERILE GLOVES

Name : ____________________ Date: ____________________

STEPS	S	U	COMMENTS
1. Wash hands or apply waterless hand antiseptic.			
2. Select a pair of wrapped gloves in a size that fit your hands snugly.			
3. Check to be certain that the gloves are sterile. a. Package intact with no signs of dampness? b. Seal of sterility?			
4. Place package on a clean, dry, flat surface.			
5. Open the wrapper, handling only the outside.			
6. Use your left hand to pick up the right glove. Touch only the inside folded cuff. Do not touch the outside of the glove!			
7. Put the glove on your right hand.			
8. Use your gloved right hand to pick up the left glove: a. Place the finger of your gloved right hand under the cuff of the left glove. b. Lift the glove up and away from the wrapper, and pull it onto your left hand. c. Continue pulling left glove up to wrist. Be certain that the gloved right thumb does not touch your skin or clothing.			
9. With your gloved left hand, place fingers under the cuff of the right glove and pull it up over your right wrist.			
10. Adjust the fingers of the glove as necessary.			
11. If either glove tears or becomes soiled, remove them both and begin the procedure again with another pair.			

Charting:

____

____

____

____

Date of Satisfactory Completion ____________________

Instructor's Signature ____________________

PROCEDURE 6-10: OPENING A STERILE PACKAGE

Name : ____________________ Date: ____________________

STEPS	S	U	COMMENTS
1. Wash hands.			
2. Assemble the equipment and supplies a. Sterile gloves b. Sterile package			
3. Check to be certain all supplies are sterile a. Package intact, with no signs of dampness? b. Seal of sterility?			
4. Place the package on dry, flat, clean work surface. Position the package so that the first edge to be unfolded is pulled away from you. The outer wrap of the package serves as a sterile field to work on.			
5. Slowly pull the corners at the right and left of the package. This exposes the inside of the package.			
6. Carefully pull back the corner pointing toward you.			
7. If you are going to add sterile items to your field, do so now. Remember that the edge (1" around) of your sterile field, and anything hanging over the edge of your work area, is contaminated.			
8. Do not touch anything inside your sterile package or sterile field until you have put your sterile gloves on.			

Charting:

____

____

____

____

Date of Satisfactory Completion ____________________

Instructor's Signature ____________________

PROCEDURE 6-11: APPLYING A DRY NON-STERILE DRESSING

Name : ______________________ Date: ______________________

STEPS	S	U	COMMENTS
1. Wash hands.			
2. Assemble the equipment and supplies as directed by the nurse. a. Clean, non-sterile gloves (2 pairs) b. Personal protective equipment (PPE) as needed c. Dressing materials d. Tape or Montgomery ties e. Dressing set f. Cleaning solution g. Gauze pads for cleaning h. Plastic bag			
3. Put on PPE and non-sterile gloves. This protects you from coming into contact with body fluids.			
4. Remove the old dressing by pushing the skin away from the adhesive tape. If it is stuck, you may moisten it with a small amount of warm water or saline solution.			
5. Place the old dressing in the plastic bag.			
6. Observe the wound looking for any redness, bleeding, color of drainage and odor, if any.			
7. Gently clean the wound, as directed, using clean gauze pads moistened with saline. Clean starting from the wound with a single stroke outward away from the wound. Repeat, as needed, using a clean moistened gauze pad with each stroke.			
8. Remove your gloves and discard them in the plastic bag.			
9. Wash your hands.			
10. Open the new dressings and cut the length of tape needed.			
11. Put on clean gloves.			
12. Cover the wound with a bandage or gauze pad large enough to cover the wound and enough surrounding skin to protect the wound from being exposed. Be sure to touch only the edges of the dressing material that will not come into direct contact with the wound.			
13. Use tape (or Montgomery ties) to secure the dressing in place. Do not cover the entire dressing with tape or circle the entire wound with tape. Rather, apply tape at the top, middle, and bottom of the dry dressing so that it extends several inches beyond both sides of the dressing.			

14. Remove your gloves and discard them in the plastic bag. Put the plastic bag in the appropriate trash receptacle.			
15. Wash your hands.			
16. Report and record your observations.			

Charting:

____

____

____

____

Date of Satisfactory Completion ______________

Instructor's Signature ______________

7

Safety

Key Terms Review

Match the key terms in the right column with the definitions in the left column by placing the letter of each correct answer in the space provided.

____ **1.** The act of walking.

____ **2.** A regulating device that controls the amount of oxygen delivered to a patient.

____ **3.** A type of oxygen delivery device that consists of two prongs that fit into the nostrils.

____ **4.** An odorless, tasteless, non-visible gas that makes up 21% of room air.

____ **5.** A mat used with bed or chair alarms that senses when the patient's weight is displaced.

____ **6.** A device used to provide protection for a patient.

____ **7.** A device or technique used to control behavior without physically limiting the movement of a patient.

____ **8.** Any device that the patient cannot remove on his own; used to physically limit the movement of the patient.

____ **9.** A type of alarm that sounds when a patient's weight is removed from a bed; this indicates the patient is getting out of bed.

____ **10.** A type of alarm that sounds when a patient's weight is removed from a chair; this indicates the patient is attempting to get out of the chair.

Terms

A. Gait training

B. Gait

C. Restraint alternative

D. Restraints

E. Pressure-sensitive mat

F. Protective device

G. Bed alarm

H. Chair alarm

I. Flow meter

J. Oxygen

K. Nasal cannula

L. Ambulation

_____ **11.** Speed and rhythm of walking (ambulation).

_____ **12.** A training program developed by physical therapists to assist patients in reaching the highest level of independence in walking.

MULTIPLE-CHOICE QUESTIONS

Circle the letter next to the word or statement that best completes the sentence or answers the question.

1. **RACE** stands for
   a. **R**un **A**way and **C**all **EMS**.
   b. **R**emove yourself **A**nd **C**all for **E**mergency help.
   c. **R**un **A**nd **C**orrect the **E**mergency.
   d. **R**emove the patient; **A**ctivate the fire alarm; **C**ontain the fire; **E**xtinguish the fire if safe to do so.

2. When the patient is using oxygen via a nasal cannula, the area where skin irritation may occur is
   a. any area where the plastic cannula touches the skin.
   b. only behind the ears.
   c. the nostrils and eyelids.
   d. behind the neck and on the cheeks.

3. _______ is the number one cause of fires in health care institutions.
   a. A sleeping patient
   b. A broken electrical cord
   c. Too much oxygen
   d. Smoking

4. A fire extinguisher may be labeled
   a. A for all; B for wood; C for combustion.
   b. only A for paper fires and B for electrical fires.
   c. ABC for industrial kitchen fires.
   d. ABC for use on any type of fires.

5. Always place used disposable razors
   a. in a red wastebasket located in most bathrooms.
   b. in approved sharps containers.
   c. in a recycling bin.
   d. where they can be used later.

6. Room cleaning supplies should
   a. be left at the patient's bedside at all times.
   b. be labeled and dated before leaving them in patient's bathroom.
   c. be stored away from the patient's area.
   d. be kept behind the nurse's station and under the desk.

7. Electrical equipment must never come in contact with
   a. heat, fuel, or oxygen.
   b. patients.
   c. the nursing assistant.
   d. water.

8. Elderly patients who tend to wander should be
   a. restrained so they do not try to escape or harm themselves or others.
   b. allowed to move about safely as much as possible during the day so they sleep better throughout the night.
   c. medicated so they can sit quietly and not fall.
   d. humored.

9. A cane should be
   a. used on the stronger side to help the person balance.
   b. used on the weaker side to stabilize weight evenly.
   c. replaced with a walker because canes can increase falls in the elderly.
   d. held so the patient's arm is straight.

10. What comment is accurate in regards to a cane, a walker, and a crutch?
a. Patients can learn to use these devices safely by themselves.
b. All patients must use these devices regardless of their condition.
c. They do not have to be fitted to each individual.
d. None should be used to help a patient stand but rather they should be used as an aid when walking.

11. When using a cane or walker, the patient's elbows must be
a. contracted.
b. bent at a 180-degree angle.
c. locked.
d. slightly flexed.

12. The patient's hands must rest on the ________ of the crutches.
a. handrails
b. top
c. hand rests
d. tips

13. In order for facilities to ensure safety,
a. deadbolt locks must be placed on all doors and stay bolted at all times.
b. the nursing assistant should place disposable razors immediately in the wastebasket when finished using them.
c. handrails must be installed in bathrooms.
d. staff must keep wheelchairs and stretchers stored in the hallways at all times.

14. Which patient is at the greatest risk for falling?
a. An 80-year-old man who ambulates without any assistive devices.
b. A 72-year-old woman who is confused and agitated.
c. A teenage patient who wears contact lenses.
d. An infant who is sleeping in a crib with the crib rails up.

15. A patient complains of dizziness when he stands. The nursing assistant should
a. stay with him when he stands and assist him back to bed if the dizziness continues, then report his complaint.
b. ignore the complaint because in a few seconds the dizziness will go away.
c. allow him to walk until the dizziness goes away.
d. sit him in a chair and tell him everything will be all right.

16. What is the correct statement about mitts when used as a restraint?
a. They can be used for long periods of time because they are soft.
b. They are never used.
c. They are usually used when a person is at risk for pulling tubes out after surgery occurs.
d. They are used only in extreme emergency situations and when the patient is under the influence of mood-altering medications.

17. A patient is on oxygen therapy. The nursing assistant should
a. allow the patient to go outside with a portable oxygen tank to smoke.
b. observe for any skin breakdown around the ears, nostrils, and cheeks.
c. place a small amount of petroleum jelly by the nostrils to prevent skin breakdown.
d. kink the tubing to make sure air flow is delivered correctly.

18. Wrist restraints
a. must be removed every 2 hours and a drink and food must be offered.
b. must be reordered by the nurse every 72 hours.
c. are safe and soft and cannot hurt the patient.
d. can be applied at night to any person that is considered a fall risk.

19. A fire is discovered in a patient's wastebasket. What is the first thing the nursing assistant should do?
a. Bring a fire extinguisher to the room.

b. Close the door to the room and rescue other patients on the unit.
c. Remove the patient from the room.
d. Report the fire at once to the supervisor.

20. Some facilities identify patients at risk for falling by
a. pinning a note on the patient's back that reads "At Risk for Falling."
b. placing brightly colored non-slip socks on the patient.
c. always restraining them in a chair next to the nurses' desk.
d. all of the above.

21. Snowstorms, tornadoes, floods, and ________ are considered natural disasters that cannot be avoided or prevented.
a. transportation crashes
b. earthquakes
c. riots
d. chemical warfare

22. A bed alarm
a. sometimes works with pressure mats to ensure optimal safety.
b. should be checked immediately when the alarm sounds.
c. should not be used for patients who weigh less than 100 pounds.
d. all of the above.

23. Which measure helps keep the child safe?
a. Make sure all chemicals are placed under the sink in a locked cabinet.
b. Teach children that medicine is candy.
c. Keep windows unlocked for easy escape should a fire occur.
d. Keep crib side rails down.

24. When dealing with a combative and verbally abusive patient, remember that
a. the team leader is the one who should redirect all visitors and patients away from the disruptive patient.
b. members of the staff should all talk at once to help deescalate the negative behavior.
c. restraining the patient should occur only if trying other strategies fails and if the person becomes a threat to himself.
d. a debriefing should occur before any behavior management strategy begins.

25. An example of a training program developed by physical therapists that assists patients in reaching the highest level of independence in walking is
a. gait training
b. fine-motor coordination.
c. repositioning program.
d. bowel and bladder training.

TRUE OR FALSE QUESTIONS

Determine whether each question is true or false. In the space provided, write "T" for true and "F" for false. If the statement is false, rewrite it on the line provided to make it a true statement.

____ **1.** It takes three things for a fire to continue to burn: heat, fuel, and oxygen.

____

____ **2.** The Omnibus Budget Reconciliation Act (OBRA) calls any device a restraint that keeps a patient from moving freely or keeps the patient from reaching part of her body.

____

____ **3.** It is important to practice your facility's evacuation plan so everyone knows what to do in case a real emergency occurs.

____

____ **4.** Sometimes, restraints cause even more injury, and in some cases may even cause death.

____

____ **5.** It is the nursing assistant's job to administer oxygen to the patient.

____

____ **6.** Some facilities place a sign on the door and over the bed that states "Oxygen in Use" so everyone is aware that the patient is receiving oxygen.

____

____ **7.** Enhanced 911 can find out where an emergency is located when a call is made from a cell phone.

____

____ **8.** It is the nursing assistant's responsibility to stay until all the flames are extinguished completely.

____

____ **9.** Bedridden patients are at high risk for falling.

____

____ **10.** Every 4 hours, provide care and continue to monitor the patient who has a bed alarm.

____

FILL-IN-THE-BLANK QUESTIONS

Provide the meaning of the following abbreviations.

1. OBRA ______________________________
2. A (type of fire extinguisher) ______________________________
3. B (type of fire extinguisher)______________________________
4. C (type of fire extinguisher)______________________________
5. K (type of fire extinguisher)______________________________
6. ABC (type of fire extinguisher) ______________________________
7. PASS ______________________________
8. RACE ______________________________

EXERCISE 7-1

Objective: To recognize safety issues and immediate actions to be taken.

Directions: Place the correct letters that apply to the situation next to the matching phrase, then circle the correct response you should take immediately. More than one set of letters can be selected for each situation.

OS—oxygen safety
RS—restraint safety
CS—child safety
FS—fire safety
AS—ambulation safety
PS—patient safety

1. Your patient has nasal oxygen on at 3 liters and there is a NO SMOKING—OXYGEN IN USE sign on the wall above his bed. His wife is preparing to light a candle at the bedside and say a prayer for his recovery. What should you do?
   a. You grab the fire extinguisher and Pull the pin, Aim low, Squeeze the handle, and Sweep from side to side, aiming at the base of the candle.
   b. You put out the candle and explain to her that open flames are dangerous when oxygen is running. You offer to show her where the chapel is located.
   c. You turn off the oxygen for 20 minutes until she is done praying.
   d. You ignore the situation because such a small flame is harmless.
2. You are ready to leave for the day and stop in to say goodbye to your patient. She tells you that the floor in the bathroom is wet. You realize that the housekeeping staff has gone home for the day. What should you do?
   a. You clean up the floor immediately, or get someone else to do it.
   b. You leave immediately, because you must take your sick child to the doctor.
   c. You provide the patient with a call light and instruct her to ask someone on the new shift to do it because you are leaving.
   d. You tell the patient to stay out of the bathroom until someone else comes to clean it up.
3. You are coming on your new shift and notice that one of your patients is wearing a chest restraint that is on backward. The patient is sleeping at this time. What should you do?
   a. Let him sleep for now.
   b. Make a note to change the restraint later on when you have more time.
   c. Leave a call light within reach.
   d. Check with your immediate supervisor to determine if help is needed when changing the restraint, based on the patient's condition and reason for wearing the restraint. You change the restraint immediately.
4. You notice that your patient, a 7-year-old, is picking at the IV site on his arm. What should you do?
   a. You restrain him immediately.
   b. You report this to your immediate supervisor.
   c. You sit with the child, give him some toys to play with, and report this to your immediate supervisor later that day.
   d. You report this to your supervisor immediately. You stop by often to distract him as you sit with him, give him some toys, and explain how important it is to not disturb the IV.
5. When getting a patient up to sit at the bedside in a reclining chair, you notice the chair's wheel brakes do not work well. This causes the chair to slide backward about 6 inches across the floor as the patient sits down. The patient is not injured. What should you do?
   a. Make out a work repair form and send it to the proper person.
   b. Notify your immediate supervisor, and tell your coworkers to be careful.

c. Get another chair for your patient. Get help transferring him to the new chair, and remove the broken chair from the patient care area after labeling it "Broken." Report this to your immediate supervisor.

d. Make sure the chair is always up against the wall in the future when you transfer the patient to it, so that he will not be injured when it moves.

6. As you prepare to take Mr. O'Shea for a walk, you notice that the walker he brought from home to use in the hospital has two rubber tips missing from the feet. What should you do?

a. Make a note to have the medical equipment staff take a look at it next time they are in.

b. Obtain another walker that is the same size and that has all four rubber tips in place before you ambulate him.

c. Tell his wife to buy some new tips for the walker.

d. Let him use it this time because he is too impatient to wait for his walk, and you don't want him to complain to the immediate supervisor about you.

EXERCISE 7-2

Directions: On the line provided under each illustration, write what you should do in order to work the fire extinguisher and put out a fire.

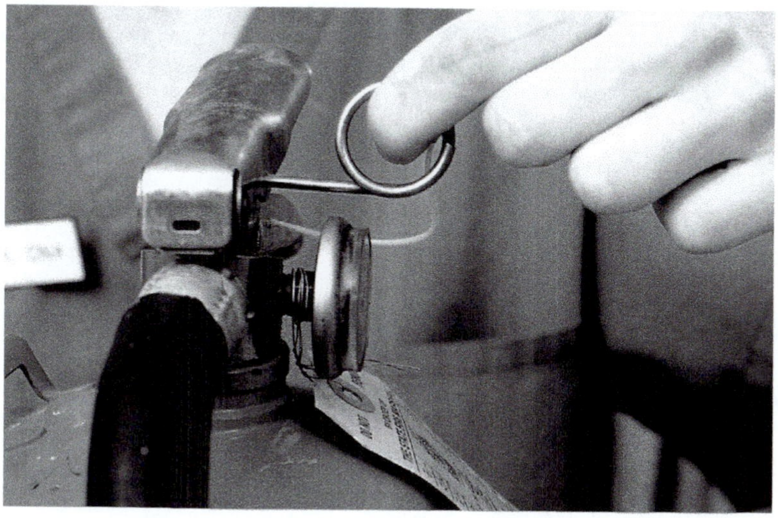

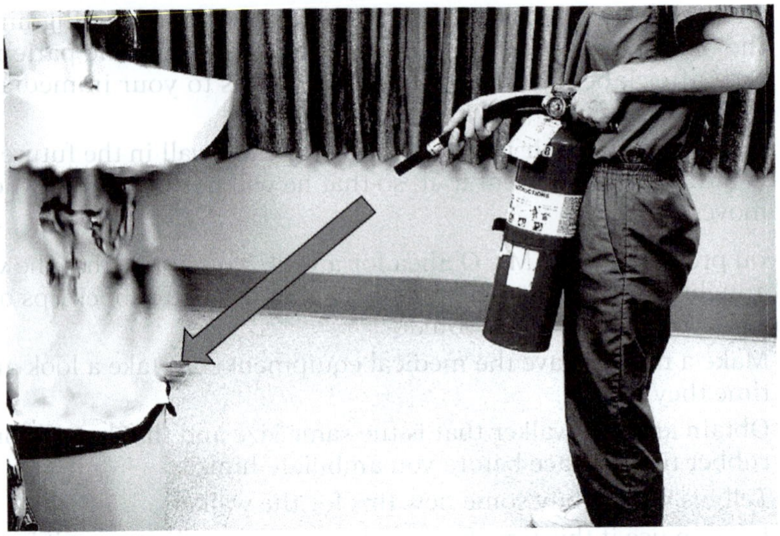

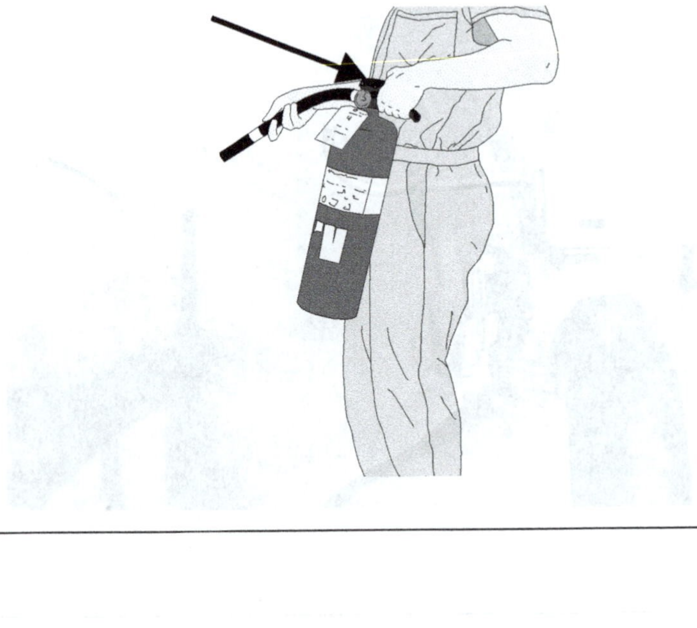

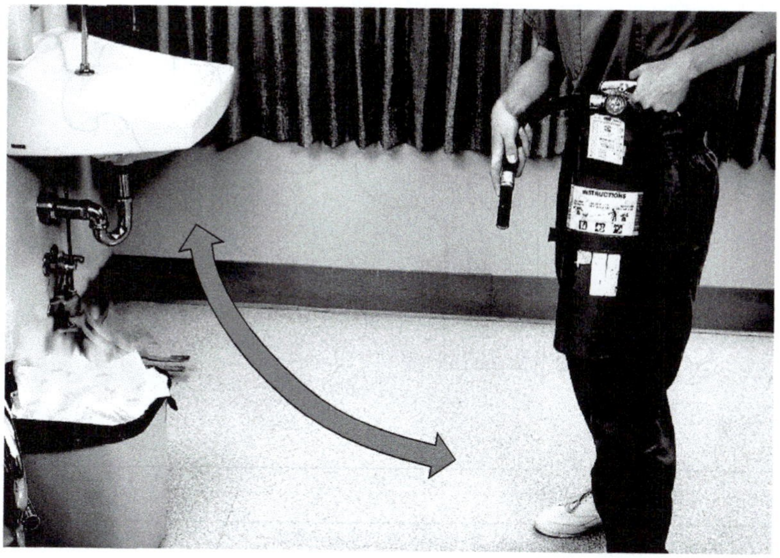

EXERCISE 7-3

Directions: On the line provided under each illustration, write what you should do in order to put a fire out and make sure patients are safe.

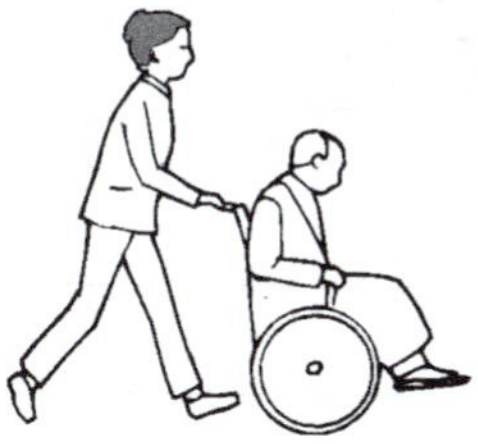

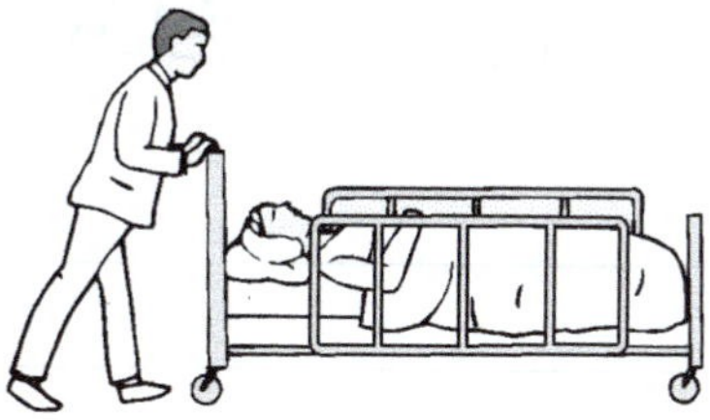

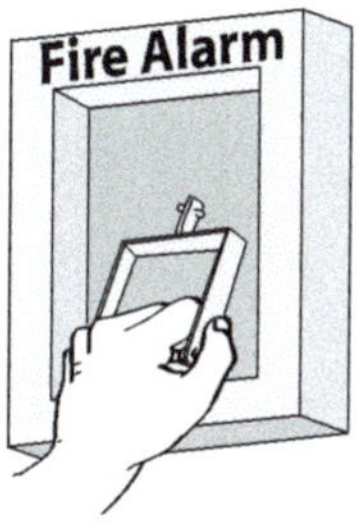

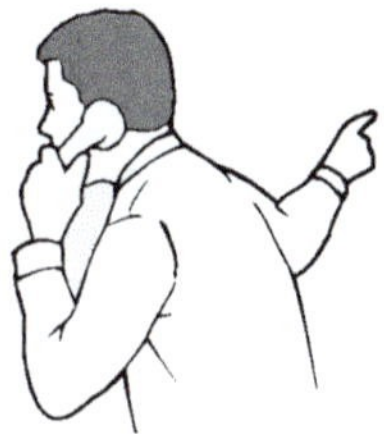

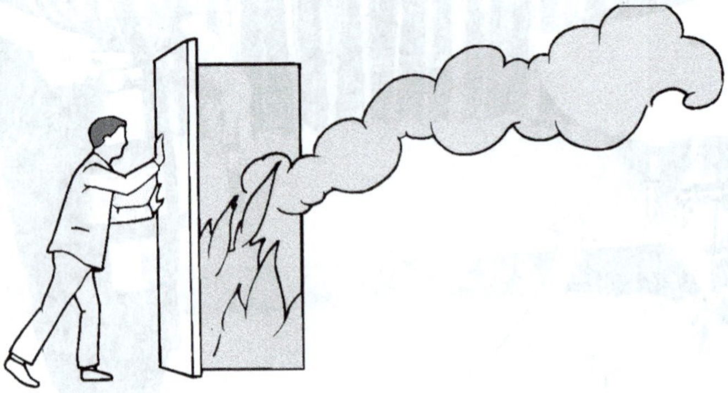

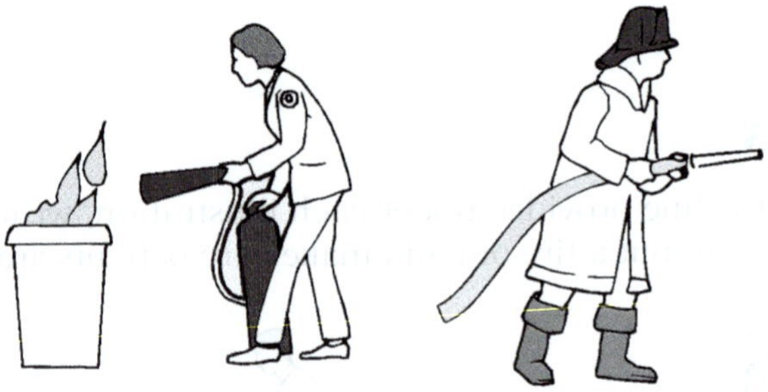

EXERCISE 7-4

Directions: Draw a line from column A and find the fire extinguisher that is best used for the type of fire described in column B.

Fire Extinguisher	Type of Fire
Type A	Any type of fire
Type B	Paper products, wood, and household garbage
Type C	Electrical fires
Type ABC	Kitchen fires; used in restaurants and large, industrial kitchens
Type K	Burnable liquids such as oil or grease

LEARNING ACTIVITIES

1. Develop a fire evacuation plan for your home that helps everyone know how to escape if a fire occurs. Every 3 months, practice the plan using different scenarios. Make sure everyone in the family knows a safe place to meet outside should a fire really happen.
2. Review your facility's disaster plan and participate in an evacuation day if you are able to do so.

PROCEDURE CHECKLISTS

PROCEDURE 7-1: USING A FIRE EXTINGUISHER

Name: ______________________ Date: ______________________

STEPS	S	U	COMMENTS
1. Follow the acronym RACE as previously outlined.			
2. Remove all persons from the area.			
3. Only fight the fire if it is safe to do so and if you are trained to use the appropriate fire extinguisher.			
4. Locate the fire extinguisher. These should be located in visible areas in all health care facilities. Be sure you have obtained the appropriate type of fire extinguisher. ABC fire extinguishers can be used on all types of fires. These are the ones used most commonly in health care settings.			
5. Pull the safety pin on the upper handle.			
6. Aim low. Point the nozzle at the base of the fire. Squeeze the handle releasing the extinguisher's agent.			
7. Sweep from side to side, aiming at the base of the fire until the fire goes out or is extinguished.			
8. Ensure the fire is completely extinguished and there are no smoking embers.			
9. Report to your supervisor. Fill out appropriate incident reports.			
10. Follow your facility's policy for disposing of and restocking the fire extinguisher that was used.			

Charting:

____

____

____

____

Date of Satisfactory Completion ______________________

Instructor's Signature ______________________

PROCEDURE 7-2: APPLYING BED AND CHAIR ALARMS

Name: ______________________ Date: ______________________

STEPS	S	U	COMMENTS
1. Assemble equipment.			
2. Identify the correct patient.			
3. Explain the procedure to the patient, and explain why the alarm is necessary.			
4. Wash your hands.			
5. Set up the chair alarm.			
a. Position the pressure-sensitive mat across the back of the chair.			
b. Plug the wire connection from the mat into the control unit.			
c. Attach the control unit to the back of the chair, out of the patient's sight or reach.			
d. Seat the patient in the chair.			
e. Test the alarm system daily.			
6. Set up the bed alarm.			
a. Position the pressure-sensitive mat across the width of the bed, directly on top of the mattress, and under the patient's buttocks.			
b. Plug the wire connection from the mat into the control unit.			
c. Attach the control unit to the bed frame.			
d. Plug the control unit into a wall outlet.			
e. Plug the nurse call light cord into the adaptor for the wall call system.			
f. Set the alarm for a 3-second delay.			
g. Place the patient in bed.			
h. Test the alarm system daily.			
7. Follow the manufacturer's product information guidelines for the on/off and reset mechanisms.			
8. Wash hands and document and report the results of the procedure to the RN or supervisor. Include the patient's response to the alarm.			
9. Provide care, and continue to monitor the patient every 15 minutes to 1 hour, per facility policy.			
10. When necessary, clean the mat with approved disinfectant solution.			

Charting:

____

____

____

____

Date of Satisfactory Completion ________________

Instructor's Signature ________________

8

Body Mechanics: Positioning, Moving, and Transporting Patients

Key Terms Review

Match the key terms in the right column with the definitions in the left column by placing the letter of each correct answer in the space provided.

_____ **1.** To walk or move about.

_____ **2.** Unable to walk.

_____ **3.** Unable to get out of bed.

_____ **4.** Unable to move without assistance.

_____ **5.** Special ways of standing and moving one's body to make the best use of strength and avoid fatigue.

_____ **6.** The correct or anatomical positioning of a patient's body; also the arrangement of the body in a straight line.

_____ **7.** A piece of canvas or fabric that goes around a person's waist to allow better steadying and assistance while walking.

_____ **8.** A covering used to provide privacy during an examination or operation.

_____ **9.** Covering a patient or parts of a patient's body with a sheet, blanket, bath blanket, or other material during a physical examination or prior to surgery.

_____ **10.** Small sheet made of cotton or a moisture-resistant material placed across the middle of the bed to cover and protect the bottom sheet and assist in moving the patient.

11. The skin remaining in one place while the underlying structures slide downward.

Terms

A. Trendelenburg position

B. Dorsal lithotomy position

C. Side-lying (lateral) positions

D. Semi-Fowler's position

E. Fowler's position

F. Knee–chest position

G. Prone position

H. Supine position

I. Transporting

J. Stretcher

K. Shearing

L. Ambulation

M. Immobile

N. Bedridden

O. Nonambulatory

P. Body alignment

Q. Proper/protective body mechanics

R. Draw sheet

12. A narrow rolling table or cart with or without a mattress used to transport patients; may be called a *gurney*.
13. Moving something or someone from one place to another.
14. Position in which the bed on which a patient is lying is tilted to the patient's head is about one foot below the level of his knees, to allow more blood flow to the head.
15. The position in which a patient lies on the back, with legs spread apart and knees bent.
16. Lying down or reclining; refers to the back or back part of an organ.
17. Lying on one's back.
18. Positioning the body on the right or left side, often done for comfort, to relieve pressure, and prevent skin breakdown.
19. The position in which the head of the bed is at a 30 to 45 degree angle
20. Lying on one's stomach.
21. The position in which the head of the bed is at a 45- to 90-degree angle.
22. A bent posture with the knees and chest touching the examination table, sometimes used for examination of the rectum or for women who have recently given birth to allow the uterus to fall forward into its natural position.

S. Drape
T. Draping
U. Gait belt
V. Dorsal recumbent position

MULTIPLE-CHOICE QUESTIONS

Circle the letter next to the word or statement that best completes the sentence or answers the question.

1. The term *body mechanics* refers to
   a. the correct positioning of the patient's body.
   b. the bones and joints.
   c. special ways of standing and moving one's body.
   d. rolling the patient like a log.
2. The purpose of good body mechanics is to
   a. rest comfortably in a hospital bed.
   b. make the best use of your own strength and avoid injury.
   c. avoid friction and irritation to the patient's skin.
   d. become stronger and more agile.
3. When an action requires physical effort, you should
   a. get close to the load that is being lifted.
   b. twist your back from side to side.
   c. try to use the smallest muscles in your arms and hands at all times.
   d. all of the above.
4. When lifting an object, the nursing assistant should
   a. keep her feet slightly more than hip width apart.
   b. squat close to the load.
   c. maintain the natural curves in her back.
   d. all of the above.

5. When the nursing assistant must move a heavy object,
   a. he should use a piece of equipment that can help him lift it.
   b. it is better to roll it than to carry it.
   c. he should ask another nursing assistant to help him.
   d. all of the above.

6. The correct positioning of a patient's body is referred to as
   a. body mechanics.
   b. body alignment.
   c. body position.
   d. body arrangement.

7. When using a gait belt, the nursing assistant should position herself
   a. about 12" from the patient.
   b. in front of the patient's stronger side.
   c. in the dorsal recumbent position.
   d. slightly behind the weaker side of the patient.

8. If a patient begins to fall when the nursing assistant is ambulating him, the nursing assistant should
   a. bend her back and lower herself to the floor.
   b. quickly drop to the floor to cushion the patient's fall with her body.
   c. bend her knees and flex her arms.
   d. bend her knees and lower her body to the floor with the patient.

9. Which is an acceptable position the nursing assistant can place a patient?
   a. Anterior
   b. Supine
   c. Foley's
   d. Caudal

10. Before moving the patient, all ___________ must be placed where they will not be pulled.
    a. visitors
    b. sheets
    c. tubing (such as catheters and IVs)
    d. pillows

11. A general rule when moving patients is to
    a. drop the arms and legs over the edge of the stretcher.
    b. pull with a quick, jerky movement.
    c. remove all catheters and other tubing.
    d. give the most support to the heaviest parts of the body.

12. Before moving any patient, the nursing assistant should
    a. explain what he is doing to the patient.
    b. rest by taking a break.
    c. notify his immediate supervisor.
    d. be fitted for a gait belt.

13. Before helping the patient move up in bed, the nursing assistant should first
    a. raise the head of the bed to semi-Fowler's position or higher and encourage the patient to reposition himself.
    b. introduce herself and explain what it is you want the patient to do to help with the move.
    c. raise the bottom of the bed and let the patient slide up to the headboard.
    d. hold the patient as far away from herself as possible.

14. When moving a patient in bed, the nursing assistant should
    a. place the draw sheet under the patient's head to protect him from hitting the headboard.
    b. turn the patient on his side before the move occurs.
    c. ask a colleague to assist with the move and then use the draw sheet to help prevent friction and irritation to the patient's skin from occurring.
    d. tie the patient to the frame of the bed using the draw sheet so the patient does not fall out of bed.

15. The nursing assistant sits the patient up on the side of the bed to dangle. The nursing assistant should report
    a. any complaint of dizziness
    b. if the patient is weak on one side of the body
    c. how well the patient tolerated the change in position
    d. all of the above

16. When transferring a patient from the bed to a wheelchair, the nursing assistant should
   a. remove the patient's robe so it does not get caught in the wheels.
   b. position the locked wheelchair so it touches the bed frame
   c. do all the work when lifting to make sure the patient does not hurt himself.
   d. avoid using an assistive device such as a gait belt or mechanical lift.

17. When transferring a patient from the bed to a stretcher, the nursing assistant should
   a. raise the bed height even with the height of the stretcher.
   b. never ask for help from any colleagues as she can do this herself with help from the patient.
   c. keep the patient's bed in the lowest height and closest to the ground so a fall does not happen while the transfer occurs.
   d. avoid locking both the bed and the stretcher.

18. When moving a stretcher, the nursing assistant should
   a. position herself at the foot of the stretcher.
   b. leave the rails down.
   c. enter an elevator by moving the head of the stretcher in first.
   d. stay at the head of the stretcher when going down a ramp.

19. Which position is commonly used when a vaginal examination occurs?
   a. Sims' position
   b. Dorsal lithotomy
   c. Fowler's
   d. Trendelenburg

20. Trendelenburg position is used in which type of situation?
   a. A teenager needs to rest in bed after his chemotherapy treatment is finished.
   b. An elderly man experiences shortness of breath from his respiratory problems.
   c. A patient faints.
   d. An enema needs to be administered.

21. Which position should be used when offering a back rub?
   a. Prone
   b. Supine
   c. High-Fowler's
   d. Trendelenburg

22. Mrs. Lopez complains of having difficulty breathing when lying on her back. The nursing assistant repositions her to a ________ position, and then report her complaint to the nurse.
   a. Sims'
   b. side-lying
   c. Trendelenburg
   d. Fowler's

23. How many drapes are offered when a patient is in knee–chest position?
   a. One
   b. Two
   c. Three
   d. None

24. In an effort to avoid ________, it is best to lift a patient rather than to pull a patient up in bed.
   a. shearing
   b. friction
   c. tension
   d. pressure sores

25. When moving an immobile comatose patient to one side of the bed, the nursing assistant should
   a. move the shoulders, then the legs, and then the middle portion of the body.
   b. move the shoulders, then the middle portion of the body, and leave the legs for last.
   c. logroll the patient.
   d. ask the patient to assist him.

TRUE OR FALSE QUESTIONS

Determine whether each question is true or false. In the space provided, write "T" for true and "F" for false. If the statement is false, rewrite it on the line provided to make it a true statement.

____ **1.** A stretcher should be pushed with the patient's head moving first.

____

____ **2.** When moving a patient in a wheelchair down a steep ramp, you should push the chair down frontward.

____

____ **3.** Many conditions and injuries make it dangerous for a patient to be in certain positions.

____

____ **4.** Before getting a patient from a bed to a chair, it is common courtesy to ask whether they need to use the bedpan or have any pain.

____

____ **5.** Trendelenburg position is used for rectal examinations.

____

____ **6.** The Joint Commission allows the use of side rails when a person has been sedated and is waiting to go into surgery.

____

____ **7.** The Joint Commission suggests that side rails should be avoided for patients with seizure disorder.

____

____ **8.** If a patient falls in the hallway, you should slide him to the ground, protect his head, make sure he is not hurt, and then get him back on his feet immediately.

____

____ **9.** When ambulating a patient, it is important to encourage the patient to walk with his head up.

____

____ **10.** When a patient is in dorsal lithotomy position, she is placed on her back with her legs and her knees slightly bent.

____

EXERCISE 8-1

Objective: To demonstrate an understanding of correct body mechanics to use when lifting or changing position.

Directions: Circle the letters of the pictures in Figure 8-1 that illustrate correct body mechanics.

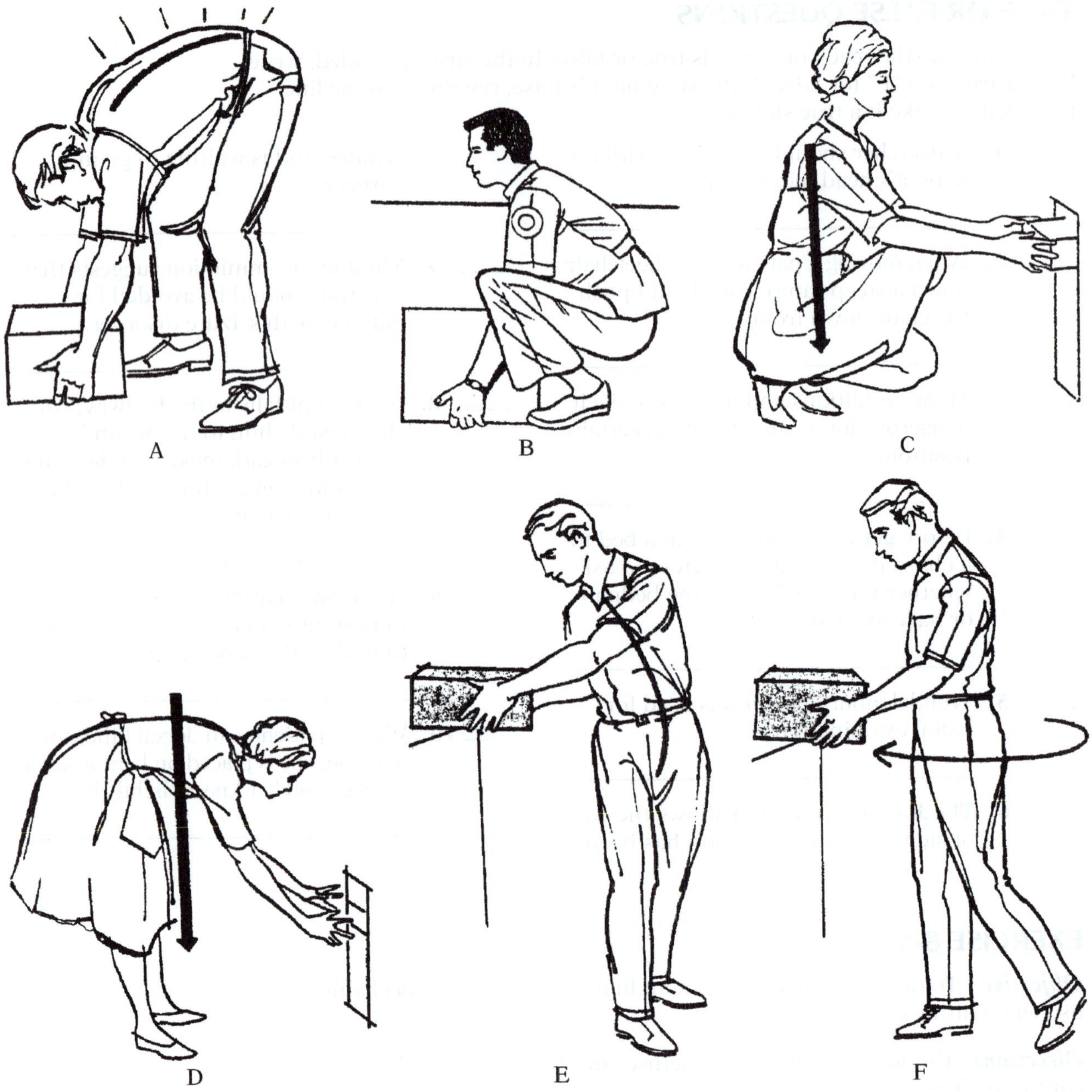

FIGURE 8-1

EXERCISE 8-2

Objective: To recognize methods of moving a patient using proper body mechanics.

Directions: Label the pictures in Figure 8-2 with the correct letter from the following list that describes the type of moving procedure shown.

A. Turning a patient on his side away from you.

B. Moving the mattress to the head of the bed with the patient's help.

C. Moving a helpless patient to one side of the bed on his back.

D. Moving the non-ambulatory patient up in bed.

E. Turning a patient on his side toward you.

F. Moving a patient up in bed with his help.

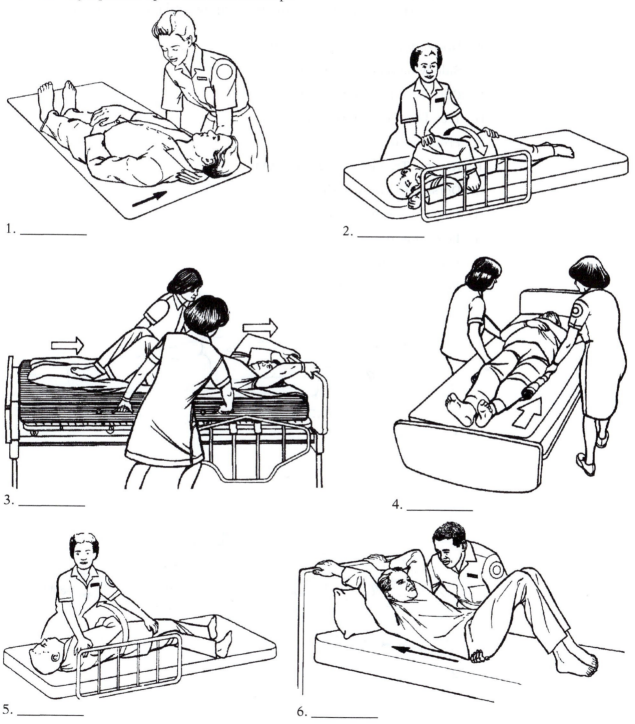

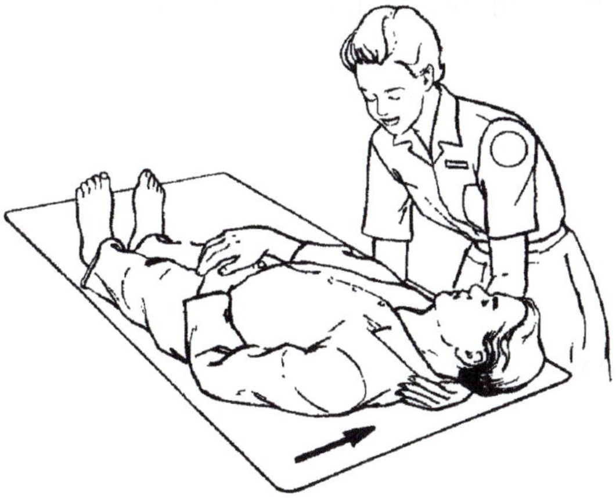

1. ________

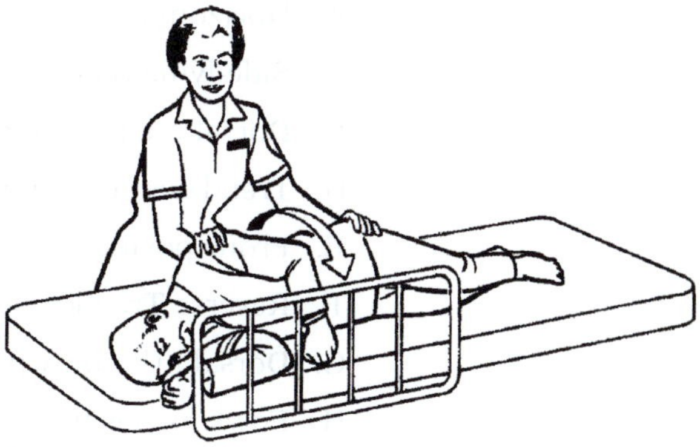

2. ________

3. ________

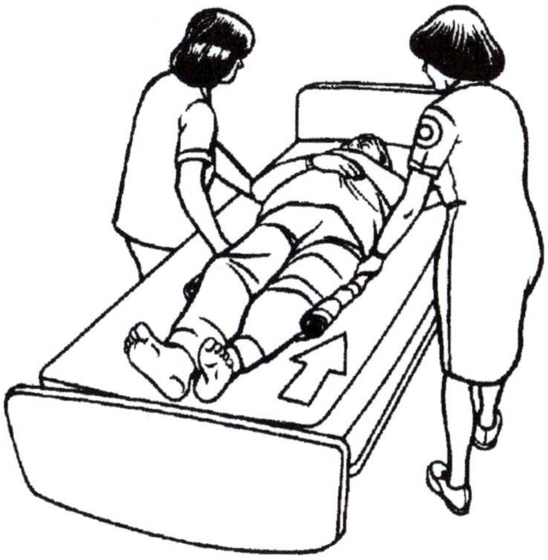

4. ________

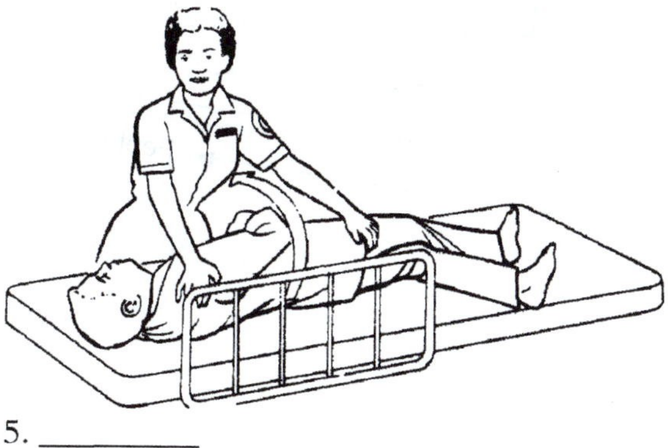

5. ________

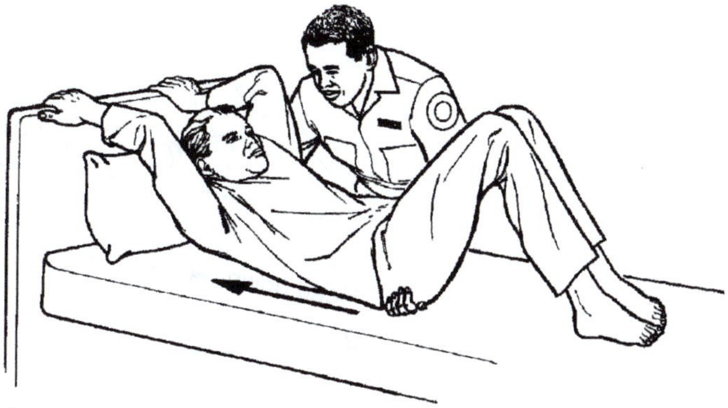

6. ________

FIGURE 8-2

EXERCISE 8-3

Objective: To recognize the proper methods of draping and positioning the patient.

Directions: Label the pictures in Figure 8-3 with the letter from the following list that describes the correct method of draping and positioning the patient.

A. Horizontal recumbent position
B. Side-lying (lateral) position
C. Dorsal recumbent position
D. Trendelenburg's position
E. Prone position
F. Reverse Trendelenburg's position
G. Dorsal lithotomy position
H. Fowler's position at 45 degrees
I. Left Sims' position
J. Knee–chest position
K. Left lateral position

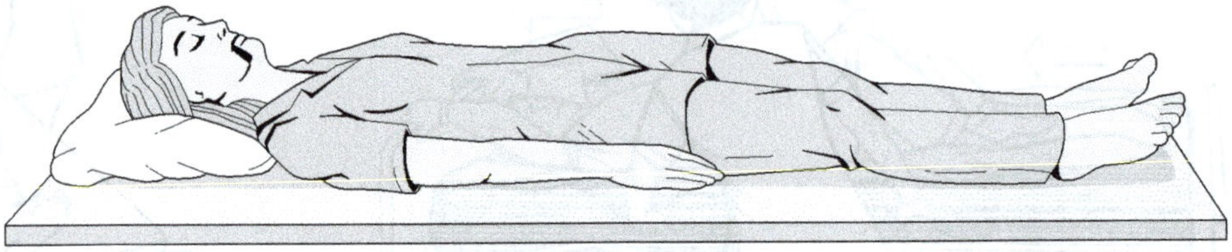

1. ___________

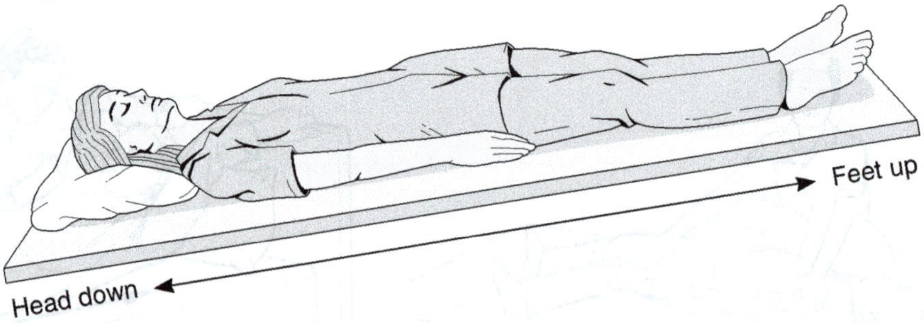

2. ___________

FIGURE 8-3

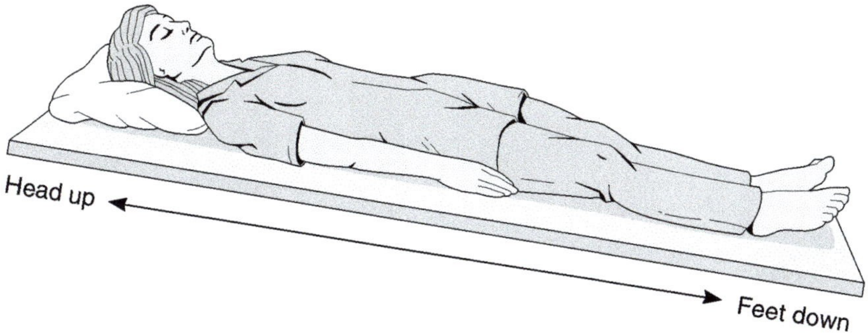

3. ___________

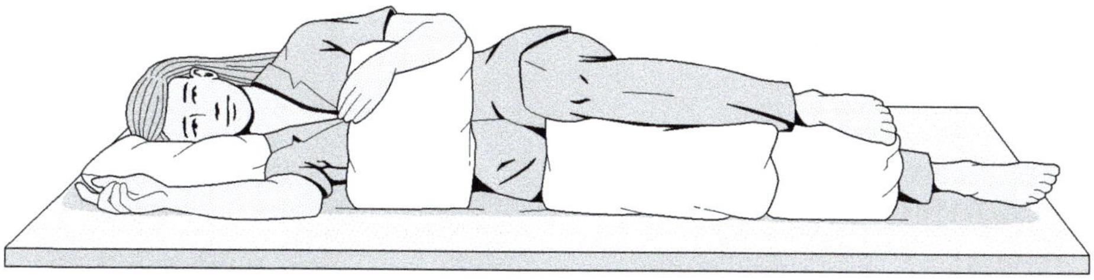

4. ___________

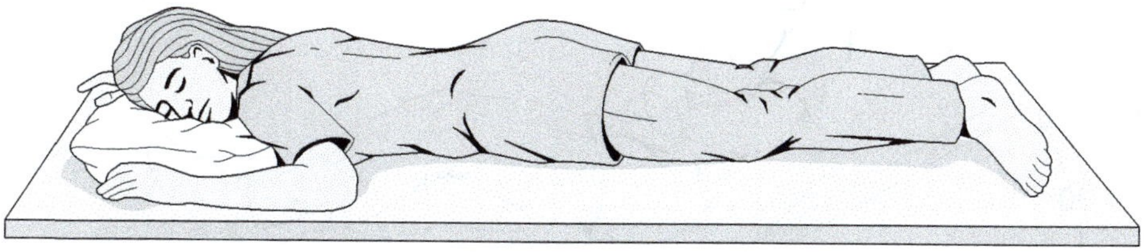

5. ___________

FIGURE 8-3 (cont.)

6. ___________

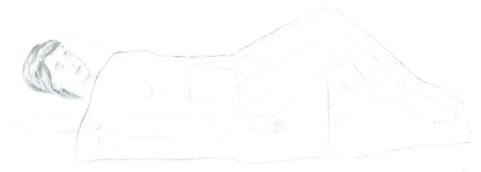

7. ___________

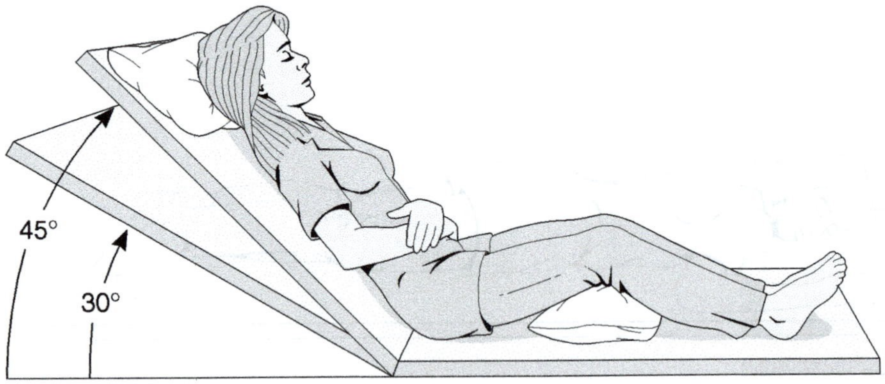

8. ___________

FIGURE 8-3 (cont.)

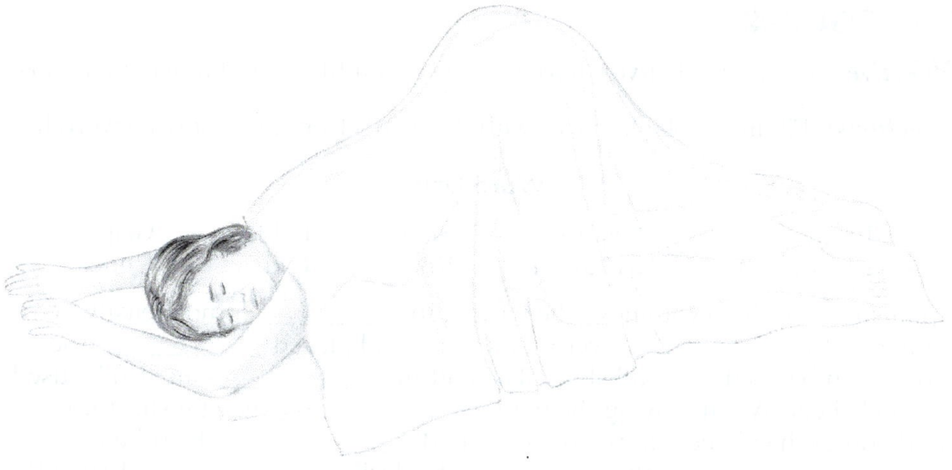

9. __________

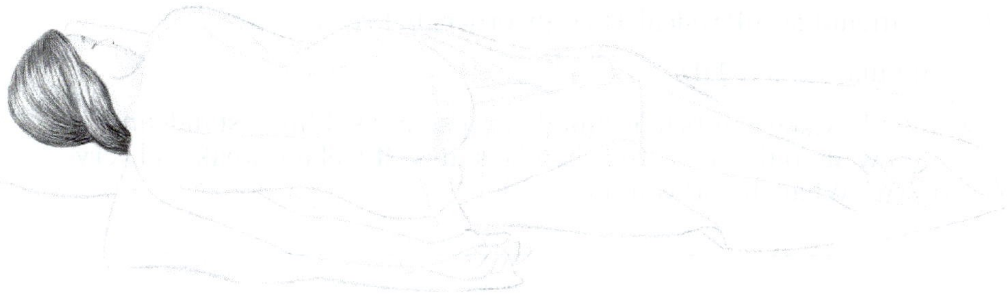

10. __________

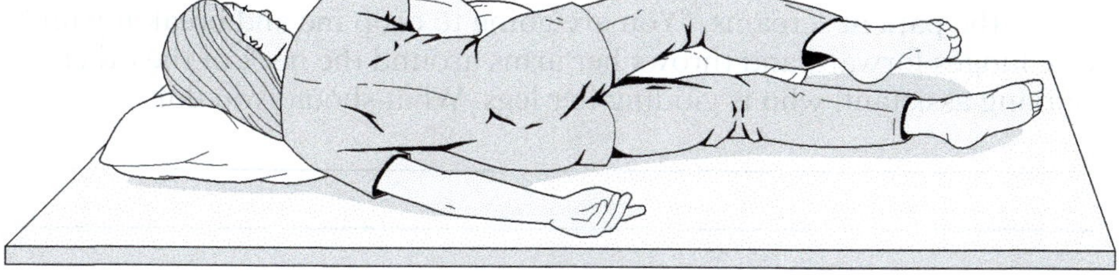

11. __________

FIGURE 8-3 (cont.)

EXERCISE 8-4

Objective: To apply what you have learned about lifting and moving patients.

Directions: Fill in the blank spaces with the words from the following word list.

Word List

Friction	Position	Slide	Folded	Grip
Draw sheet	Irritation	Roll	Bed	Under

A pull sheet can help you move the patient in ____________ more easily. A regular sheet ____________ over many times and placed ____________ the patient can be used as a pull sheet. The cotton ____________ can also be used as a pull sheet. When moving the patient, ____________ the pull sheet up tightly on each side next to the patient's body. ____________ the rolled portion to ____________ the patient into the desired ____________. Use of the pull sheet avoids ____________ and ____________ to the patient's skin that touches the bedding.

THE NURSING ASSISTANT IN ACTION

1. A patient has a Physical Therapy order that reads

   Ambulate 150 ft TID.

   You place the gait belt around his waist, assist him to stand, and you both walk to the doorway when he states, "I feel too weak and very dizzy." What should you do?

   ____

   ____

   ____

   ____

2. Another nursing assistant is helping you assist a patient using a mechanical lift. You have placed the sling under the patient, adjusted and secured the straps, and proceed to lift the patient. Halfway to the chair, the patient screams, "You are going to drop me and break my hip!" She lunges forward and throws her arms around the neck of the other nursing assistant, who is guiding her legs. What should you do?

   ____

   ____

   ____

   ____

3. You check on a patient who is in a wheelchair and notice she is slipping down near the edge of the seat. What should you do?

   ____

   ____

4. A patient with respiratory problems tends to slide to the foot of the bed and complains frequently he is uncomfortable. What should you do?

5. An operating room nurse returns your patient to the unit on a stretcher after his surgery is completed. She asks you to help her return this patient to his bed. He is semi-conscious. What should you do?

LEARNING ACTIVITIES

1. With a friend, practice lifting and transferring using the various methods described in the textbook. What was difficult about the procedure? How did it feel to have someone perform the skill on you? Discuss.
2. In your own bed or a practice lab, practice placing yourself into some of the positions you learned from the textbook. Identify what was uncomfortable or embarrassing for you. Then think about what kinds of things you must do to ensure privacy, make the patient feel comfortable, and provide safe care.

PROCEDURE CHECKLISTS

PROCEDURE 8-1: PLACING A PATIENT IN SUPINE POSITION

Name: ____________________ Date: ____________________

STEPS	S	U	COMMENTS
1. Wash your hands.			
2. Identify the patient by checking the identification bracelet.			
3. Ask visitors to step out of the room, if this is facility policy.			
4. Tell the patient that you are going to position her lying on her back.			
5. Provide privacy for the patient.			
6. Gently position the patient flat on her back. Use pillows to prop arms and legs as needed.			
7. Ensure patient comfort and ease of breathing (some patients with respiratory conditions have problems breathing while in this position).			
8. Cover the patient as appropriate.			
9. Lower the bed to a position of safety and comfort.			
10. Raise the side rails when ordered or indicated.			
11. Place the call light within easy reach of the patient.			
12. Wash your hands.			
13. Report to your supervisor			
• The patient has been placed in supine position.			
• The time the patient's position was changed.			
• How the patient tolerated the procedure.			
• Any abnormal or unusual observations.			

Charting:

____

____

____

____

Date of Satisfactory Completion ____________________

Instructor's Signature ____________________

PROCEDURE 8-2: PLACING A PATIENT IN SIMS' POSITION

Name: ____________________ Date: ____________________

STEPS	S	U	COMMENTS
1. Wash your hands.			
2. Identify the patient by checking the identification bracelet.			
3. Ask visitors to step out of the room, if this is facility policy.			
4. Tell the patient that you are going to position her in a partial side-lying and partial prone position.			
5. Provide privacy for the patient.			
6. Gently position the patient lying partially on her side and partially on her stomach. Use pillows to prop arms and legs as needed.			
7. Ensure patient comfort and ease of breathing (some patients with respiratory conditions have problems breathing while in this position).			
8. Cover the patient as appropriate.			
9. Lower the bed to a position of safety and comfort.			
10. Raise the side rails when ordered or indicated.			
11. Place the call light within easy reach of the patient.			
12. Wash your hands.			
13. Report to your supervisor			
• The patient has been placed in Sims' position.			
• The time the patient's position was changed.			
• How the patient tolerated the procedure.			
• Any abnormal or unusual observations.			

Charting:

____

____

____

____

Date of Satisfactory Completion ____________________

Instructor's Signature ____________________

PROCEDURE 8-3: PLACING A PATIENT IN SEMI-FOWLER'S POSITION

Name: ______________________ Date: ______________________

STEPS	S	U	COMMENTS
1. Wash your hands.			
2. Identify the patient by checking the identification bracelet.			
3. Ask visitors to step out of the room, if this is facility policy.			
4. Tell the patient that you are going to position him in a semi-sitting position.			
5. Provide privacy for the patient.			
6. Gently position the patient in the supine position, and adjust the head of the bed to about a 30-degree angle. Use pillows to prop arms and legs as needed.			
7. Ensure patient comfort.			
8. Cover the patient as appropriate.			
9. Lower the bed to a position of safety and comfort.			
10. Raise the side rails when ordered or indicated.			
11. Place the call light within easy reach of the patient.			
12. Wash your hands.			
13. Report to your supervisor			
• The patient has been placed in semi-Fowler's position.			
• The time the patient's position was changed.			
• How the patient tolerated the procedure.			
• Any abnormal or unusual observations.			

Charting:

____

____

____

____

Date of Satisfactory Completion ______________________

Instructor's Signature ______________________

PROCEDURE 8-4: PLACING A PATIENT IN FOWLER'S POSITION

Name: ____________________ Date: ____________________

STEPS	S	U	COMMENTS
1. Wash your hands.			
2. Identify the patient by checking the identification bracelet.			
3. Ask visitors to step out of the room, if this is facility policy.			
4. Tell the patient that you are going to position her in a sitting position.			
5. Provide privacy for the patient.			
6. Gently position the patient in the supine position, and adjust the head of the bed to about a 45-degree angle. Use pillows to prop arms and legs as needed.			
7. Ensure patient comfort.			
8. Cover the patient as appropriate.			
9. Lower the bed to a position of safety and comfort.			
10. Raise the side rails when ordered or indicated.			
11. Place the call light within easy reach of the patient.			
12. Wash your hands.			
13. Report to your supervisor			
• The patient has been placed in Fowler's position.			
• The time the patient's position was changed			
• How the patient tolerated the procedure			
• Any abnormal or unusual observations.			

Charting:

____

____

____

____

Date of Satisfactory Completion ____________________

Instructor's Signature ____________________

PROCEDURE 8-5: ASSISTING A PERSON WITH SITTING ON THE EDGE OF THE BED (DANGLING)

Name: ______________________ Date: ______________________

STEPS	S	U	COMMENTS
1. Wash your hands.			
2. Identify the patient by checking the identification bracelet.			
3. Ask visitors to step out of the room, if this is facility policy.			
4. Tell the patient that you are going to assist her with sitting on the edge of the bed.			
5. Provide privacy for the patient.			
6. Raise the head of the bed to about a 45-degree angle.			
7. Assist the patient with swinging her legs to one side while raising her shoulders off the head of the bed.			
8. Support the patient's shoulders as she lowers her legs to dangle over the side of the bed.			
9. Allow the patient to assume control of her posture as she sits on the edge of the bed. Watch the patient carefully, and be prepared to assist the patient back into a supine position if she becomes dizzy or faint.			
10. When the patient states she feels as though she can sit unassisted, remove your hands from her shoulders and allow her to sit comfortably on the side of the bed.			
11. Either assist the patient back into bed or assist to a standing position.			
12. Ensure patient comfort.			
13. Lower the bed to a position of safety.			
14. Place the call light within easy reach of the patient.			
15. Wash your hands.			
16. Report to your supervisor			
• You assisted the patient with sitting on the edge of the bed.			
• How long the patient was able to sit on the edge of the bed.			
• How the patient tolerated sitting on the edge of the bed.			
• Any abnormal or unusual observations.			

Charting:

____

____

____

____

Date of Satisfactory Completion ______________________

Instructor's Signature ______________________

PROCEDURE 8-6: MOVING THE IMMOBILE PATIENT UP IN BED

Name: ______________________ Date: ______________________

STEPS	S	U	COMMENTS
1. Ask another member of the nursing staff to work with you.			
2. Wash your hands.			
3. Identify the patient by checking the identification bracelet.			
4. Ask visitors to step out of the room, if this is facility policy.			
5. Tell the patient that you are going to move her up in bed. Do this step whether or not the patient appears to be able to hear or understand you.			
6. Provide privacy for the patient.			
7. Place the pillow from under the patient's head up against the headboard. This serves as protection for the patient's head.			
8. Lock the wheels on the bed.			
9. Raise the height of the bed to a comfortable working position.			
10. Lower the backrest and footrest, if allowed.			
11. Stand on one side of the bed, with the other member of nursing staff standing on the opposite side.			
12. Both movers should stand straight, pivoting with feet slightly toward the head of the bed and hip width apart. The foot closest to the head of the bed should be pointed in that direction. Both should bend their knees and maintain the natural curves in the back.			
13. The use of a draw sheet is always preferred for moving an immobile patient up in bed. This avoids friction on the patient's skin. Roll the sides of the sheet to be used as a draw sheet close to the patient. Each mover then grasps one side of the rolled portion of the sheet firmly so that when the patient is moved up, the sheet remains in place.			
14. You will be sliding the patient's body when you move her up in bed. Slightly bend your knees as you start to slide the patient, shifting your weight from one foot to the other.			
15. When you say "one, two, three" in unison, you and your partner move together to slide the patient gently toward the head of the bed or to the desired position.			

16. Ensure patient comfort.			
17. Replace pillows as requested by the patient.			
18. Lower the bed to a position of safety.			
19. Raise the side rails where ordered, indicated, and appropriate for patient safety.			
20. Place the call light within easy reach of the patient.			
21. Wash your hands.			
22. Report to your supervisor			
• The patient has been repositioned.			
• The time the position was changed.			
• How the patient tolerated the procedure.			
• Observations of anything else unusual.			

Charting:

____

____

____

____

Date of Satisfactory Completion ______________

Instructor's Signature ______________

PROCEDURE 8-7: MOVING A PATIENT UP IN BED WITH THE PATIENT'S HELP

Name: ____________________ Date: ____________________

STEPS	S	U	COMMENTS
1. Wash your hands.			
2. Identify the patient by checking the identification bracelet.			
3. Ask visitors to step out of the room, if this is facility policy.			
4. Tell the patient that you are going to move him up in bed. Before you begin, ask your supervisor if the patient is allowed to use exertion to assist with moving			
5. Provide privacy for the patient.			
6. Lock the wheels on the bed.			
7. Raise the height of the bed to a comfortable working position.			
8. Lower the backrest and footrest, if allowed.			
9. Remove the pillow from under the patient's head. Put the pillow at the top of the bed against the headboard. This protects the patient's head from hitting the headboard.			
10. Put the side rails in the up position on the far side of the bed.			
11. Put one hand under the patient's shoulder. Put your other hand under the patient's hip. Provide assistance to the weaker side of the patient.			
12. Ask the patient to bend his knees and brace his feet firmly on the mattress. Have your feet hip width apart. The foot closest to the head of the bed should be pointed in the direction of the head of the bed.			
13. Bend your knees and maintain the natural curves of your back.			
14. Bend your body from your hips and pivot slightly toward the head of the bed.			
15. At the count of "one, two, three," have the patient push toward the head of the bed with his hands and feet.			
16. At the same time, help the patient move toward the head of the bed by sliding the patient with your hands and arms as you shift weight from back foot to foot closest to the head of the bed.			
17. Replace the pillows under the patient's head and shoulders.			

18. Ensure patient comfort.			
19. Lower the bed to a position of safety.			
20. Raise the side rails if indicated to provide patient safety.			
21. Place the call light within easy reach of the patient.			
22. Wash your hands.			
23. Report to your supervisor			
• The patient position has been changed.			
• The time the position was changed.			
• How the patient tolerated the procedure.			
• Your observations of anything unusual.			

Charting:

____

____

____

____

Date of Satisfactory Completion ____________________

Instructor's Signature ____________________

PROCEDURE 8-8: MOVING THE MATTRESS TO THE HEAD OF THE BED WITH THE PATIENT'S HELP

Name: ____________________ Date: ____________________

STEPS	S	U	COMMENTS
1. Wash your hands.			
2. Ask another team member to help you.			
3. Identify the patient by checking the identification bracelet.			
4. Ask visitors to step out of the room, if this is facility policy.			
5. Tell the patient that you are going to move the mattress to the head of the bed.			
6. Provide privacy for the patient.			
7. Lock the wheels on the bed.			
8. Raise the height of the bed to a comfortable working position.			
9. Lower the head of the bed, if permitted.			
10. If you are working alone, put the side rail in the up position on the far side of the bed.			
11. If you are working with a partner, each of you should stand at opposite sides of the bed and loosen the sheets.			
12. Lock arms with the patient and remove the pillow.			
13. Ask the patient to grasp the headboard with both hands.			
14. Ask the patient to bend her knees and brace her feet firmly on the mattress.			
15. Grasp the mattress loops, or the sides of the mattress.			
16. At the count, "one, two, three," have the patient pull with her hands toward the head of the bed and push with her feet against the mattress.			
17. At the same time, both movers slide the mattress toward the head of the bed, keeping knees bent and backs straight.			
18. Lock arms with the patient and put the pillow back in place.			
19. Ensure patient comfort.			
20. Lower the bed to a position of safety for the patient.			
21. Raise the side rails if indicated or appropriate for patient safety.			

22. Place the call light within easy reach of the patient.			
23. Wash your hands.			
24. Report to your supervisor			
• The mattress was moved to the head of the bed with the patient's help.			
• The time the mattress was moved.			
• How the patient tolerated the procedure.			
• Your observations of anything unusual.			

Charting:

____

____

____

____

Date of Satisfactory Completion ____________________

Instructor's Signature ____________________

PROCEDURE 8-9: MOVING AN IMMOBILE PATIENT TO ONE SIDE OF THE BED ON THE PATIENT'S BACK

Name: ____________________ Date: ____________________

STEPS	S	U	COMMENTS
1. Wash your hands.			
2. Identify the patient by checking the identification bracelet.			
3. Ask visitors to step out of the room, if this is facility policy.			
4. Tell the patient that you are going to move him to one side of the bed on his back without turning him.			
5. Provide privacy for the patient.			
6. Lock the wheels on the bed.			
7. Raise the height of the bed to a comfortable working position.			
8. Lower the head of the bed, if permitted.			
9. Put the side rail on the far side of the bed in the "up" position.			
10. Loosen the top sheets, but don't keep the patient covered.			
11. With one leg slightly in front of the other and the front knee slightly bent, slide both your arms under the patient's back to his far shoulder. Slide the patient's shoulders toward you on your arms as you shift weight from front leg to back leg, while straightening the front leg.			
12. Slide both your arms as far as you can under the patient's hips and slide his hips toward you, again shifting weight from front leg to back leg. If possible, use a draw sheet.			
13. Place both your arms under the patient's lower legs and slide them toward you on your arms, again, shifting your weight from one leg to the other.			
14. Adjust the pillow, if necessary.			
15. Remake the top of the bed.			
16. Ensure patient comfort.			
17. Lower the bed to a position of safety.			
18. Raise the side rails if indicated or appropriate.			
19. Place the call light within easy reach of the patient.			

20. Wash your hands.			
21. Report to your supervisor			
• The patient has been moved to one side of the bed on his back.			
• The time the patient position was changed.			
• How the patient tolerated the procedure.			
• Observations of anything unusual.			

Charting:

____

____

____

____

Date of Satisfactory Completion ____________________

Instructor's Signature ____________________

PROCEDURE 8-10: LOGROLLING A PATIENT

Name: ____________________ Date: ____________________

STEPS	S	U	COMMENTS
1. Wash your hands.			
2. Identify the patient by checking the identification bracelet.			
3. Ask visitors to step out of the room, if this is facility policy.			
4. Explain to the patient that you are going to roll him like a log to his side.			
5. Provide privacy for the patient.			
6. If necessary, get additional help.			
7. Lock the wheels on the bed.			
8. Raise the height of the bed to a comfortable working position.			
9. Raise the side rail on the far side of the bed.			
10. If permitted and patient condition allows, remove the pillow from under the patient's head. Position the patient's arm across the chest.			
11. Position your legs so that one is in front of the other, with the front knee slightly bent.			
12. Slide both your arms under the patient's back to his far shoulder, and then slide the patient's shoulders toward you on your arms as you shift your weight from the front leg to the back leg while straightening your front knee.			
13. Grasp the patient under the knees and ankles. Shift your weight from your back foot to the foot closest to the bed as you bend the patient's hips and knees. Place the patient's feet flat on the bed. If needed, place a pillow between the patient's legs.			
14. Grasp the patient under the knees and ankles. Shift your weight from your back foot to the foot closest to the bed as you bend the patient's hips and knees. Place the patient's feet flat on the bed. If needed, place a pillow between the patient's legs.			
15. Replace the pillow under the patient's head, if permitted.			
16. Use pillows against the patient's back to keep the body in proper alignment.			
17. Replace linens on the top of the bed.			
18. Ensure patient comfort.			

19. Lower the bed to a position of safety.			
20. Raise the side rails if ordered or indicated.			
21. Place the call light within easy reach of the patient.			
22. Wash your hands.			
23. Report to your supervisor			
• The patient's position was changed by log-rolling.			
• The time the patient's position was changed.			
• How the patient tolerated the procedure.			
• Observations of anything unusual.			

Charting:

____

____

____

____

Date of Satisfactory Completion ____________________

Instructor's Signature ____________________

PROCEDURE 8-11: TURNING A PATIENT ONTO THE PATIENT'S SIDE TOWARD YOU

Name: ____________________ Date: ____________________

STEPS	S	U	COMMENTS
1. Wash your hands.			
2. Identify the patient by checking the identification bracelet.			
3. Ask visitors to step out of the room, if this is facility policy.			
4. Explain to the patient that you are going to turn him on his side.			
5. Provide privacy for the patient.			
6. Lock the wheels on the bed.			
7. Raise the height of the bed to a comfortable working position.			
8. Lower the head and foot of the bed, if permitted.			
9. Put the side rail on the far side of the bed in the "up" position.			
10. Loosen the top sheets, but do not expose the patient.			
11. When you are turning the patient toward you, cross the patient's arms over the chest and bend the knees, placing the feet on the bed.			
12. With one leg slightly in front of the other and the front knee slightly bent, reach across the patient and put one hand behind the far shoulder, shifting your weight to the front leg as you do so.			
13. Place your other hand behind the patient's far hip, gently roll the patient toward you again as you shift your weight from the front leg to the back leg.			
14. Fold a pillow lengthwise and place it against the patient's back for support.			
15. Place a pillow under the patient's head.			
16. Place the patient's arms and legs in a comfortable position. Be sure the arm resting on the mattress is free from pressure.			
17. Replace linens on the top of the bed.			
18. Ensure patient comfort.			
19. Lower the bed to a position of safety.			
20. Raise the side rails if ordered or indicated.			
21. Place the call light within easy reach of the patient.			

22. Wash your hands.			
23. Report to your supervisor			
• The patient's position has been changed.			
• How the patient tolerated the procedure.			
• Any unusual observations.			

Charting:

____

____

____

____

Date of Satisfactory Completion ____________________

Instructor's Signature ____________________

PROCEDURE 8-12: TURNING A PATIENT ONTO THE PATIENT'S SIDE AWAY FROM YOU

Name: ______________________ Date: ______________________

STEPS	S	U	COMMENTS
1. Wash your hands.			
2. Identify the patient by checking the identification bracelet.			
3. Ask visitors to step out of the room, if this is facility policy.			
4. Explain to the patient that you are going to turn him on the other side.			
5. Provide privacy for the patient.			
6. Lock the wheels on the bed.			
7. Raise the height of the bed to a comfortable working position.			
8. Lower the head and foot of the bed, if permitted.			
9. Put the side rail on the far side of the bed in the "up" position.			
10. Loosen the top sheets without exposing the patient.			
11. With one leg positioned in front of the other, slide both your arms under the patient's back to the far shoulder as you shift your weight from the back leg to the front leg. Slide the patient's shoulders toward you on your arms as you shift your weight from the front leg to the back leg.			
12. Slide both of your arms as far as you can under the patient's hips toward you, again, as you shift your weight from the back leg to the front leg.			
13. Place both your arms under the patient's lower legs and slide them toward you on your arms as you shift your weight from the front leg to the back leg.			
14. Cross the patient's arms over the chest and bend the patient's knees, placing the feet on the bed.			
15. Place one hand on the patient's shoulder near you.			
16. Put your other hand along the hip/thigh nearest you.			
17. Turn the patient gently on his side, facing away from you.			
18. Fold a pillow lengthwise. Place it against the patient's back for support.			
19. Place a pillow under the patient's head.			

20. Make sure the patient's arms and legs are in a comfortable position. A pillow may be placed between the knees of the patient if needed. Be sure the arm resting on the mattress is free from pressure.			
21. Remake the top of the bed.			
22. Lower the bed to a position of safety.			
23. Ensure patient comfort.			
24. Raise the side rails if ordered or indicated.			
21. Place the call light within easy reach of the patient.			
22. Wash your hands.			
23. Report to your supervisor			
• The patient's position has been changed.			
• How the patient tolerated the procedure.			
• Any unusual observations.			

Charting:

____

____

____

____

Date of Satisfactory Completion ____________________

Instructor's Signature ____________________

PROCEDURE 8-13: REPOSITIONING A PATIENT IN A WHEELCHAIR

Name: ______________________ Date: ______________________

STEPS	S	U	COMMENTS
1. Place the patient's feet flat on the floor.			
2. Bend your knees and place one foot in front of the other.			
3. Bend the patient at the waist and gently rock the patient onto the left or right hip, while sliding the other side of the patient's body back into the chair. Repeat for the other side.			
4. An alternate technique to adjust the patient's position is to stand behind the patient in the wheelchair and lift the patient up.			
5. Replace footrests.			
6. Ensure patient comfort and safety.			

Charting:

____

____

____

____

Date of Satisfactory Completion ______________________

Instructor's Signature ______________________

PROCEDURE 8-14: MOVING THE NONAMBULATORY PATIENT INTO A WHEELCHAIR OR ARM CHAIR FROM THE BED

Name: ____________________ Date: ____________________

STEPS	S	U	COMMENTS
1. Assemble equipment			
• Wheelchair or arm chair			
• Blanket or sheet			
• Gait belt, if needed			
• Robe, if desired			
2. Wash your hands.			
3. Identify the patient by checking the identification bracelet.			
4. Ask visitors to step out of the room, if this is your facility's policy.			
5. Explain to the patient that you are going to assist him into a wheelchair.			
6. Provide privacy for the patient.			
7. Lock the wheels on the bed.			
8. Spread a blanket or sheet on the chair. Have the corner of the blanket between the handles over the back so the opposite corner will be at the patient's feet.			
9. Ask another nursing assistant to help you.			
10. Put the patient's robe and nonslip shoes on while she is in bed.			
11. Move the patient to the edge of the bed			
a. Slide both of your arms under the patient's back to the shoulder, then slide the patient's shoulders toward you on your arms.			
b. Slide both your arms as far as you can under the patient's hips and slide the hips toward you. Use a draw sheet if possible.			
c. Place both of your arms under the patient's lower legs and slide them toward you on your arms.			
12. Raise the side rail.			
13. Lower the bed to its lowest horizontal position so that when you dangle the patient, her feet touch the floor when she sits up.			
14. Raise the backrest so that the patient is in a sitting position in bed.			
15. Lower the side rail on the side where you and the other nursing assistant are working.			

16. Place both hands under the patient's legs and turn them to the dangling position. The patient's feet should be firmly on the floor. One nursing assistant supports the patient's back and head and raises them at the same time. The other nursing assistant places her arm around the patient's shoulders to support the patient's back while the patient is in the dangling position. Give the patient a minute or so to adjust. Observe how the patient is tolerating sitting.			
17. Place a gait belt around the patient's waist per facility policy.			
18. Assist the patient in sliding forward to the side of the bed. Place the patient's feet flat on the floor. Support the patient behind the shoulders so that she is sitting upright.			
19. Place the wheelchair at the bedside with the back of the chair in line with the middle of the bed. Lock the wheels on the chair.			
20 Fold up the footrests of the wheelchair so they are out of the way. If the wheelchair has leg rests, adjust them to hang straight down, or remove them.			
21. Lock the brakes on the wheelchair.			
22. Ask the patient to hug you in front, around your waist. Then block the patient's knees between your knees and grasp the gait belt at the patient's sides.			
23. The second nursing assistant, or helper, should be positioned with one knee on the bed.			
24. The first assistant, in front, should gently pull the patient forward into the wheelchair while the second assistant guides the patient's hips onto the chair.			
25. Fasten the safety straps around the patient, if applicable, to prevent the patient from falling out of the chair.			
26. Arrange the blanket snugly but firmly around the patient. Make sure no part of the blanket can get caught in the wheels.			
27. Adjust the footrests so the patient's feet are resting comfortably on them.			
28. Use the signal cord to call your immediate supervisor and take the patient's pulse and blood pressure if any of the following is observed:			
a. The patient becomes very pale.			
b. The patient seems to be perspiring heavily.			
c. The patient complains of feeling weak or dizzy.			
29. Adjust the chair to a comfortable angle.			

30. Put a pillow behind the patient's back or shoulders if needed.			
31. Wash your hands.			
32. Report to your supervisor			
• The patient has been moved out of bed into a chair or wheelchair.			
• The time the patient's position was changed.			
• How the patient tolerated the procedure.			
• Any unusual observations.			

Charting:

____

____

____

____

Date of Satisfactory Completion ____________________

Instructor's Signature ____________________

PROCEDURE 8-15: HELPING A NONAMBULATORY PATIENT BACK INTO BED FROM A WHEELCHAIR OR ARMCHAIR

Name: ____________________ Date: ____________________

STEPS	S	U	COMMENTS
1. Ask another nursing assistant to help you.			
2. Wash your hands.			
3. Identify the patient by checking the identification bracelet.			
4. Ask visitors to step out of the room, if this is your facility's policy.			
5. Explain to the patient that you are getting him back into bed.			
6. Place a draw sheet on the bottom sheets; fan-fold from the top of the bed to the foot.			
7. Lock the wheels on the bed.			
8. Raise the head of the bed as high as it will go to a sitting position.			
9. Lower the bed to its lowest horizontal position.			
10. Raise the side rail on the far side of the bed.			
11. Bring the wheelchair with the patient to the bedside.			
12. Position the wheelchair so that the seat of the chair is in line with the middle of the bed. The chair should be positioned so the patient is transferred from the patient's strongest side.			
13. Lock the brakes on the wheelchair.			
14. Raise the footrests of the wheelchair, lifting the patient's feet off them and onto the floor at the same time. Remove the footrests if possible.			
15. Open up the blanket and safety straps that are on the patient in the wheelchair.			
16. Assist the patient in moving forward in the seat. Place the patient's feet flat on the floor. Support the patient behind the shoulder so that the patient is sitting upright.			
17. Place a gait belt around the patient's waist.			
18. Ask the patient to hug you in front, around your waist. Then block the patient's knees between your knees and grasp the gait belt at the patient's sides.			
19. The second nursing assistant should be positioned with one knee on the bed behind the wheelchair.			
20. The first assistant, in front, should gently pull the patient forward and up while the second assistant guides the patient's hips onto the bed.			

21. Raise the side rail.			
22. Raise the bed to waist height.			
23. One nursing assistant is positioned at the far side of the bed.			
24. Lower the side rail.			
25. Slide both of your arms under the patient's back to the shoulder; then slide the patient's shoulders toward you on your arms.			
26. Slide both of your arms as far as you can under the patient's hips and slide the hips toward you. Use a draw sheet whenever possible.			
27. Keep your knees bent and your back straight as you slide the patient.			
28. Place both of your arms under the patient's lower legs and slide them toward you on your arms.			
29. Both nursing assistants then roll the draw sheet toward the patient and slide the patient up in bed using the draw sheet, with a side-to-side weight shift.			
30. Place a pillow under the patient's head.			
31. Remake the top of the bed.			
32. Ensure patient comfort.			
33. Lower the bed to a position of safety for the patient.			
33. Raise the side rails if ordered or indicated.			
34. Place the call light within easy reach of the patient.			
35. Wipe the wheelchair with disinfectant solution and return the chair to its proper location.			
36. Wash your hands.			
37. Report to your supervisor			
• The patient has been put back into bed.			
• The time the patient was put back into bed.			
• How the patient tolerated the procedure.			
• Any unusual observations.			

Charting:

____

____

____

____

Date of Satisfactory Completion ____________________

Instructor's Signature ____________________

PROCEDURE 8-16: HELPING AN AMBULATORY PATIENT WHO CAN STAND BACK INTO BED FROM A CHAIR OR WHEELCHAIR

Name: ____________________ Date: ____________________

STEPS	S	U	COMMENTS
1. Wash your hands.			
2. Identify the patient by checking the identification bracelet.			
3. Ask visitors to step out of the room, if this is your facility's policy.			
4. Explain to the patient that you are getting her back into bed.			
5. Provide privacy for the patient.			
6. Raise the footrest of the wheelchair or remove them. Place the patient's feet on the floor.			
7. Lock the wheels on the bed.			
8. Bring the wheelchair close to the bed so the patient's strongest side is closest to the bed.			
9. Lock the brakes on the wheelchair.			
10. Raise the head of the bed to a sitting position.			
11. Lower the bed to its lowest horizontal position.			
12. Open up the safety straps on the wheelchair, if applicable.			
13. Help the patient out of the wheelchair to stand, pivot, and sit on the side of the bed. The patient's feet should be resting firmly on the floor.			
14. Lean the patient against the raised head of the bed.			
15. Put one arm around the patient's shoulders for support. Put your other arm under the patient's knees.			
16. Swing the patient's body slowly around, helping the patient lift his legs onto the bed.			
17. Raise the side rail.			
18. Lower the head of the bed.			
19. Help the patient move to the center of the bed.			
20. Place a pillow under the patient's head.			
21. Remove the patient's robe and nonskid shoes or slippers.			
22. Remake the top of the bed.			
23. Make the patient comfortable, and place the call light within easy reach.			

24. Set the bed to a position of safety for the patient.			
25. Raise the side rails where ordered or indicated.			
26. Clean the wheelchair with an approved disinfectant solution and return it to its proper place.			
27. Wash your hands.			
28. Report to your supervisor			
• You helped the patient back into bed.			
• The time you helped the patient back into bed.			
• How the patient tolerated the procedure.			
• Any unusual observations.			

Charting:

____

____

____

____

Date of Satisfactory Completion ____________________

Instructor's Signature ____________________

PROCEDURE 8-17: USING A PORTABLE MECHANICAL LIFT TO MOVE THE IMMOBILE PATIENT

Name: ________________ Date: ________________

STEPS	S	U	COMMENTS
1. Assemble equipment: mechanical patient lift and sling.			
2. Wash your hands.			
3. Identify the patient by checking the identification bracelet.			
4. Ask visitors to step out of the room, if this is your facility's policy.			
5. Explain to the patient that you are going to get him out of bed using the mechanical patient lift.			
6. Provide for privacy.			
7. Get another member of the patient care team to assist.			
8. Position the chair next to the bed with the back of the chair in line with the headboard of the bed. Lock the wheels of the bed and of the lift.			
9. Cover the chair with a blanket or sheet.			
10. Slide the sling under the patient by turning the patient from side to side on the bed.			
11. Attach the sling to the mechanical lift with the hooks in place through the metal frame. (Some lifts have color-coded straps.) Secure the sling to the lift following the manufacturer's instructions. If hooks are used, be sure to apply hooks with open, sharp ends away from the patient.			
12. Have the patient fold both arms across his chest, if possible.			
13. Using the crank, lift the patient from the bed.			
14. Have your partner guide the patient's legs.			
15. Lower the patient into the chair.			
16. Remove the hooks from the frame of the lift.			
17. Wrap the patient with a blanket.			
18. Leave the patient safe and comfortable in the chair for the proper amount of time, as instructed.			
19. To get the patient back to bed, put the hooks through the metal frame of the sling, which is still under the patient.			
20. Raise the patient by using the crank on the mechanical patient lift. Lift him from the chair to the bed.			
21. Lower the patient into the center of the bed.			

22. Remove the hooks from the frame.			
23. Remove the sling from under the patient by having the patient turn from side to side on the bed.			
24. Put a pillow under the patient's head.			
25. Remake the top of the bed.			
26. Ensure patient comfort.			
27. Lower the bed to a position of safety.			
28. Raise the side rails if ordered or indicated.			
29. Place the call light within easy reach of the patient.			
30. Clean the mechanical patient lift using an approved disinfectant solution and return the lift to its proper place.			
31. Wash your hands.			
32. Report to your supervisor			
• The patient was taken out of bed by means of the portable mechanical patient lift.			
• The time the patient was taken out of bed.			
• The prescribed length of time the patient sat in the chair.			
• The patient was put back into bed by means of the portable mechanical patient lift.			

Charting:

____

____

____

____

Date of Satisfactory Completion ____________

Instructor's Signature ____________

PROCEDURE 8-18: MOVING A PATIENT FROM THE BED TO THE STRETCHER

Name: ____________________ Date: ____________________

STEPS	S	U	COMMENTS
1. Assemble your equipment			
a. Stretcher			
b. Sheet or blanket			
2. Ask another member of the patient care team to assist you. The two of you should work in unison to move the patient from the bed to the stretcher.			
3. Wash your hands.			
4. Identify the patient by checking the identification bracelet.			
5. Tell the patient that you are going to move him from the bed to a stretcher.			
6. Ask visitors to step out of the room, if this is your facility's policy.			
7. Provide privacy for the patient.			
8. Loosen the top sheets.			
9. Cover the patient with a blanket or sheet.			
10. Move the stretcher next to the bed.			
11. Raise the bed so that it is the same height as the stretcher. Lock the wheels on the bed.			
12. Lock the wheels on the stretcher.			
13. You stand on the far side of the bed, using your body to hold the bed in place.			
14. Your partner stands on the far side of the stretcher, using her body to hold the stretcher in place.			
15. Position your legs so that one is in front of the other, bend your knees, and maintain the natural curves in your back.			
16. At the signal, "one, two, three," push, pull, and slide the patient from the bed to the stretcher, while shifting your weight from the front leg to the back leg, or from the back leg to the front leg. Use a draw sheet whenever possible.			
17. Support the patient's head and feet, keeping the body loosely covered with a blanket or sheet.			
18. Fasten the stretcher straps around the patient at the hips and shoulders.			
19. Put the side rails of the stretcher in the "up" position for the patient's safety.			

20. Wash your hands.			
21. Report to your supervisor			
• You moved the patient from the bed to a stretcher.			
• The time you moved the patient to the stretcher.			
• How the patient tolerated the procedure.			
• Any unusual observations.			

Charting:

____

____

____

____

Date of Satisfactory Completion ____________

Instructor's Signature ____________

PROCEDURE 8-19: APPLYING A TRANSFER OR GAIT BELT

Name: ____________________ Date: ____________________

STEPS	S	U	COMMENTS
1. Assemble equipment: gait belt and nonslip shoes.			
2. Identify the patient by checking the identification bracelet.			
3. Explain to the patient that you will be placing a belt around his waist to better assist him with walking.			
4. Wash your hands.			
5. Provide privacy for the patient.			
6. Lower the bed to the lowest position.			
7. Assist the patient to a sitting position with legs dangling.			
8. Place the gait belt around the patient's waist, ensuring a snug, but not tight, fit.			
9. Secure the belt according to manufacturer's instructions.			
10. Ensure that the belt is secure. Grasp the front of the belt and gently assist the patient to a standing position.			
11. Hold the back of the belt to maintain control of the patient while ambulating.			
12. Assist the patient back to bed or chair.			
13. Remove the gait belt according to manufacturer's instructions.			
14. Assist the patient into a position of comfort.			
15. Lower the bed to a position of safety.			
16. Place the call light within easy reach of the patient.			
17. Wash your hands.			
18. Report to your supervisor			
• You used the gait belt to assist a patient with ambulating.			
• How the patient tolerated ambulating.			

Charting:

____

____

____

____

Date of Satisfactory Completion ____________________

Instructor's Signature ____________________

PROCEDURE 8-20: HELPING A PATIENT WALK

Name: ______________________ Date: ______________________

STEPS	S	U	COMMENTS
1. Assemble equipment: Robe, nonskid slippers, and gait belt.			
2. Identify the patient by checking the identification bracelet.			
3. Explain to the patient that you will assist him with walking.			
4. Wash your hands.			
5. Lower the bed to the lowest position.			
6. Assist the patient to a sitting position with feet dangling over the side of the bed.			
7. Help the patient put on robe and slippers.			
8. Observe for dizziness and check for decreased blood pressure if this is the first time the patient has attempted ambulation since illness or injury.			
9. Apply the gait belt around the patient's waist.			
10. Assist the patient to a standing position.			
a. Stand facing the patient.			
b. Grasp the gait belt with both hands.			
c. Place your knee against the patient's knee and place your right foot between the patient's feet.			
d. Assist the patient by pulling him into a standing position as you straighten your knees.			
e. Keep your hands on the gait belt as you move behind or beside the patient and wait for the patient to gain his balance.			
f. Instruct the patient to stand up straight and hold his head up.			
11. Assist the patient with walking. Provide support as you walk slightly behind the patient.			
12. Walk the required distance or whatever the patient can tolerate. Do not rush or hurry the patient, and provide encouragement.			
13. Return the patient to his bed and assist him with getting into bed.			
14. Remove gait belt, robe, and slippers.			
15. Ensure patient comfort.			
16. Lower the bed to a position of safety for the patient.			
17. Raise the side rails if ordered or interested.			

18. Place the call light within easy reach of the patient.			
19. Report to your supervisor			
• You assisted the patient with ambulation.			
• How far the patient ambulated.			
• You helped the patient back into bed.			
• How the patient tolerated the procedure.			
• Any unusual observations.			

Charting:

____

____

____

____

Date of Satisfactory Completion ____________________

Instructor's Signature ____________________

PROCEDURE 8-21: ASSISTING A FALLING PATIENT

Name: ____________________ Date: ____________________

STEPS	S	U	COMMENTS
1. If a patient begins to fall, move your feet apart to increase your stability, bend your knees, and lower your body to the floor with the patient. Keep the patient's body close to yours.			
2. Hold onto the patient from behind, placing your arms under the patient's arms and placing your hands on his gait belt to help ease him to the floor.			
3. Maintain the natural curves in your back.			
4. If the patient is next to a wall when he begins to fall, use the wall to assist in easing the patient to the floor.			
5. Protect the patient's head from injury.			
6. Stay with the patient, call for help, and do not move the patient until you are instructed to do so.			
7. Always ask for assistance to help the patient back into a standing position.			
8. Report the details to your supervisor and complete an incident report.			

Charting:

____

____

____

____

Date of Satisfactory Completion ____________________

Instructor's Signature ____________________

Personal Care of the Patient

9

Key Terms Review

Match the key terms in the right column with the definitions in the left column by placing the letter of each correct answer in the space provided.

_____ **1.** Activities that a patient can perform himself.

_____ **2.** Those activities that a patient performs daily, such as bathing, dressing, washing, or toileting.

_____ **3.** A sheet in a patient's chart that allows certain activities to be checked off as the activities are performed.

_____ **4.** A partial or complete set of false teeth for the upper and/or lower jaw.

_____ **5.** Cleaning of the mouth and teeth.

_____ **6.** A container that a male patient uses to collect urine.

_____ **7.** The opening of the urethra on the body through which urine is passed.

_____ **8.** To pass urine through the urethra.

_____ **9.** To pass fecal waste through the anus.

_____ **10.** Inability to control one's bowel or bladder function.

_____ **11.** A pan used by patients who must defecate or urinate while in bed.

_____ **12.** A moveable chair enclosing a bedpan with an opening that can fit over a toilet.

_____ **13.** A shallower, flatter bedpan that is used for patients with very limited mobility.

Terms

A. Bedpan
B. Fracture pan
C. Commode
D. Defecate
E. Urinate
F. Incontinence
G. Urinal
H. Urinary meatus
I. Perineal area
J. Perineum
K. Dentures
L. Oral hygiene
M. Activities of daily living
N. Self-care
O. Flow sheet

____14. The genital area between the vulva and anus in a woman, and between the scrotum and the anus in a man.

____15. The area between the thighs.

MULTIPLE-CHOICE QUESTIONS

Circle the letter next to the word or statement that best completes the sentence or answers the question.

1. Patient care must be unhurried and _____ to meet each patient's special needs.
   a. uninterrupted
   b. fast
   c. personalized
   d. worthwhile

2. A patient who is comatose should
   a. perform oral care only after eating.
   b. perfom oral care using a mouth care swab.
   c. never have mouth care done.
   d. perform mouth care only in the morning and evening.

3. ______ should be worn when brushing and flossing a patient's teeth.
   a. A mask
   b. Disposable gloves
   c. Gloves and a mask
   d. Gloves, mask, and a gown

4. Perineal care is done for which of the following reasons?
   a. To cleanse the perineal area
   b. To prevent skin breakdown
   c. To promote healing of perineal stitches
   d. All of the above

5. Perineal care is specific care given to the
   a. arms and legs.
   b. periorbital arches.
   c. ears and mouth.
   d. external genitalia and rectal area.

6. If the patient's fingernails or toenails need trimming,
   a. follow the policy of your institution regarding care of the patient's nails.
   b. tell the patient to cut her own nails.
   c. soak them in warm water for a minimum of 2 minutes.
   d. do nothing because this is not part of personal care.

7. Giving the patient hair care will make him
   a. hungry and tired.
   b. slim and trim.
   c. look and feel better.
   d. want to go home.

8. Before shaving a patient's face,
   a. get advice from his wife.
   b. get permission from the patient and your immediate supervisor.
   c. make sure he is sleeping.
   d. wait until he is eating breakfast.

9. Each patient is to be treated
   a. as if he were family.
   b. according to the flow sheet.
   c. to a reward if he follows orders.
   d. as an individual.

10. Providing personal care for the patient in a skillful and respectful manner will
    a. take too much time.
    b. prevent avoidance of ADLs.
    c. increase her comfort and well-being.
    d. decrease her appetite.

11. Babies lose body heat more quickly than adults, so be sure to
    a. turn the air conditioning on.
    b. dry their skin quickly.
    c. keep them undressed until the skin is dry to the touch.
    d. bathe them only when they look dirty.

12. Adults and geriatric patients like to
   a. have all personal care performed for them.
   b. maintain control over their care.
   c. have the nursing assistant make all decisions for them.
   d. give up as much freedom to choose their care as possible.

13. Signs of skin problems that should be reported when offering a bath include
   a. rashes.
   b. blisters.
   c. redness over a bony area.
   d. all of the above.

14. When dressing a patient with right-side weakness, the nursing assistant should
   a. ask him to stand up near the bed so dressing will be faster for both the patient and nursing assistant and prevent back injury for the nursing assistant.
   b. first, remove the old soiled gown from his right arm, then undress his left arm and then place his clean shirt on his left arm.
   c. first, remove the old soiled gown from his left arm, then undress his right arm and then place his clean shirt on his right arm.
   d. allow him the privacy he needs to do everything himself in the bathroom.

15. When cleaning dentures, the nursing assistant should
   a. line the sink with a towel to prevent damage should they fall.
   b. clean them over the emesis basin at the bedside.
   c. use a toothbrush, toothpaste, and hot water to kill bacteria.
   d. rinse them with mouthwash and give them back to her.

16. When offering foot care, it is best to
   a. dry between the toes well to prevent bacteria from growing.
   b. place lotion on the feet and between the toes to reduce drying and cracking.
   c. cut the toenails of a diabetic.
   d. all of the above.

17. The bath water must be changed
   a. when it becomes dirty.
   b. when it becomes cold or soapy.
   c. after the arms and legs are washed and before giving perineal care.
   d. all of the above.

18. The proper way to cleanse a female patient's perineal area is to
   a. use a wet, soapy washcloth and wipe from the front toward the anus.
   b. use a wet, soapy washcloth and scrub back and forth around the perineal area.
   c. allow air to dry the perineal area, because she may have had stitches and drying with a towel could be painful.
   d. clean the anus first, because this is usually the dirtiest area.

19. When shaving a male patient's face, the nursing assistant should
   a. never use shaving cream.
   b. apply aftershave lotion to all patients.
   c. shave in the direction of hair growth.
   d. all of the above.

20. A patient on Coumadin should
   a. use an electric razor when shaving.
   b. never be shaved by a nursing assistant.
   c. have constant pressure applied to any nicks that are caused by shaving.
   d. be advised to use upward strokes when shaving the cheeks.

21. Frequent mouth care is essential for patients who
   a. take certain medications that leave a bad taste.
   b. are in a coma.
   c. are NPO.
   d. all of the above.

22. When providing mouth care for an unconscious patient, the nursing assistant should
   a. continue to talk to them.
   b. encourage them to spit into the emesis basin.
   c. place her finger in their mouth to open it.
   d. all of the above.

23. For which patient should cutting nails be avoided?
a. Diabetic patient
b. Patient who just had open-heart surgery
c. Patient living with right-side weakness
d. All of the above

24. A commode is
a. another name for a mechanical lift.
b. a portable toilet.
c. a room where linens are stored.
d. another name for the overbed table.

25. A backrub
a. is not a part of the evening care routine.
b. should be done using long, firm, circular strokes.
c. will make the patient anxious.
d. is not allowed for a patient who is waiting to go to surgery.

TRUE OR FALSE QUESTIONS

Determine whether each question is true or false. In the space provided, write "T" for true and "F" for false. If the statement is false, rewrite it on the line provided to make it a true statement.

_____ **1.** Bath water should never be changed once you have started the bath.

_____

_____ **2.** Incontinent patients should be checked to see if they are clean and dry only at the beginning and at the end of each shift.

_____

_____ **3.** Decubitis ulcers can result if the patient's skin is not kept clean and dry.

_____

_____ **4.** Mouth care is needed only when the patient is expecting visitors.

_____

_____ **5.** When performing personal care for the small child, include the parent or have them remain close by.

_____

_____ **6.** When performing perineal care, clean from the front to the back.

_____

_____ **7.** A patient on blood thinners like aspirin should use an electric razor.

_____

_____ **8.** Before giving a bath, the nursing assistant should make sure the temperature of the bath water is comfortable.

_____

_____ **9.** When performing perineal care on a male patient, the nursing assistant should place the foreskin back over the glans of the penis when care is completed.

_____

_____ **10.** Shampooing a patient's hair can increase circulation while improving general well-being and appearance for the patient.

_____

FILL-IN-THE-BLANK QUESTIONS

Provide the meaning of the following abbreviations.

1. ADL _____

2. NPO _____

EXERCISE 9-1

Objective: To recognize when to discuss a change in patient condition or activity with your immediate supervisor. Example: Patient requires a change in the bathing procedure.

Directions: For each of the following situations, identify the change in bathing procedure you think should be considered and discussed with your immediate supervisor. Place the correct letters next to the situation described.

CBB—complete bed bath
PBB—partial bed bath
TB—tub bath
S—shower

____**1.** Mr. Thompson has had a partial bed bath ordered for the last 2 days. He will be discharged soon, and he walks to the bathroom and in the hallway with assistance. He tells you he usually takes showers at home.

____**2.** Mrs. James will be going home tomorrow with her new baby. Yesterday, she received a partial bed bath. She is able to use the bathroom and dress herself with no difficulty today.

____**3.** Mrs. Sun, a new nursing home resident, tells you that at home she liked to take tub baths. You check your list and see that you have been assigned to have her take a shower.

____**4.** You are assigned to give Mr. Sims a partial bath. You notice that he does not wash himself thoroughly and complains of being very tired today.

____**5.** Mrs. Walls likes to walk in her bare feet and has to be reminded frequently to put on her slippers. Her feet and toenails are quite dirty, and she has many calluses. She says that at home she likes to put a chair in the tub to sit on while she soaks her feet and washes. She has been taking partial bed baths.

EXERCISE 9-2

Directions: Using the following case scenario, practice documenting the care you gave to your patient and use the patient care flow sheet provided.

Scenario: Mrs. Smith was admitted at 8:00 am from the OR on January 20 to room 203 B. Vital signs are taken and recorded as: T 98.6° F orally, P 86, R 12 and BP 120/80 mg/dL. She is on I&O, has an IV to her left lower forearm, a urine catheter which is intact. When drained record 800 mL of clear amber urine. Her doctor orders read: BR × 8 hours then BRP with assist × 1 as tol, clear fluid diet, daily wt, antiembolitic stockings bilaterally and encourage use of an incentive spirometer q 2°. Assist c̄ personal oral care and face hygiene is offered. She refused a bed bath and asked if this could be done at night instead. Her wt is recorded at 140 lbs via bedscale. Assist c̄ meal prep offered and intake of fluids is recorded as 540 mL at breakfast. She is in Fowler's position with bed rails down and a call bell in her hand.

Catherine McAuley Health System

St. Joseph Mercy Hospital
5301 East Huron River Drive
P.O. Box 995
Ann Arbor, Michigan 48106

8765-004 N 4/93

Patient Care Flow Sheet

Admission Date	OP Date	POD

Date		MIDNIGHTS								DAYS								AFTERNOONS							
		24	01	02	03	04	05	06	07	08	09	10	11	12	13	14	15	16	17	18	19	20	21	22	23
VITAL SIGNS	Temperature																								
	Pulse																								
	Respiratory Rate																								
	Blood Pressure																								
	CVP																								

		MIDNIGHTS	CREDITS	DAYS	CREDITS	AFTERNOONS	CREDITS
FLUID INTAKE	Oral						
	Feeding/NG						
	IV/IVPB						
	Hyperal/Lipids						
	Blood						
	Total 8°						
						24° Total	
FLUID OUTPUT	Urine						
	Emesis						
	Nasogastric Tube						
	Total 8°						
						24° Total	

ACTIVITY	Safety Code				EVENING SHIFT			
	Progession Weight							
	SCDs / TEDs							
SAFETY / RESTRAINT	Type of restraint and				DAY SHIFT			
	Location of restraint							
	Observation ql°							
	Turn/ROM q2°				MIDNIGHT SHIFT			
	Fluids offered							
	Toilet patient q2°							
	Skin status under restraint checked							
	Circulation checked							

Date		24	01	02	03	04	05	06	07	08	09	10	11	12	13	14	15	16	17	18	19	20	21	22	23
GI / GU	Diet and Amount	BREAKFAST								LUNCH								SUPPER							
	Weight																								
	Stool character and number																								
	Guaiac and date of last stool																								
	Bowel sounds																								
	Bladder																								
RESPIRATORY	Assessment																								
	Cough/Deep Breathe																								
INTEGUMENT	Surgical incision/Dressing																								
	Drains/characteristics																								
	Wound Care																								
TESTS AND SPECIMENS	Test results (mg/dL)																								
	Treatment/Medications																								
BLOOD GLUCOSE	Patient response																								
	ACCU-CHECK Instrument No.																								
	Date of last quality check																								
	CHEMSTRIP Lot No.																								
	Same as Calibration Lot (Yes, No)																								
	Sample type (cap, venous)																								
	Initials																								
NEUROLOGICAL	Assessment																								
	Best Eye Opening																								
	Best Verbal Response																								
	Best Motor Response																								
	Total Score																								
	Grasp																								
	Leg Lift/Foot Presses																								
	Pupils R																								
	L																								
HYGIENE	AM Care/HS Care																								
	Foley Care/Perineal Care																								
	Oral Care																								

KEY

Bowel Sounds:
✓ = Present in all 4 quadrants

Bladder:
✓ = Able to empty bladder Urine clear and yellow
F = Foley to DD
F✓ = Foley to DD, urine clear and yellow

Respiratory Assessment:
✓ = Bilateral breath sounds clear and respirations quiet and regular
☆ = See description

Surgical Incision:
I✓ = incision well approximated no drainage
D✓ = dressing dry/intact
★ = See description

Best Motor Response:
6 = Obeys commands
5 = Localizes pain
4 = Flexion withdrawal
3 = Flexion abnormal
2 = Extension abnormal
1 = No response

Grasp and Leg Lift
R = L, R > L, or R < L
and
W = Weak
S = Strong

Pupils
Record size in mm and
R = reactive to light
NR = nonreactive to light

Neurological Assessment:
✓ = Alert and oriented X3
☆ = See description

Best Eye Opening:
4 = spontaneous
3 = to speech
2 = to pain
1 = no response

Best Verbal Response
5 = Oriented to time, person, place
4 = Confused
3 = Inappropriate words
2 = Incomprehensible sounds
1 = no response

EXERCISE 9-3

Directions: Look at the following pictures and decide the correct order they should go in when offering a bed bath to a patient. Place the letter of the picture in the first column. In the second column, explain what is happening in the picture. Finally, in the last column, offer your explanation as to why you should do this step in the order you suggested.

STEPS Decide which order the pictures should go to offer the best care.	**Explain what is happening in the picture.**	**Explain why this step should occur.**
Example: Picture C (demo handwashing)	Handwashing	You should wash your hands before doing any skill, like offering a bed bath, to make sure you do not transfer germs to the patient.
Picture		
Picture		
Picture		
Picture		
Picture		
Picture		
Picture		

Picture A

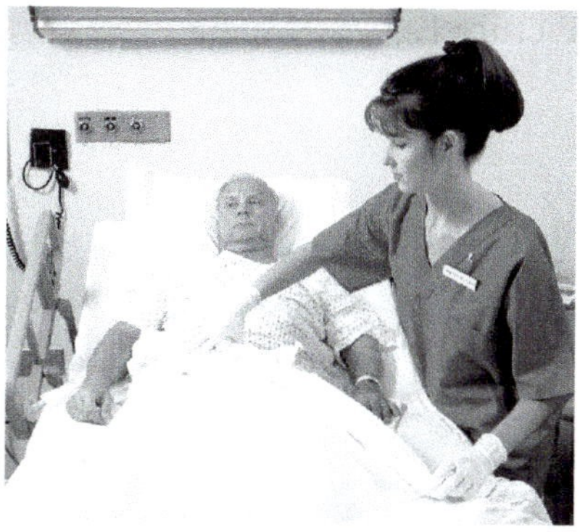

Picture B

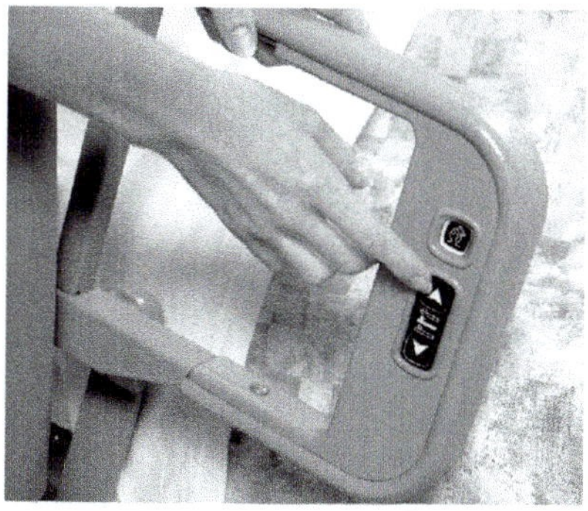

Picture C

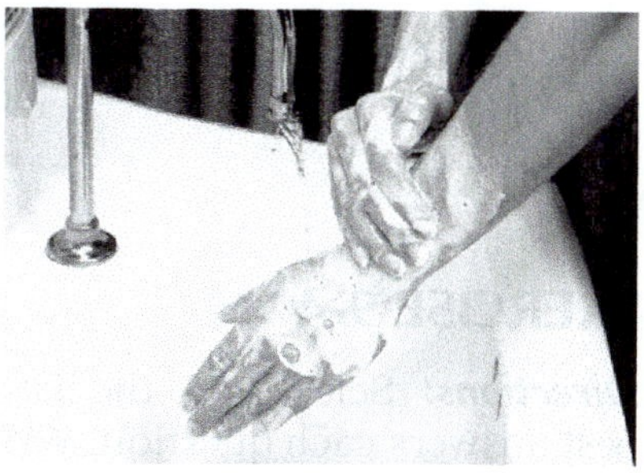

Picture D

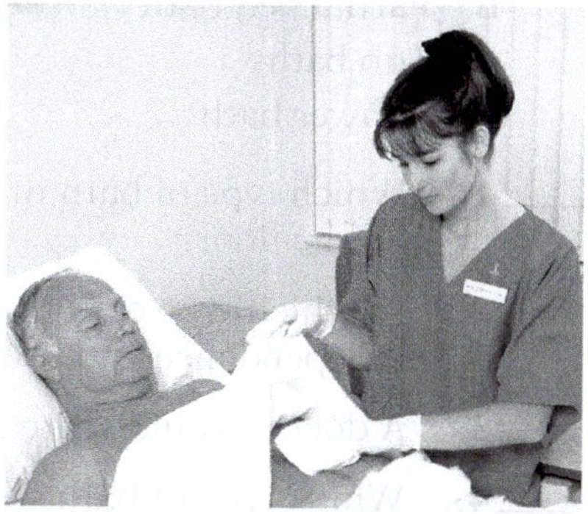

Picture E

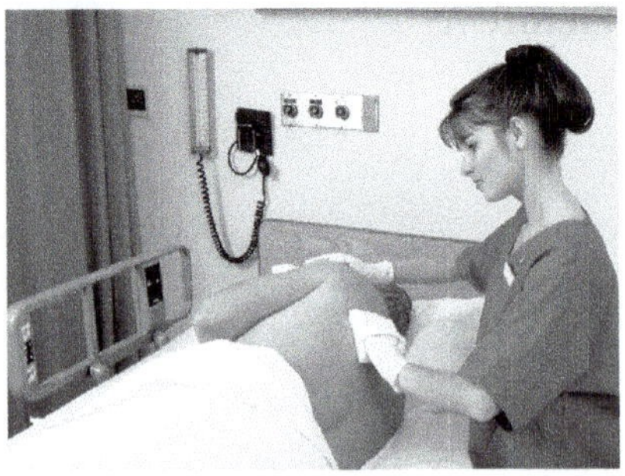

Picture F

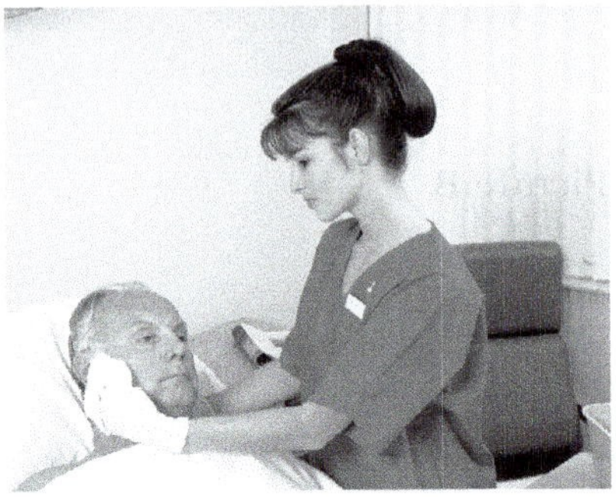

Picture G

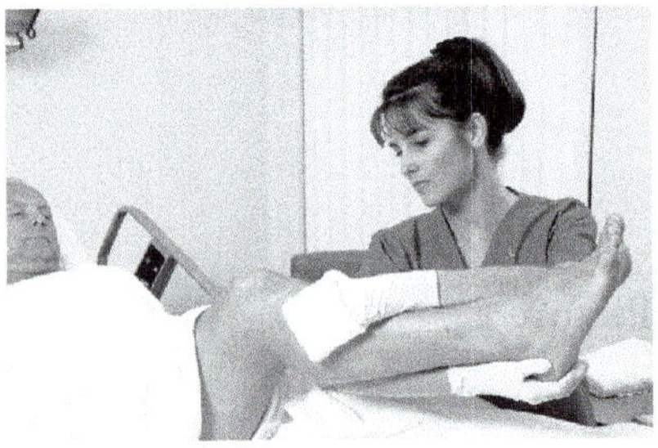

EXERCISE 9-4

Directions: Select from the list of procedures the letter of the procedure that best answers each question. Write the correct letter(s) on the blank line next to the question.

A. Complete bed bath
B. Partial bed bath
C. Tub bath
D. Shower bath

____**1.** Which type of bath might require that a bath mat or towel be placed on the floor?

____**2.** In which type of bath should a nursing assistant encourage as much independence and involvement from the patient?

____**3.** A doctor would write an order for which type of bath?

____**4.** Which type of bath should be offered to a comatose patient?

THE NURSING ASSISTANT IN ACTION

1. While giving a bath, you notice new bruises on a patient's back. What should you do?

____

____

____

____

2. You are almost finished giving a bed bath. You roll the patient to his side to wash his back and notice he was incontinent of stool. What should you do?

____

____

____

____

3. Your patient refuses to have a partial bath given to her in the morning. What should you do?

____

____

____

____

4. You find a male patient who is on Coumadin, a blood thinner, shaving with a straight razor. What should you do?

____

____

____

____

5. You enter a patient's room and find a colleague ending a bed bath by washing the perineal area of an elderly patient. She is not wearing gloves. Before you can get to the bedside and ask to speak with her, she reaches into the patient's mouth and removes his dentures. She still is not wearing gloves and did not wash her hands after washing this patient. What should you do?

____

____

____

____

LEARNING ACTIVITIES

1. Pretend you have right-side weakness. Take a front-buttoning sweater or a zip-up sweatshirt and practice dressing yourself. Consider the difficulties and frustrations you experienced while performing this task. Using a piece of paper, write down as many things that you can think of that could help your patient who cannot dress himself be more successful when performing this task, or ways you can help him when dressing.
2. Using the Internet, identify those cultures or religions that place significance on having facial or body hair. Educate yourself about why hair maybe important to them.

PROCEDURE CHECKLISTS

PROCEDURE 9-1: ORAL HYGIENE

Name: ____________________ Date: ____________________

STEPS	S	U	COMMENTS
1. Assemble equipment a. Mouthwash b. Fresh water c. Disposable cup d. Toothbrush e. Toothpaste f. Emesis basin g. Face towel h. Disposable gloves i. Dental floss j. Face mask k. Towel or paper towels			
2. Identify the patient by checking the ID bracelet.			
3. Inform the patient that you will help her clean her teeth and mouth.			
4. Provide privacy and comfort for the patient.			
5. Wash your hands and put on gloves.			
6. Raise the bed to a comfortable working height.			
7. Place the patient in a sitting position, if condition permits.			
8. Spread the towel across the patient's chest to protect the gown and top sheets.			
9. Mix one-half cup of water with one-half cup of mouthwash in the disposable cup.			
10. Let the patient take a mouthful from the cup and rinse her mouth.			
11. Hold the emesis basin under the patient's bottom lip so she can spit out the mouthwash solution.			
12. Put toothpaste on the wet toothbrush.			
13. If the patient can do it, let her brush her own teeth. If she cannot, brush teeth for her.			
14. Help the patient rinse the toothpaste out of her mouth, using the mouthwash solution or fresh water.			

15. Floss the patient's teeth using a 12- to 14-inch piece of dental floss. Wear a facemask while flossing, because there is potential for gums bleeding and your face will be in close proximity. • Wrap the ends of the dental floss around your middle fingers. • Ask the patient to open her mouth. • As you hold the dental floss between your thumb and forefingers, gently insert the floss between each tooth, down to but not into the gum. • When finished, offer mouthwash or water so the patient can rinse her mouth.			
16. Clean and put equipment in its proper place.			
17. Discard any disposable equipment.			
18. Make the patient comfortable and replace the call light.			
19. Dispose of your gloves and wash your hands.			
20. Lower the bed to a position of safety for the patient.			
21. Raise the side rails when ordered or indicated.			
22. Report to your supervisor • That you assisted the patient with oral hygiene • How the patient tolerated the procedure • Any unusual observations			

Charting:

____

____

____

____

Date of Satisfactory Completion ____________________

Instructor's Signature ____________________

PROCEDURE 9-2: CLEANING DENTURES

Name: ____________________ Date: ____________________

STEPS	S	U	COMMENTS
1. Assemble equipment a. Paper towel b. Mouthwash c. Disposable cup d. Emesis basin e. Toothbrush or denture brush f. Towels (2) g. Denture toothpaste h. Disposable gloves (2)			
2. Identify the patient by checking the ID bracelet.			
3. Inform the patient that you are going to clean his dentures.			
4. Provide privacy and comfort for the patient.			
5. Wash your hands and put on gloves.			
6. Raise the bed to a comfortable working height.			
7. Place the patient in a sitting position, if permitted.			
8. Spread the towel across the patient's chest to protect the gown.			
9. Ask the patient to remove his dentures. Assist the patient if needed.			
10. Take the dentures to the sink in an emesis basin lined with a paper towel.			
11. Place a paper towel or washcloth in the bottom of the sink to protect the dentures from being broken or scratched. Fill the sink with water.			
12. Apply toothpaste or denture cleanser to the dentures. With the dentures in the palm of your hand, brush all surfaces until they are clean.			
13. Rinse dentures thoroughly under cool running water.			
14. Fill the clean denture cup with cool water, mouthwash, or denture solution. Place the dentures in the cup and close the lid.			
15. Help the patient rinse his mouth with water or mouthwash.			

16. Have the patient replace the dentures in his mouth, if desired. Be sure dentures are moist before replacing them.			
17. Leave the labeled denture cup with clean solution on the bedside table where the patient can reach it.			
18. Clean and replace all your equipment. Discard disposable equipment in the proper container.			
19. Make the patient comfortable.			
20. Dispose of your gloves and wash your hands.			
21. Lower the bed to a position of safety.			
22. Raise the side rails when ordered or indicated.			
23. Place the call light within easy reach of the patient.			
24. Report to your supervisor • That you cleaned the patient's dentures • Your observations of anything unusual			

Charting:

____

____

____

____

Date of Satisfactory Completion ______________

Instructor's Signature ______________

PROCEDURE 9-3: ORAL HYGIENE FOR THE UNCONSCIOUS PATIENT (SPECIAL MOUTH CARE)

Name: ____________________ Date: ____________________

STEPS	S	U	COMMENTS
1. Assemble equipment a. Towel b. Emesis basin c. Special disposable mouth care kit of commercially prepared swabs (if available) d. Disposable gloves			
2. Identify the patient by checking the ID bracelet.			
3. Inform the patient that you are going to clean his mouth. Even if a patient is not responsive, he still may be able to hear you.			
4. Provide privacy and comfort for the patient.			
5. Wash your hands and put on gloves.			
6. Raise the bed to a comfortable working height.			
7. Stand at the side of the bed. Turn the patient's head to the side facing you.			
8. Put a towel on the pillow under the patient's head and under the face.			
9. Raise the head of the bed, if permitted.			
10. Place the emesis basin on the towel under the patient's chin.			
11. Tell the patient that you are going to open his mouth. Press on his cheeks or open the mouth using gentle pressure with your hand on his chin. NEVER put your fingers into the mouth of an unconscious or uncooperative patient.			
12. Open the package of mouth care swabs, if available. Wipe the patient's entire mouth with the swab.			
13. Put used swabs into the emesis basin.			
14. Dry the patient's face with a towel.			
15. Using an applicator, place a small amount of water-soluble lubricant on the patient's lips and tongue.			
16. Clean and return your equipment to its proper place. Discard any disposable equipment.			
17. Raise head of the bed, if it was lowered. Make the patient comfortable.			
18. Dispose of your gloves and wash your hands.			

19. Lower the bed when ordered or appropriate for patient safety.			
20. Raise the side rails when ordered or indicated.			
21. Place the call light within easy reach of the patient.			
22. Report to your supervisor • That you provided oral hygiene for the patient • How the patient tolerated the procedure • Any unusual observations			

Charting:

____

____

____

____

Date of Satisfactory Completion ____________________

Instructor's Signature ____________________

PROCEDURE 9-4: THE COMPLETE BED BATH

Name: ______________________ Date: ______________________

STEPS	S	U	COMMENTS
1. Assemble your equipment a. Soap and soap dish b. Washcloths c. Washbasin d. Towels e. Clean gown f. Bath blanket (if available) g. Baby powder (optional) h. Lotion i. Comb or hair brush j. Bag for soiled linen k. Clean bed linens l. Disposable gloves			
2. Identify the patient by checking the ID bracelet.			
3. Wash your hands and put on gloves.			
4. Inform the patient that you are going to give him a bath.			
5. Provide privacy and comfort for the patient.			
6. Assist the patient with oral hygiene.			
7. Offer bedpan or urinal.			
8. Place laundry bag on a chair near the bed.			
9. Raise the bed to a comfortable working position and ensure wheels are locked.			
10. Pull out all the bedding from under the mattress. Leave it in place under the patient, with all four sides on the edges of the bed.			
11. Take the bedspread and regular blanket off the bed. Place them in a chair, leaving the patient covered with a top sheet.			
12. If applicable, place the bath blanket over the top sheet.			
13. Remove the top sheet, either one part at a time, or use a bath blanket, being careful to not expose the patient. Place sheets in the laundry bag.			
14. Lower the headrest and knee rest of the bed, if permitted. The patient should be as flat as comfortably possible.			

15. Remove the patient's gown and ornamental jewelry. (It is not necessary to remove wedding rings.) Keep the patient covered with a sheet or bath blanket. Place the hospital gown in the laundry bag. If the gown belongs to the patient, put it away as requested by the patient or family.			
16. Fill the washbasin two-thirds full of warm water.			
17. Help the patient to move to the side of the bed closest to you. Always be sure to use good body mechanics.			
18. Put a towel across the patient's chest and fold a washcloth over your hand to make a mitten. Wash the patient's eyes by using a corner of the bath mitten and cleaning one eye from the inside to the outside. Then, using another section of the bath mitten, clean the remaining eye from the inside to the outside. Do not use soap when washing the eyes. Continue to wash the patient from the nose to the outside of the face. Only use soap on the patient's face if the patient requests it. Rinse and dry by patting with a bath towel.			
19. Place a towel lengthwise under the patient's arm farthest from you. This helps keep the bed dry. Support the patient's arm with the palm of your hand under his elbow. Wash his shoulder, armpit, and arm. Use long, firm, circular strokes. Rinse and dry the area well.			
20. Place the basin of water on the towel. Put the patient's hand into the water. Wash and rinse it well. Clean beneath the patient's fingernails with a brush or washcloth. Dry the hand well and place it under the bath blanket or sheet.			
21. Repeat steps 19 and 20 for the shoulder, axilla, arm, and hand closest to you.			
22. Place a towel across the patient's chest. Fold the bath blanket or sheet down the patient's stomach. Wash and rinse the patient's chest. Take not of the condition of the skin under the patient's breasts. Dry the area thoroughly.			
23. Cover the patient's entire chest with a towel. Fold the bath blanket or sheet down to the pubic area. Wash the patient's abdomen. Be sure to wash the navel and any creases in the skin. Dry the abdomen. Apply warm lotion and look for reddened areas. Then pull the bath blanket or sheet over the stomach and chest and remove the towels.			
24. Check the water temperature and clarity and change if needed.			
25. Fold the bath blanket or sheet back from the patient's leg furthest from you.			

26. Put a towel lengthwise under that leg and foot.			
27. Bend the knee and wash, rinse, and dry the leg and foot. Take hold of the heel for more support when flexing the knee or place your hand under the knee. Place the patient's foot directly into the basin to wash it.			
28. Observe the toenails and the skin between the toes. Look for redness or cracking of the skin. Dry the patient's leg and foot and between the toes. Cover the leg and foot with a bath blanket or sheet and remove the towel.			
29. Repeat steps 25–28 for the leg and foot closest to you.			
30. Cover the legs. Change the water if needed.			
31. Ask the patient to turn on his side with his back toward you. Assist the patient if needed. Raise the side rail to the up position for safety. Return to your working side of the bed.			
32. Put the towel lengthwise on the bottom sheet near the patient's back. Wash, rinse, and dry the back of the neck, back, and buttocks with long, firm, circular strokes. Provide a backrub with warm lotion. Rub the back for at least a minute and a half. Give special attention to bony areas, such as the shoulder blades and hipbones. Look for reddened areas. Remove the towel and turn the patient on his back.			
33. Check the water for temperature and clarity. Change if needed. Water should always be changed before providing perineal care.			
34. Place a clean gown on the patient.			
35. Comb the patient's hair if he cannot do it himself.			
36. Make the patient's bed. Straighten the bedside table and remove unneeded articles. Replace any items moved during the bath.			
37. Help position the patient in good body alignment.			
38. Clean and return your equipment to its proper place. Discard used disposable equipment.			
39. Wipe off the bedside table. Check linens for personal items. Bag and discard soiled linen in the hamper.			
40. Dispose of your gloves and wash hands.			
41. Raise the backrest and knee rest to suit the patient, if this is permitted. Lower the bed to a position of safety.			
42. Raise the side rails if ordered or appropriate for the patient.			

43. Place call light within easy reach of the patient.			
44. Report to your supervisor • That you gave the patient a bed bath • How the patient tolerated the bath • Any unusual observations			

Charting:

____

____

____

____

Date of Satisfactory Completion ____________________

Instructor's Signature ____________________

PROCEDURE 9-5: THE PARTIAL BED BATH

Name: ______________________ Date: ______________________

STEPS	S	U	COMMENTS
1. Assemble equipment a. Soap b. Washcloth c. Washbasin d. Towels e. Clean gown f. Bath blanket (optional) g. Lotion for back rub h. Comb or hair brush i. Laundry bag for soiled linen j. Clean bed linen k. Disposable gloves			
2. Identify the patient by checking the ID bracelet.			
3. Wash your hands and put on gloves.			
4. Provide privacy and comfort for the patient.			
5. Explain to the patient that you are going to help her with a bath.			
6. Raise the bed to a comfortable working height.			
7. Assist the patient with oral hygiene.			
8. Offer the bedpan or urinal or assist the patient with toileting.			
9. Place a barrier (towel or protective pad) on a chair near the bed then place the laundry bag on that chair.			
10. Pull out all bedding from under the mattress. Leave it hanging loosely at all four sides of the bed.			
11. Take the bedspread and blanket off the bed and place in a chair (or move blankets to the foot of the bed). Leave the patient covered with the top sheet.			
12. Place the bath blanket over the top sheet, if being used.			
13. Remove the patient's gown and ornamental jewelry. (It is not necessary to remove wedding rings.) Keep the patient covered with the bath blanket or sheet.			
14. Fill the washbasin two-thirds full of warm water.			
15. Ask the patient to wash the areas of her body she can easily reach.			

16. Place the call light where the patient can easily reach it. Instruct the patient to call when she has finished washing herself.			
17. Dispose of gloves and wash your hands.			
18. Leave the room, providing privacy for the patient.			
19. When the patient calls, return to the room.			
20. Wash hands and put on gloves.			
21. Replace water in the basin.			
22. Raise the rails on the opposite side of the bed and raise the bed to a comfortable working height.			
23. Wash the areas of the body that the patient was unable to reach. Follow the procedure for a complete bed bath. Be sure to wash all parts the patient could not reach.			
24. Put a clean gown on the patient.			
25. Lower the bed to a position of safety for the patient.			
26. If permitted, assist the patient to a chair.			
27. Make the bed.			
28. Raise the side rail when ordered or appropriate.			
29. Place the call light in its proper place.			
30. Clean and return your equipment to its proper place. Discard disposable equipment.			
31. Wipe off the bedside table. Place used linen in the hamper.			
32. Dispose of gloves and wash your hands.			
33. Make the patient comfortable and replace jewelry.			
34. Report to your supervisor • That you gave the patient a partial bath • How the patient tolerated the bath • Any unusual observations			

Charting:

____

____

____

____

Date of Satisfactory Completion ________________

Instructor's Signature ________________

PROCEDURE 9-6: THE TUB BATH

Name: ______________________ Date: ______________________

STEPS	S	U	COMMENTS
1. Assemble equipment a. Bath towels b. Washcloths c. Bath mat d. Soap e. Lotion f. Washbasin g. Clean gown h. Disinfectant solution i. Disposable gloves j. Disposable laundry bag k. Chair placed near the tub			
2. Wash the bathtub with disinfectant solution.			
3. Identify the patient by checking the ID bracelet.			
4. Inform the patient that you are going to assist him with a tub bath.			
5. Wash hands.			
6. Provide privacy and comfort for the patient.			
7. Help the patient out of bed. Assist him to the bathroom by walking or wheelchair.			
8. Remove all electrical appliances from near the bathtub.			
9. Place the chair next to the bathtub and assist the patient into the chair.			
10. Fill the bathtub halfway with warm water.			
11. Place one towel in the bathtub for the patient to sit.			
12. Place one towel or a bath mat on the floor where the patient will be stepping out of the tub.			
13. Assist the patient with getting undressed and getting into the bathtub.			
14. Let the patient stay in the bathtub as long as permitted, or as instructed. Do not leave the patient unattended.			
15. Put on gloves and help the patient wash himself, if needed.			
16. Put one towel across the chair.			

17. Drain the water from the tub.			
18. Help the patient out of the bathtub. Seat him on the chair.			
19. Dry the patient well by patting with a towel. Apply lotion. Assist the patient into pajamas, gown, or robe.			
20. Dispose of gloves.			
21. Help the patient return to his room and bed.			
22. Make the patient comfortable and place the call light within easy reach.			
23. Lower the bed to a position of safety for the patient.			
24. Raise the side rails when ordered or appropriate for patient safety.			
25. Return to the tub room.			
26. Put on clean gloves. Clean the bathtub with disinfectant solution.			
27. Clean the bathtub with disinfectant solution.			
28. Bag and discard soiled linen in the laundry hamper.			
29. Discard gloves and wash your hands.			
30. Report to your supervisor • That you gave the patient a tub bath • How the patient tolerated the procedure • Any unusual observations			

Charting:

____

____

____

____

Date of Satisfactory Completion ________________

Instructor's Signature ________________

PROCEDURE 9-7: ASSISTING THE PATIENT WITH A SHOWER

Name: ______________________ Date: ______________________

STEPS	S	U	COMMENTS
1. Assemble equipment a. Bath towels b. Soap c. Lotion d. Shower cap (if requested) e. Washcloth f. Bath mat g. Clean gown h. Disinfectant solution i. Laundry bag j. Disposable gloves			
2. Wash the floor of the shower with disinfectant solution.			
3. Identify the patient by checking the ID bracelet.			
4. Inform the patient that you will assist her with taking a shower.			
5. Wash hands and put on gloves.			
6. Provide privacy and comfort for the patient.			
7. Help the patient out of bed and into the bathroom.			
8. Remove all electrical appliances from the shower room.			
9. Place one towel on the floor outside of the shower.			
10. Place one towel on a chair close to the shower. Assist the patient into the chair.			
11. Turn on the shower and adjust the water temperature.			
12. Assist the patient into the shower.			
13. Give the patient soap and a washcloth to wash herself. Cue the patient to wash missed areas and let the patient know you will wash whatever areas the patient is unable to reach.			
14. Wait outside the shower in case assistance is needed.			
15. Turn off the water and assist the patient out of the shower when she is finished. Seat her on the chair.			

16. Dry the patient well by patting her with a towel.			
17. Apply lotion.			
18. Dispose of gloves and wash your hands.			
19. Assist the patient into a clean gown, pajamas, or clothes.			
20. Help the patient return to her room and into bed or chair.			
21. Make the patient comfortable and place the call light within easy reach.			
22. Lower the bed to a position of safety.			
23. Raise the side rails when ordered or appropriate for patient safety.			
24. Return to the shower room.			
25. Put on gloves. Bag and discard soiled linen in the laundry hamper.			
26. Remove gloves and wash your hands.			
27. Report to your supervisor • That you helped the patient take a shower • How the patient tolerated the procedure • Any unusual observations			

Charting:

____

____

____

____

Date of Satisfactory Completion ____________________

Instructor's Signature ____________________

PROCEDURE 9-8: PERINEAL CARE FOR THE MALE PATIENT

Name: ______________________ Date: ______________________

STEPS	S	U	COMMENTS
1. Assemble your equipment a. Bedpan or urinal b. Soap c. Bed protector d. Washbasin with warm water e. Gloves f. Washcloth and towels g. Laundry bag			
2. Identify the patient by checking the ID bracelet.			
3. Inform the patient that you are providing perineal care.			
4. Provide privacy and comfort for the patient.			
5. Provide safety with the side rail up on the opposite side of the bed.			
6. Raise the bed to a comfortable working height.			
7. Lower the side rail on the side nearest you.			
8. Position the patient on his back or side.			
9. Remove the bedspread and blanket and place on a nearby chair or table for use after the bath or move them to the foot of the bed.			
10. Cover the patient with a sheet or bath blanket.			
11. Ask the patient to raise his hips and slide a bed protector or towel under him.			
12. Put on gloves.			
13. Offer bedpan or urinal.			
14. Remove gloves and wash hands after assisting with toileting.			
15. Place washbasin with warm water on barrier on the overbed table.			
16. Ask the patient to bend his knees and separate his legs. If the patient is on his side, position a folded blanket or pillow between his knees.			
17. Slide down the sheet or blanket to expose perineal area only, keeping legs covered.			
18. Put on gloves.			
19. Wet the washcloth in the basin, form it into a mitt, and add a small amount of soap.			

20. Grasp the penis gently in one hand. Wash by starting at the urinary meatus and wash in a circular motion down to the base on each side of the penis.			
21. Uncircumcised patients require that the foreskin be pulled down gently to expose the end of the penis, which can then be washed. Remember to replace the foreskin over the glans once the penis is washed, rinsed, and dried.			
22. Wash the scrotum, lifting it to wash the perineum.			
23. Rinse the washcloth, using the mitt to rinse the area washed. It may be necessary to rinse more than once.			
24. Dry the area with a towel.			
25. Turn the patient on his side away from you, and flex the knee of his upper leg slightly, if permitted.			
26. Wet the washcloth, form into a mitt, and apply soap.			
27. Wash the anal area, using gently front to back strokes.			
28. Rinse carefully as before, and repeating if necessary.			
29. Dry gently.			
30. Reposition the patient on his back.			
31. Remove the protective pad or towel from the bed and place in laundry.			
32. Dispose of gloves.			
33. Place the spread and blanket back on the patient.			
34. Lower the bed and rails.			
35. Apply clean gloves.			
35. Remove any wet or soiled linens and discard in the laundry hamper.			
36. Empty the washbasin, clean according to policy, and store appropriately. Dispose of gloves and wash your hands.			
37. Document the procedure, noting any unusual observations.			

Charting:

____

____

____

____

Date of Satisfactory Completion ________________

Instructor's Signature ________________

PROCEDURE 9-9: PERINEAL CARE FOR THE FEMALE PATIENT

Name: ____________________ Date: ____________________

STEPS	S	U	COMMENTS
1. Assemble your equipment a. Bath blanket b. Bedpan c. Soap d. Washbasin with warm water e. Gloves f. Bed protector or towels g. Washcloth h. Laundry bag			
2. Identify the patient by checking the ID bracelet.			
3. Inform the patient that you are going to provide perineal care.			
4. Provide privacy and comfort for the patient.			
5. Place a barrier on the overbed table, then place the basin filled with warm water on the overbed table.			
6. Raise the rails and bed height to a comfortable working position.			
7. Provide safety with the side rail up on the opposite side of the bed.			
8. Lower the side rail on the side nearest you.			
9. Position the patient on her back or side.			
10. Remove the bedspread and blankets.			
11. Cover the patient with a sheet or bath blanket.			
12. Ask the patient to raise her hips and slide the bed protector or towels under her.			
13. Put on gloves. Offer the patient a bedpan. After assisting with toileting, remove gloves and wash your hands.			
14. Ask the patient to bend her knees and separate her legs. If the patient is on her side, use a pillow or folded blanket between the knees.			
15. Slide down the sheet or bath blanket to expose the perineal area only, keeping the legs covered.			
16. Put on gloves.			

17. Wet the washcloth in the basin, form it into a mitt, add a small amount of soap.			
18. Separate the labia with one hand.			
19. Wash gently • Using one mitt, stroke the outer labia once from top downward to the perineum. • Change areas on the washcloth and stroke the remaining labia from top to bottom. Place soapy washcloth on barrier. Wet new washcloth and repeat this on each stroke to rinse the area. • Discard the towel and use another washcloth with soap on it to clean from the clitoris to the anus. • Wet a new washcloth, wring out excess water, and rinse this area with one downward stroke.			
20. Rinse the washcloth, using the mitt to rinse the area washed.			
21. More than one wash or rinse may be necessary to clean the area thoroughly.			
22. Dry the area with the towel.			
23. Turn the patient on her side away from you, and bend the knee of her upper leg slightly, if permitted.			
24. Wet the washcloth, form into a mitt, and apply soap.			
25. Wash the anal area, using gentle front to back strokes.			
26. With a new washcloth, rinse carefully as before. Repeat the wash and rinse if necessary.			
27. Dry gently.			
28. Reposition the patient on her back or side.			
29. Remove the protective pad or towels and discard in the laundry hamper.			
30. Dispose of gloves and wash your hands.			
31. Place the sheet, blanket, and bedspread back on the patient.			
32. Lower bed and rails.			
33. Apply clean gloves.			
34. Remove any wet or soiled linens and discard in the laundry hamper.			

35. Empty the basin of water, place in proper storage, and dispose of washcloths and towels. Discard gloves and wash your hands.			
36. Document the procedure, noting any unusual observations.			

Charting:

____

____

____

____

Date of Satisfactory Completion ______________

Instructor's Signature ______________

PROCEDURE 9-10: GIVING NAIL AND FOOT CARE

Name: ______________________ Date: ______________________

STEPS	S	U	COMMENTS
1. Assemble your equipment a. Washbasins (3) b. Gloves c. Bed protector or towels d. Washcloth e. Soap f. Orangewood stick g. Emory board h. Nail clipper i. Lotion (non-alcohol based) j. Laundry bag			
2. Identify the patient by checking the ID bracelet.			
3. Inform the patient that you are going to provide nail and foot care.			
4. Provide privacy for the patient.			
5. Assist the ambulatory patient to a sitting position on the edge of the bed, or in a chair, with the overbed table at a comfortable level.			
6. Place emesis basin of warm water on the overbed table (or at appropriate level) for fingernail care and place two separate bath basins on a protective barrier on the floor for foot care (follow partial bed bath procedure).			
7. Check water temperature for safety and comfort.			
8. Apply clean gloves.			
9. Immerse patient's fingernails into the emesis basin for soaking. If safe to do so, you may soak the patient's feet at the same time by placing each foot into separate bath basins filled with warm water; otherwise, perform nail and foot care separately.			
10. Let the fingernails soak 5 to 10 minutes. Let the feet soak 15 to 20 minutes. Rewarm water as necessary.			
11. Apply clean gloves.			
12. Remove the emesis basin and have the patient rest her hands on a towel.			
13. Clean under the fingernails of each hand using an orange stick. Wipe the orange stick on a towel after each nail.			

14. Dry the patient's hands, especially between the fingers.			
15. If you have permission and instructions to do so, trim the nails straight across.			
16. File the nails using an emery board or nail file to shape the nails and remove rough edges.			
17. Apply lotion to the patient's hands. Wipe excess lotion off with a towel.			
18. Move the overbed table to the side.			
19. Apply soap to the washcloth.			
20. Using the washcloth, rub the dry skin from the heels of the feet and wash well between the toes.			
21. Rinse each foot.			
22. Remove each foot from the washbasins and place on protective barrier or towel.			
23. Dry the feet thoroughly, especially between the toes.			
24. Apply lotion to the top and bottom of each foot, removing any excess with a towel. (Avoid getting lotion between the toes.)			
25. Assist the patient to a position of comfort in bed, or apply non-skid footwear if the patient will be getting out of bed.			
26. Empty the basins of water, place in storage, and dispose of washcloths and towels.			
27. Remove gloves. Wash hands.			
28. Document the procedure, noting any unusual observations.			

Charting:

____

____

____

____

Date of Satisfactory Completion ____________________

Instructor's Signature ____________________

PROCEDURE 9-11: GIVING THE PATIENT A BACK RUB

Name: ____________________ Date: ____________________

STEPS	S	U	COMMENTS
1. Assemble equipment a. Towels b. Lotion c. Basin of warm water			
2. Identify the patient by checking the ID bracelet.			
3. Inform the patient that you are going to give him a back rub.			
4. Provide privacy and comfort.			
5. Wash your hands. Gloves should be applied if the patient has any skin rashes, cuts, or open sores on his back.			
6. Raise the bed to a comfortable working position.			
7. Ask the patient to turn on his side or abdomen so his back is toward you. Use the position that is most comfortable for the patient and for you.			
8. The side rail should be in the up position on the far side of the bed.			
9. Lotion may be warmed by placing the container in a basin of warm water.			
10. Open the ties on the patient's gown or remove pajama top.			
11. Pour a small amount of lotion into the palm of your hand.			
12. Rub hands together using friction to warm the lotion.			
13. Exert firm pressure as you stroke upward from the buttocks toward the shoulders. Use gentle pressure as you stroke downward from shoulders to buttocks.			
14. Keep your knees slightly bent and your back straight.			
15. Apply lotion to the entire back with the flat palms of your hands. Use firm, long strokes from the buttocks to the shoulders and back of the neck.			
16. Use circular motion on each bony area.			
17. Continue rhythmic rubbing motion for 2–3 minutes.			
18. Dry the patient's back by patting gently with a towel.			

19. Close and retie the gown.			
20. Assist the patient in turning back to a comfortable position. Replace the call light within easy reach of the patient.			
21. Arrange the top sheets of the bed neatly.			
22. Lower the bed to a position of safety for the patient.			
23. Raise the side rails when ordered or indicated for patient safety.			
24. Put your equipment back in its proper place. Discard any disposable equipment.			
25. Wash your hands.			
26. Report to your supervisor • That you gave the patient a back rub • The time it was given • How the patient tolerated the procedure • Any unusual observations			

Charting:

____

____

____

____

Date of Satisfactory Completion ____________________

Instructor's Signature ____________________

PROCEDURE 9-12: CHANGING THE PATIENT'S GOWN

Name: ______________________ Date: ______________________

STEPS	S	U	COMMENTS
1. Assemble equipment a. Clean gown b. Gloves c. Laundry hamper			
2. Identify the patient by checking the ID bracelet.			
3. Inform the patient that you are going to change his gown.			
4. Provide privacy for the patient.			
5. Wash hands and apply gloves.			
6. Raise rails on opposite side of bed.			
7. Adjust the bed to a comfortable working height.			
8. Ask the patient to turn on his side with his back toward you so you can untie the gown.			
9. Loosen the soiled gown around the patient's body.			
10. Get the clean gown ready to put on the patient. Unfold the gown and lay it across the patient's chest on top of the sheets.			
11. Take off one sleeve at a time, leaving the old gown in place on the patient.			
12. Slide each arm through one sleeve of the clean gown.			
13. If the patient cannot hold his arm up, put your hand through the sleeve. Take his hand in yours and slip the sleeve up the patient's wrist and arm. Do this for both arms. Then pull the gown down over the patient's chest.			
14. Remove the soiled gown from under the sheets.			
15. Secure the ties on the clean gown.			
16. Put the soiled gown in the laundry bag or hamper.			
17. Make the patient comfortable and replace the call light.			
18. Lower the bed to a position of safety.			
19. Raise the side rails when ordered or indicated.			
20. Remove gloves and wash your hands.			

21. Report to your supervisor • That you replaced the patient's soiled gown with a clean one • Any unusual observations			

Charting:

____

____

____

____

Date of Satisfactory Completion ____________

Instructor's Signature ____________

PROCEDURE 9-13: UNDRESSING THE PATIENT

Name: ______________________ Date: ______________________

STEPS	S	U	COMMENTS
1. Assemble equipment a. Bath blanket b. Gloves c. Laundry hamper			
2. Identify the patient by checking the ID bracelet.			
3. Inform the patient that you are going to assist with undressing.			
4. Provide privacy for the patient.			
5. Wash your hands and apply gloves.			
6. Adjust the bed to a comfortable working height.			
7. Assist the patient to a supine position.			
8. Remove upper body clothing a. Raise the head and shoulders or turn patient to the side facing away from you. b. Undo buttons, ties, zippers, snaps, or other clothing fastenings. c. If the clothing opens all the way in the back, bring the sides of the clothing to the sides of the patient. d. Assist the patient to roll to a supine position. e. Remove the clothing from the strong (unaffected) arm first and then from the weak arm, maintaining caution not to force or overextend the arms. f. Remove clothing from the patient's extremities or bring the clothing up to the patient's neck and remove over the head. g. If the patient will be staying in bed, assist with gown.			
9. Remove lower body clothing a. Remove shoes, slippers, and socks b. Undo buttons, ties, zippers, snaps, or buckles. c. Remove the belt. d. Ask the patient to bend at the knees and lift the buttocks off the bed. Grasp the top of the pants with both hands and slide the pants over the buttocks and down toward the knees. If the patient is unable to assist, you may roll the patient from side to side to lower the pants.			

e. Slide the pants down the legs. f. Remove the clothing from the strong (unaffected) leg first and then from the weak (affected) leg, maintaining caution not to force or overextend the legs.			
10. Make the patient comfortable and replace the call light.			
11. Lower the bed to a position of safety.			
12. Raise the side rails when ordered or indicated.			
13. Place dirty clothing in laundry hamper.			
14. Remove gloves and wash your hands.			
15. Report to your supervisor • That you assisted the patient with undressing • Any unusual observations			

Charting:

____

____

____

____

Date of Satisfactory Completion ____________________

Instructor's Signature ____________________

PROCEDURE 9-14: DRESSING THE PATIENT

Name: ______________________ Date: ______________________

STEPS	S	U	COMMENTS
1. Assemble equipment a. Bath blanket b. Gloves c. Clothes			
2. Identify the patient by checking the ID bracelet.			
3. Inform the patient that you are going to assist with dressing.			
4. Ask the patient what he or she would like to wear.			
5. Provide privacy for the patient.			
6. Wash hands and apply gloves.			
7. Raise rails on opposite side of bed.			
8. Adjust the bed to a comfortable working height.			
9. Assist the patient to a supine position.			
10. Cover the patient with a bath blanket.			
11. Undress the patient.			
12. Put on upper-body clothing a. For clothes that open in the back i. Slide the clothing onto the arm and shoulder of the weak (affected) arm first and then dress the strong (unaffected) arm. ii. Raise the patient's head and shoulders. iii. Bring the sides of the garment to the back. iv. Assist the patient to a sitting position in bed (or roll from side to side) to fasten buttons, ties, zippers, and snaps. v. Position the patient supine. b. For clothes that open in the front i. Slide the clothing onto the arm and shoulder of the weak (affected) arm. ii. Raise the patient's head and shoulders. iii. Bring the sides of the garment to the back. iv. Lower the patient's head and shoulders and slide the patient's strong (unaffected) arm through the garment. v. Fasten buttons, ties, zippers, and snaps.			

c. For pullover clothes i. Assist the patient to a supine position. ii. Put the neck of the garment over the patient's head. iii. Slide the arm and shoulder of the weak (affected) arm into the garment. iv. Raise the patient's head and shoulders while pulling the garment down to the waist. v. Slide the arm and shoulder of the strong (unaffected) arm through the garment. vi. Fasten buttons, ties, zippers, and snaps.			
13. Put on lower-body clothing a. Slide the pants over and up the legs. b. Ask the patient to bend at the knees and lift the buttocks off the bed. Grasp the top of the pants with both hands and slide the pants over the hips and buttocks toward the waist. If the patient is unable to assist you, you may roll the patient from side to side to pull up the pants. c. Fasten buttons, ties, zippers, and snaps.			
14. Put socks and shoes or non-skid footwear on the patient, making certain the socks are smooth without wrinkles.			
15. Help the patient get out of bed. If the patient will be staying in bed, then do not place shoes on the patient. Cover the patient.			
16. Make the patient comfortable and replace the call light.			
17. Lower the bed to a position of safety.			
18. Raise the side rails when ordered or indicated.			
19. Place dirty clothing in laundry hamper.			
20. Remove gloves and wash your hands.			
21. Report to your supervisor • That you assisted the patient with dressing • Any unusual observations			

Charting:

____

____

____

____

Date of Satisfactory Completion ____________________

Instructor's Signature ____________________

PROCEDURE 9-15: SHAMPOOING THE PATIENT'S HAIR

Name: ____________________ Date: ____________________

STEPS	S	U	COMMENTS
1. Assemble equipment a. Basin of warm water b. Pitcher of warm water c. Shampoo trough or tray (basin) d. Bed protector or towels e. Garbage can with clean liners (may be used) f. Pillow with waterproof case g. Towels h. Washcloth i. Paper cup j. Gloves k. Cotton l. Laundry bag or hamper			
2. Identify the patient by checking the ID bracelet.			
3. Inform the patient that you are going to give her a shampoo.			
4. Provide privacy and comfort.			
5. Wash your hands and put on gloves.			
6. Raise rails on the opposite side of the bed.			
7. Raise the bed to a comfortable working height.			
8. Brush the patient's hair thoroughly.			
9. Put a large basin or garbage can with new liners on a chair. Place the chair at the side of the bed near the patient's head, with the back of the chair touching the mattress.			
10. Place a towel on the chair. Put the large basin in the chair.			
11. Place a small amount of cotton or 2 × 2s into the patient's ears to prevent water getting into the ears.			
12. Ask the patient to move to your side of the bed.			
13. Remove the pillow from under the patient's head. Place the pillow between the shoulder blades so that the head tilts back when the patient lies down.			
14. Place the bed protector on the mattress under the patient's head.			

15. Place the shampoo trough under the patient's head. A trough can be made by rolling over the three sides of the plastic sheet three times. This makes a channel for the water to run off. Put the end of the channel under the patient's head. Have the other end hanging over the side of the bed and into the basin, or, use a shampoo tray/trough if available.			
16. Loosen the patient's gown at the neck.			
17. Dampen the washcloth and ask the patient to hold the washcloth over her eyes.			
18. Fill the basin with warm water and place on the bedside table with the paper cup.			
19. Fill the pitcher with warm water.			
20. Fill the paper cup with water from the basin. Pour it over the hair, repeating until the hair is completely wet.			
21. Apply a small amount of shampoo, and using both hands, wash the hair and massage the patient's scalp with your fingertips.			
22. Rinse the soap off the hair by pouring water from the cup over the hair. Repeat until the hair is free of shampoo.			
23. Dry the patient's forehead and ears with a towel.			
24. Remove the cotton from the ears.			
25. Raise the patient's head and wrap the head with a bath towel.			
26. Rub the patient's hair to dry it as much as possible			
27. Remove your supplies from the bed. Change linens if necessary. Change the patient's gown, if necessary.			
28 Comb or style the patient's hair. If a dryer is available, it may be used according to facility policy. If the patient prefers, leave a towel wrapped around the head or spread a towel on the pillow until the hair is dry.			
29. Cover the patient with the sheet, blanket, and bedspread, if the patient wishes.			
30. Make the patient comfortable and replace the call light within easy reach.			
31. Lower the bed to a position of safety.			
31. Raise the side rails if ordered or indicated.			
32. Clean and return equipment and discard disposable equipment.			
33. Remove gloves and wash your hands.			

34. Report to your supervisor • That you gave the patient a shampoo • How the patient tolerated the procedure • Any unusual observations			

Charting:

____

____

____

____

Date of Satisfactory Completion ____________________

Instructor's Signature ____________________

PROCEDURE 9-16: COMBING THE PATIENT'S HAIR

Name: ____________________ Date: ____________________

STEPS	S	U	COMMENTS
1. Assemble equipment a. Towel b. Comb or brush c. Hand mirror, if available d. Disposable gloves e. Laundry bag or hamper			
2. Wash hands and put on gloves.			
3. Identify the patient by checking ID bracelet.			
4. Provide privacy and comfort for the patient.			
5. Inform the patient that you are going to brush or comb her hair.			
6. Raise rails on the opposite side of bed.			
7. Raise the bed to a comfortable working height.			
8. If possible, comb the patient's hair after the bath and before you make the bed.			
9. Place a towel across the pillow under the patient's head. If the patient can sit up in bed, drape the towel around her shoulders.			
10. Part the hair as the patient usually parts her hair.			
11. Brush or comb the patient's hair carefully, gently, and thoroughly, combing small sections at a time.			
12. If the patient has very long hair, suggest braiding the hair to keep it from getting tangled.			
13. Be sure you brush the back of the head.			
14. Remove the towel when finished.			
15. Let the patient use the mirror.			
16. Make the patient comfortable and place the call light within easy reach.			
17. Lower the bed to a position of safety.			
18. Raise the side rails when ordered or indicated.			
19. Clean and return your equipment to its proper place.			
20. Remove gloves and wash your hands.			

21. Report to your supervisor • That you combed the patient's hair • How the patient tolerated the procedure • Any unusual findings				

Charting:

____

____

____

____

Date of Satisfactory Completion ____________________

Instructor's Signature ____________________

PROCEDURE 9-17: SHAVING THE PATIENT'S BEARD

Name: ______________________ Date: ______________________

STEPS	S	U	COMMENTS
1. Assemble equipment a. Face towel b. Basin of warm water c. Shaving brush, shaving cream, and safety razor or electric razor d. Disposable gloves e. Laundry bag or hamper			
2. Identify the patient by checking the ID bracelet.			
3. Inform the patient that you are going to shave his beard.			
4. Provide privacy and comfort for the patient.			
5. Wash your hands and put on gloves.			
6. Raise rail on opposite side of bed.			
7. Raise the bed to a comfortable working height.			
8. Adjust a light so that it shines on the patient's face.			
9. Raise the head of the bed, if permitted.			
10. Spread the face towel under the patient's chin.			
11. Dampen the patient's face with warm water on a washcloth.			
12. Apply shaving cream or soap generously to the face (if using a safety razor).			
13. With the fingers of one hand, hold the skin tight as you shave in the direction that the hair grows. Start under the sideburns and work downward over the cheeks. Continue carefully over the chin. Work upward on the neck under the chin. Use short, firm strokes.			
14. Rinse the safety razor often.			
15. Areas under the nose and around the lips are sensitive; use special care in these areas.			
16. If you accidentally nick the patient's skin, report this to your supervisor.			
17. Wash off the remaining shaving cream or soap when you have finished.			
18. Pat on aftershave lotion or powder, as the patient prefers.			
19. Ensure patient comfort and place the call light within reach.			

20. Lower the bed to a position of safety for the patient.			
21. Raise the side rails if ordered or indicated.			
22. Clean and return your equipment.			
23. Discard gloves and wash your hands.			
24. Report to your supervisor • That you shaved the patient's beard • How the patient tolerated the procedure • Any unusual observations			

Charting:

____

____

____

____

Date of Satisfactory Completion ____________________

Instructor's Signature ____________________

PROCEDURE 9-18: TRANSFERRING THE PATIENT TO AND FROM THE TOILET

Name: ____________________ Date: ____________________

STEPS	S	U	COMMENTS
1. Assemble equipment a. Non-skid footwear b. Wheelchair c. Gait (transfer) belt d. Gloves e. Toilet paper (tissue) f. Washcloth			
2. Identify the patient by checking the ID bracelet.			
3. Tell the patient you will assist them to the toilet.			
4. Provide privacy for the patient.			
5. Wash your hands and put on gloves.			
6. Ensure patient is wearing non-skid footwear or shoes.			
7. Position the wheelchair next to the toilet.			
8. Lock the wheelchair wheels.			
9. Remove the wheelchair footplates (or raise and swing them out of the way).			
10. Make sure patient's feet are flat on floor.			
11. Apply gait belt securely over clothing or gown.			
12. Provide instructions to patient to assist in standing, communicating the signal when to stand ("on the count of three").			
13. Stand facing the patient.			
14. On signal, gradually assist patient to stand by grasping gait belt on both sides and drawing patient forward to standing position.			
15. Provide support, as needed, as patient moves in front of the toilet.			
16. Ask patient to reach for grab bars for support.			
17. Assist patient to move gown or clothing out of the way and lower undergarments.			
18. Using the transfer belt, lower the patient onto the toilet, making certain patient is sitting securely on toilet.			
19. Remove gait belt.			
20. Close the bathroom door to provide for privacy if safe to do so.			

21. Ask patient to use bathroom call signal when finished, or stay near bathroom and listen for patient to call you.			
22. Assist patient with wiping and perineal care as needed by assisting the patient stand. Wrap toilet paper around your gloved hand and wipe the perineal area from the pubic area to the anal area. Repeat with clean toilet paper until clean.			
23. Assist with flushing and hand hygiene as needed.			
24. Dispose of your gloves and wash your hands.			
25. Apply gait belt.			
26. Using gait belt, assist patient to a standing position and to the wheelchair.			
27. Lower patient into wheelchair.			
28. Assist patient to lift legs onto the wheelchair footplates.			
29. Wheel patient away from the toilet to patient's preferred location.			
30. Lock the wheelchair wheels.			
31. Place the call light within easy reach of the patient.			
32. Report to your supervisor • That the patient voided or defecated • Any unusual observations			

Charting:

____

____

____

____

Date of Satisfactory Completion ____________________

Instructor's Signature ____________________

PROCEDURE 9-19: ASSISTING WITH USING THE PORTABLE/BEDSIDE COMMODE

Name: ______________________ Date: ______________________

STEPS	S	U	COMMENTS
1. Assemble equipment a. Portable bedside commode b. Bedpan and cover c. Toilet paper (tissue) d. Basin of warm water e. Soap f. Towel g. Disposable gloves			
2. Identify the patient by checking the ID bracelet.			
3. Tell the patient you will assist him onto the bedside commode.			
4. Provide privacy for the patient.			
5. Wash your hands and put on gloves.			
6. Put the commode next to the patient's bed. Open the cover and insert bedpan under toilet, if a pan is not already in place.			
7. Help the patient put on his slippers, and then help him out of bed and onto the commode.			
8. Put toilet tissue and the call light where the patient can reach them easily.			
9. Ask the patient to signal when he is finished.			
10. Dispose of your gloves and wash your hands. Leave the room to give the patient privacy, if patient condition allows.			
11. When the patient signals, return to the room and wash your hands and put on gloves.			
12. Assist patient with wiping and perineal care as needed by assisting the patient stand. Wrap toilet paper around your gloved hand and wipe the perineal area from the pubic area to the anal area. Repeat with clean toilet paper until clean.			
13. Assist the patient back to bed.			
14. Close the cover on the commode.			
15. Help the patient wash his hands in the basin of water.			
16. Make the patient comfortable.			

17. Remove the bedpan or basin from under the commode. Cover it and carry it to the patient's bathroom.			
18. Check the feces or urine for abnormal appearance.			
19. Measure output and collect a specimen, if ordered or indicated.			
20. Empty the bedpan into the toilet.			
21. Follow facility policy for cleaning the bedpan or basin.			
22. Place the clean commode in the proper place.			
23. Dispose of your gloves and wash your hands.			
24. Lower the bed to a position of safety for the patient			
25. Raise the side rails when ordered or appropriate for patient safety.			
26. Place the call light within easy reach of the patient.			
27. Report to your supervisor • That the patient has voided or defecated • If a specimen was collected • How the patient tolerated the procedure • Any unusual observations			

Charting:

____

____

____

____

Date of Satisfactory Completion ____________________

Instructor's Signature ____________________

PROCEDURE 9-20: ASSISTING A PATIENT WITH A BEDPAN/FRACTURE PAN

Name: ______________________ Date: ______________________

STEPS	S	U	COMMENTS
1. Assemble your equipment a. Bedpan and cover or towel b. Toilet tissue c. Washbasin with warm water d. Soap e. Towels f. Disposable bed protector g. Gloves			
2. Identify the patient by checking the ID bracelet.			
3. Ask the patient if she would like to use the bedpan.			
4. Provide privacy and comfort for the patient.			
5. Wash your hands and put on gloves.			
6. Raise rail on opposite side of bed.			
7. Raise the bed to a comfortable working position.			
8. Ready the bedpan. Apply powder to the surface of the bedpan to reduce friction.			
9. Fold back the top sheets so that they are out of the way.			
10. Raise the patient's gown, but keep the lower part of the body covered.			
11. Ask the patient to bend her knees and put her feet flat on the mattress if she is able. Then ask the patient to raise her hips. Put a protective pad on the bed and put the bedpan against the patient's buttocks.			
12. If the patient is unable to lift her hips to get on or off the bedpan, turn the patient on her side facing away from you, put the bedpan against the buttocks, and then turn the patient onto her back, with the bedpan under her.			
13. Replace covers on the patient.			
14. Raise the backrest and knee rest if permitted, so the patient is in a sitting position.			
15. Place toilet tissue and the call light within the patient's reach.			
16. Ask the patient to call when she is finished.			
17. Raise the side rails for safety.			

18. Dispose of gloves and wash your hands. Leave the room to allow privacy, if patient condition allows.			
19. When the patient signals, return to the room.			
20. Wash your hands and put on gloves.			
21. Help the patient raise her hips and remove the bedpan. Lower the head of the bed and hold the bedpan as the patient rolls to the side away from you.			
22. Cover the bedpan immediately with a disposable pad or towel.			
23. Help the patient (if she is unable to) clean herself and remove pad.			
24. Take the bedpan to the patient's bathroom or toilet area.			
25. Collect a specimen and measure intake and output if ordered or indicated.			
26. Check feces for abnormal appearance.			
27. Empty the bedpan into the patient's toilet.			
28. Follow your facility's policy for cleaning and storing the bedpan.			
29. Remove gloves and wash hands. Don new gloves.			
30. Help the patient wash her hands in the basin of water.			
31. Dispose of your gloves and wash your hands.			
32. Make the patient comfortable and replace the call light within easy reach.			
33. Lower the bed to a position of safety for the patient.			
34. Raise the side rails if ordered or indicated.			
35. Report to your supervisor • That the patient urinated or defecated • If a specimen was collected • How the patient tolerated the procedure • Any unusual observations			

Charting:

____

____

____

____

Date of Satisfactory Completion ____________________

Instructor's Signature ____________________

PROCEDURE 9-21: ASSISTING A PATIENT WITH THE URINAL

Name: ____________________ Date: ____________________

STEPS	S	U	COMMENTS
1. Assemble your equipment a. Urinal and cover b. Basin with warm water c. Soap d. Towel e. Disposable gloves			
2. Identify the patient by checking the ID bracelet.			
3. Ask the patient if he would like to use the urinal.			
4. Wash your hands and put on gloves.			
5. Give the urinal to the patient.			
6. Place the call light within easy reach.			
7. Ask the patient to signal when he is finished.			
8. Dispose of your gloves and wash your hands. Leave the room and provide privacy, if patient condition allows.			
9. When the patient signals, return to the room, wash your hands, and put on gloves.			
10. Cover the urinal and take it to the bathroom or toilet area.			
11. Check urine for abnormal or unusual appearance.			
12. Measure the urine and collect a specimen, if ordered or indicated.			
13. Empty the urinal into the toilet, and wash and rinse the urinal.			
14. Place the clean urinal back in the patient's bedside table.			
15. Remove the gloves and wash your hands.			
16. Don new gloves and help the patient wash his hands in the basin of water.			
17. Remove gloves and wash hands.			
18. Make the patient comfortable and replace the call light.			
19. Lower the bed to a position of safety.			
20. Raise the side rails if ordered or indicated.			

21. Report to your supervisor • That the patient urinated • If a specimen was collected • How the patient tolerated the procedure • Any unusual observations			

Charting:

____

____

____

____

Date of Satisfactory Completion ____________________

Instructor's Signature ____________________

The Patient's Room

10

Key Terms Review

Match the key terms in the right column with the definitions in the left column by placing the letter of each correct answer in the space provided.

_____ **1.** The space for one patient, including the hospital bed, bedside table, chair, and other equipment.

_____ **2.** Equipment designed to be used one time only or for one patient only and then thrown away.

_____ **3.** Reusable equipment that can be cleaned; often purchased or rented when needed to provide care in a patient's home.

_____ **4.** Materials, tools, devices, supplies, furnishings, and necessary items used to perform a task.

_____ **5.** A pan used for catching material that a patient spits out, vomits, or coughs up (expectorates).

_____ **6.** A type of bedpan designed for use with immobile or fracture patients; used often with female patients as a urinal.

_____ **7.** A pan used by patients who must defecate or urinate while in bed.

_____ **8.** A portable container given to male patients in bed so they can urinate without getting out of bed.

_____ **9.** A stable frame made of metal tubing used to support the unsteady patient while walking; the patient holds the walker while taking a step, moves it forward, and takes another step.

Terms

A. Emesis basin
B. Fracture pan
C. Bedpan
D. Urinal
E. Durable medical equipment
F. Equipment
G. Disposable equipment
H. Wheelchair
I. Intravenous pole
J. Bed cradle
K. Specialty bed
L. Stretcher
M. Alternating-pressure mattress
N. Patient lift
O. Patient unit
P. Flammable
Q. Walker

_____ **10.** A chair on wheels used to transport patients.

_____ **11.** A tall pole, also called an *IV pole,* that attaches to a bed or is on rollers or casters; this pole is used to hold the containers or tubes needed, for example, during a blood transfusion.

_____ **12.** A mechanical device with a sling seat used for lifting a patient into and out of such equipment as the hospital bed, bathtub, or wheelchair.

_____ **13.** A narrow rolling table with or without a mattress or simply a canvas stretched over a frame used to transport patients; may also be called a *litter, gurney,* or *cart.*

_____ **14.** A bed that constantly changes pressure under the patient; used to minimize pressure points in the treatment of or to prevent pressure ulcers.

_____ **15.** A pad similar to an air mattress that can be placed beneath the patient to reduce pressure on the head, shoulders, back, heels, elbows, and bony prominences.

_____ **16.** A frame shaped like a barrel cut in half lengthwise used to keep bed linens off a part of the patient's body.

_____ **17.** Capable of burning quickly and easily.

MULTIPLE-CHOICE QUESTIONS

Circle the letter next to the word or statement that best completes the sentence or answers the question.

1. When the nursing assistant is unfamiliar with the equipment used, he must ask for assistance from the nurse or

a. must ask the patient how others have used it.

b. make a wild guess and try to figure it out by himself.

c. quickly try to get the equipment to work.

d. review instructions prior to working with the item.

2. When working in a patient's home, the nursing assistant should

a. disturb the patient's personal things.

b. respect the patient's differences in food, cleanliness, or lifestyle.

c. perform heavy labor like window washing.

d. not move items that are a safety risk.

3. A primary goal is to make the patient feel

a. comfortable in the hallway.

b. comfortable in her environment.

c. more important than other patients.

d. busy and occupied after surgery.

4. If the patient has belongings from home, the nursing assistant

a. should respect these items.

b. can borrow the articles if another patient needs them.

c. can rearrange them the way she thinks he would like them.

d. should instruct the family to take them back home.

5. The nursing assistant should create a

a. safe environment for his patients.

b. complex and busy environment for the patient.

c. list of environmental rules for the patient and family to follow.
d. risky environment to keep the patient alert to danger.

6. The unit should be arranged
a. for the comfort of the nursing assistant.
b. for the convenience of the patient.
c. by the immediate supervisor only.
d. in a complex and mazelike pattern.

7. A key word to remember when rearranging furniture is
a. anticipation.
b. drudgery.
c. speed.
d. obstacle course.

8. If the patient is right handed, place the call light near the
a. doorway.
b. left ear.
c. telephone.
d. right hand.

9. The two most important factors that determine how a pediatric unit is arranged and the equipment needed are
a. the ages of the child and the parents.
b. the diagnosis only.
c. the age of the nursing assistant.
d. the age of the child and the reason for hospitalization.

10. In long-term care settings it is recommended that room temperature remains
a. between 71° and 81° F.
b. approximately 0° to 32° C.
c. comfortable for all patients.
d. between 65° and 74° F.

11. The best way to assist an elderly patient who complains she is chilly is
a. turn up the air conditioning in her room.
b. turn the floor fan on and direct in toward her.
c. cover her with an extra blanket or offer her a sweater or robe.
d. suggest she take a long walk on a sunny day to get warm.

12. Frayed electric cords should be
a. fixed by using electrical tape immediately.
b. reported immediately.
c. placed into an extension cord.
d. cut.

13. Plugs that are not properly ______ are fire hazards.
a. grounded
b. mounted
c. taped
d. labeled

14. Smoking in a hospital
a. should be highly encouraged.
b. is not permitted.
c. can only occur in a patient's bathroom with the fan turned on.
d. can only occur at the end of every hallway.

15. Flammable cleaning rags, mops, and brooms should be
a. tied up in plastic bags and placed in closets.
b. removed from the facility to prevent fire from occurring.
c. cleaned and then placed in a well-ventilated area.
d. stored in a metal container.

16. A patient is at high risk for developing pressure sores. The best thing to do is
a. use an alternating-pressure mattress on his bed.
b. place a binder on his abdomen.
c. pad his bed with many draw sheets.
d. use a patient lift at all times.

17. Another name for a stretcher is a
a. gurney.
b. litter.
c. cart.
d. all of the above.

18. Footboards
a. help support the foot from dropping.
b. help keep the patient's feet aligned correctly.

c. are placed at the foot of the bed.
d. all of the above.

19. ________ aid the patient when walking.
a. Wheelchairs
b. Walkers
c. Footboards
d. Stretchers

20. Which of the following can cause falls to occur?
a. Scatter rugs
b. Hallways that are cluttered
c. Stairwells that do not have enough light
d. All of the above

21. Which is something a nursing assistant can do in order to promote safety and comfort?
a. Keep wheelchairs unlocked to increase mobility.
b. Decrease the volume on the telephone so a person with hearing problems does not have to be disturbed.
c. Remove extra blankets to reduce clutter in a cool room.
d. Increase the lighting in the room for a person who is high risk for falling.

22. When arranging a patient's room, it is the nursing assistant's responsibility to
a. administer medications on time.
b. wait for the patient to ask for a toothbrush, toothpaste, and comb.
c. remove obstacles that could cause a patient to trip.
d. give a female patient a urinal to use and hang it from the bedrail for convenience.

23. Mr. Jameson is blind. It is important to
a. make sure his telephone is placed on his nightstand.
b. turn on the lights as you enter the room.
c. knock before entering the room.
d. talk louder because he may not be able to identify who you are.

24. Offer a ________ to a patient who broke his pelvic bone when he must urinate or defecate.
a. fracture pan
b. bedpan
c. urinal
d. emesis basin

25. If a patient must use large equipment when returning home, it can be suggested that
a. a doctor can order some equipment so insurance companies can reimburse the patient for the cost of the equipment.
b. renting the equipment might be cheaper and more convenient.
c. Medicare and Medicaid may be able to reimburse the patient for the cost of the equipment.
d. all of the above.

TRUE OR FALSE QUESTIONS

Determine whether each question is true or false. In the space provided, write "T" for true and "F" for false. If the statement is false, rewrite it on the line provided to make it a true statement.

____ **1.** Disposable equipment requires washing and disinfecting.

____

____ **2.** Disposable equipment may be reused by other patients if it is washed in hot, soapy water.

____

____ **3.** An emergency phone list should include the police and fire departments, the patient's physician, and the responsible family member.

____

____ **4.** A unit designed for a child is the same as for an adult.

____

____ **5.** If there is more than one bed in a room, draw curtains can be used for privacy.

____

____ **6.** Air-pressure mattresses are used for all patients.

____

____ **7.** It is a nursing assistant's job to perform all heavy cleaning like waxing the kitchen floor if assigned to work in a client's home.

____

____ **8.** A bed cradle is a piece of equipment that might be used to keep bed linens from touching a patient who has been burned.

____

____ **9.** Persons admitted for a hospital stay are referred to as *patients*.

____

____ **10.** Persons admitted to stay in a long-term care facility are referred to as *clients*.

____

FILL-IN-THE-BLANK QUESTIONS

Provide the meanings of the following abbreviations.

1. A-P (mattress) ______________________________

2. IV ______________________________

EXERCISE 10-1

Objective: To recognize important actions to take in accident prevention and reporting.

Directions: The five categories shown next are about accident prevention and reporting. For each of the specific safety items listed below, select an appropriate category. You may select more than one category for each item.

HFS—home fire safety
HSH—home safety hazards
CFH—calling for help
RET—reporting an emergency by telephone
BP—burn prevention

____ **1.** If a fire occurs, get the patient out of the area.

____ **2.** The fire department emergency number is kept near the telephone.

____ **3.** Cluttered hallways and walkways.

____ **4.** Loose rugs that slip or do not have a nonskid backing.

____ **5.** Avoid using flammable liquids.

____ **6.** Check the temperature of water before using it on the patient.

____ **7.** Wet floor.

____ **8.** Have handy the telephone number of the poison control center.

_____ **9.** Give the name of the patient and identify your location, room number, or address.

_____ **10.** Dimly lit hallways and walkways.

_____ **11.** Give your name first when you call.

_____ **12.** Keep matches away from children and confused adults.

_____ **13.** Sharp objects such as knives, razors, and hypodermic needles.

_____ **14.** Poisons (such as cleaning solutions).

_____ **15.** Clearly state the problem: Objectively state exactly what has happened or what help you need.

_____ **16.** Faulty or uneven stairs or loose debris on stairs.

_____ **17.** Have the number of your home care supervisor near the telephone.

EXERCISE 10-2

Directions: Study the following picture and find the safety issues. Write what you believe to be safety issues in the lines provided.

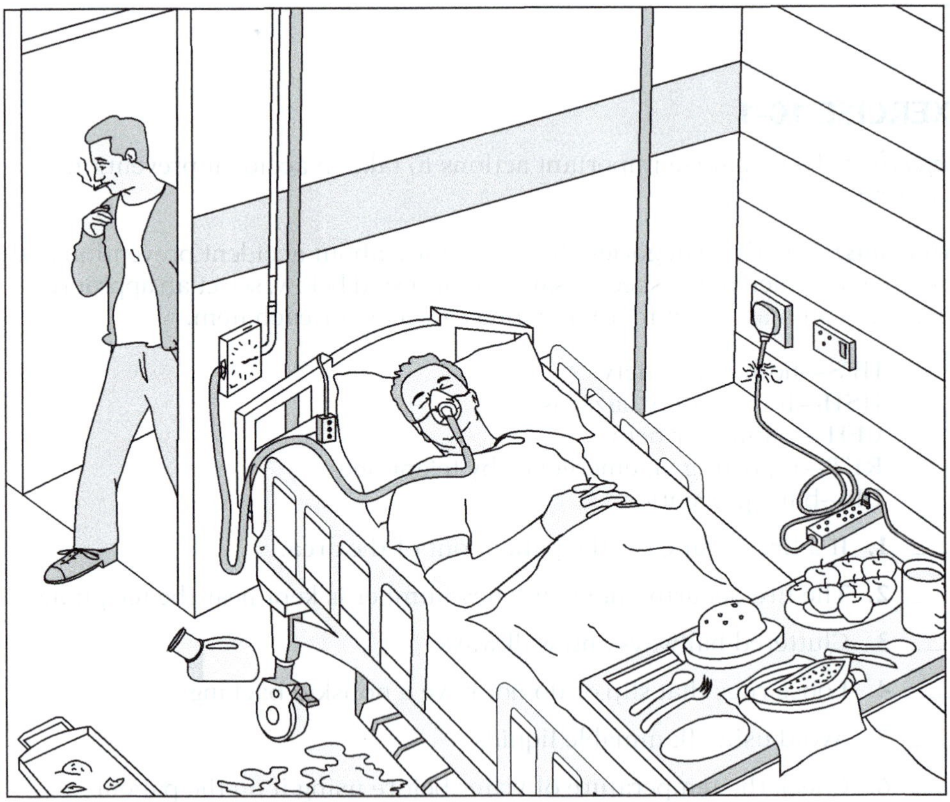

1. ______________________ 6. ______________________
2. ______________________ 7. ______________________
3. ______________________ 8. ______________________
4. ______________________ 9. ______________________
5. ______________________ 10. ______________________

EXERCISE 10-3

Directions: Using the words provided, place the correct word on the line under the following pictures depicting patient care equipment.

Word Bank

Emesis basin	Walker	Urinal
Wheelchair	Fracture pan	Patient lift
IV pole	Bedpan	Stretcher

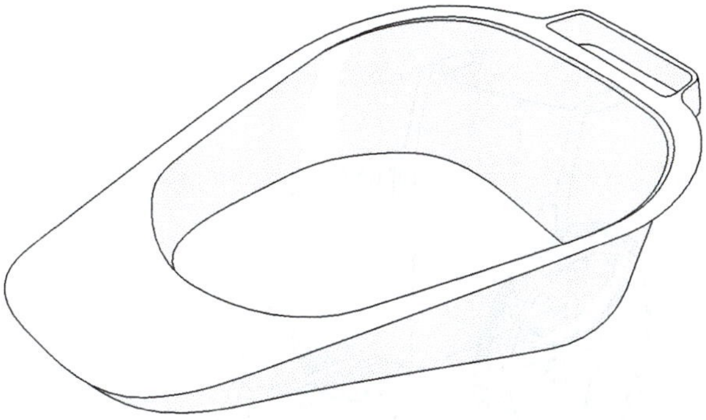

____

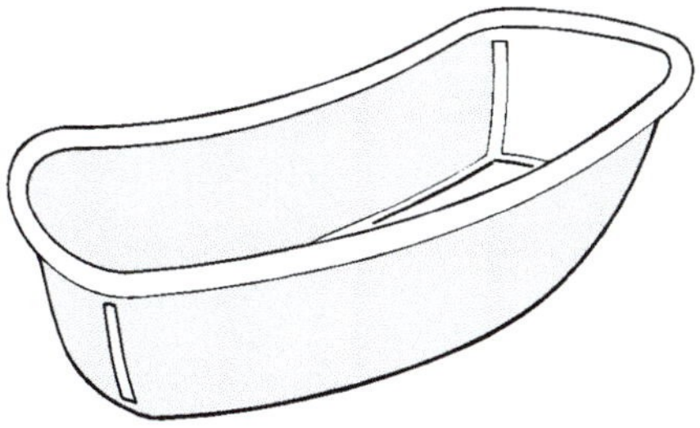

____

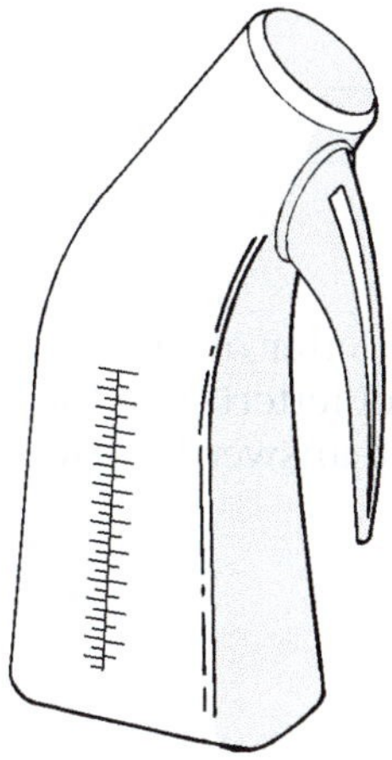

____

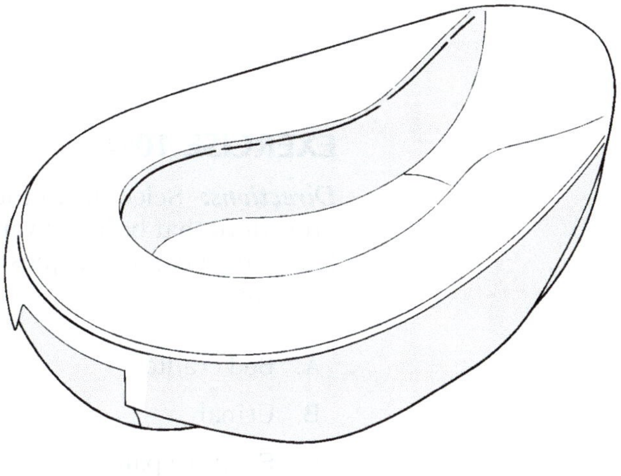

____

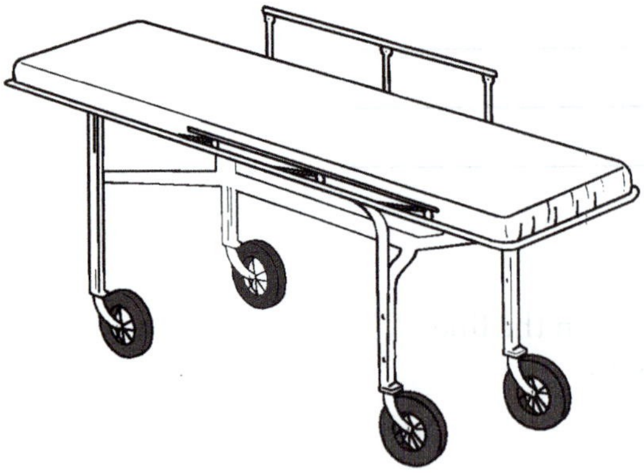

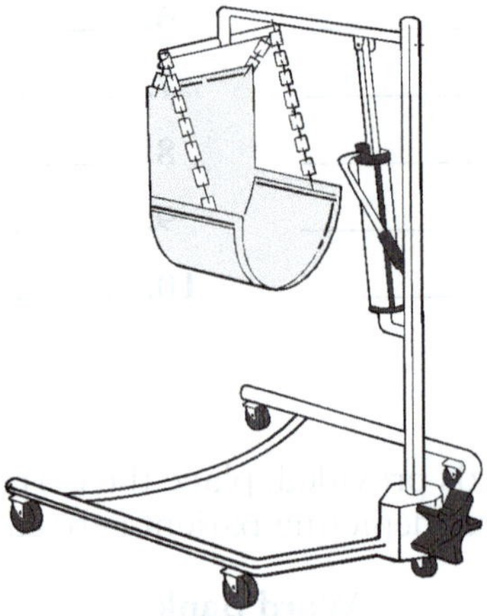

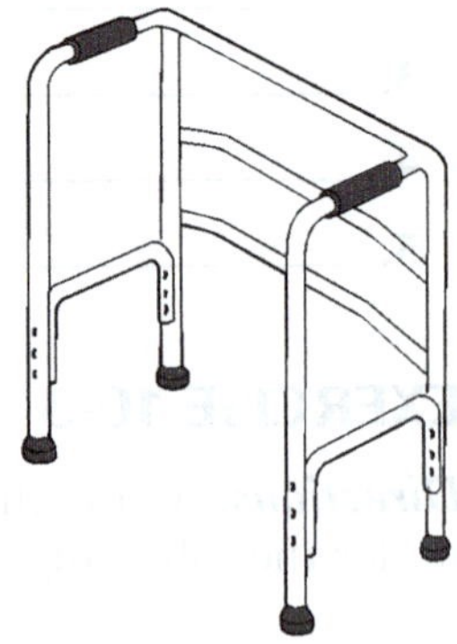

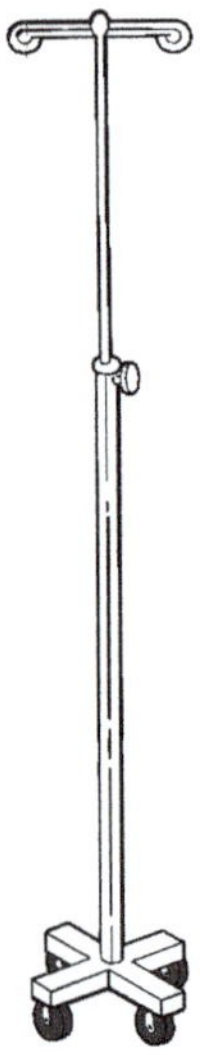

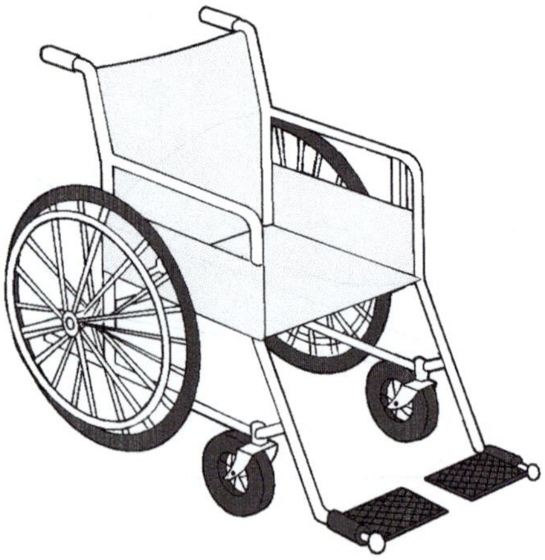

EXERCISE 10-4

Directions: Select from the following list of procedures the letter of the procedure that best answers each question. Write the correct letter(s) on the blank line next to the question. There may be more than one answer for each question.

A. Bed cradle

B. Urinal

C. Fracture pan

D. Walker

E. Emesis basin

F. Wheelchair

G. Specialty bed

H. Air-pressure mattress

I. Intravenous pole

J. Bedpan

_____ 1. Which equipment should be made available to a patient who is in a full-body cast?

_____ 2. Which equipment should be offered to an elderly man who is bedridden?

_____ 3. A patient who had toe surgery comes to your unit with a urinary catheter and an IV in her right arm. She has bathroom privileges. Which equipment might she need?

_____ 4. Which equipment helps patients ambulate or be transported?

THE NURSING ASSISTANT IN ACTION

1. You report to your unit and find that your coworker has not done her job to clean many patients' rooms. There are wet towels and linens in the shower, dirty overbed tables, and plastic wrappings left from two new admissions. This is the third time this week that you had to clean up after her. What should you do?

____

____

____

____

2. You are taking care of a person who is being treated for obsessive compulsive disorder (OCD). She likes everything just the way she places it on her side bed table, her overbed table, and in her bathroom. However, there is no room for you to place her meal tray or bathing equipment. What should you do?

____

____

____

____

3. You are working as a home health aide and your patient falls between the toilet and the wall. You cannot get her up and suspect she has broken her hip. What should you do?

____

____

____

____

4. Mr. Rogers has a cast on his right arm. How should you arrange his room and equipment to ensure optimal care and comfort measures are offered?

____

____

____

____

5. You are assigned to take care of Mrs. Jazewski, an elderly woman who is bedridden, in her home. Mrs. Jazewski's daughter left a note on the kitchen counter of all the things she wants you to do before she returns home from work. Some of the things on the list include wash the kitchen floor, bleach a load of laundry, fold laundry in the dryer, and cook dinner. What should you do?

____

____

____

____

LEARNING ACTIVITIES

1. Go through your home and identify then reduce any safety hazards. Correct the problem if possible by reducing the amount of scatter rugs, changing light bulbs to make for a brighter area, getting rid of or fixing frayed electric cords, reducing the number of extension cords, fixing broken stairs, and adding handrails in bathrooms and hallways.
2. Go through the closets and cabinets in your home. Remove any outdated chemicals, liquids, or medications. Initiate ways to make your home safer by placing locks on cabinets that hold chemicals and medications or keep flammable items in an area where there is better ventilation.

PROCEDURE CHECKLIST

PROCEDURE 10-1: CALLING FOR HELP

Name: ______________________ Date: ______________________

STEPS	S	U	COMMENTS
1. Determine what help you need.			
2. Have the address or be able to provide your location, room, or apartment number accurately.			
3. Give your name.			
4. Give the name of the patient and identify your location, room number, or address.			
5. State the problem clearly. State objectively exactly what has happened or what help you need. If calling a city emergency number, give the above information, as well as the phone number of the patient's physician to the person who answers the phone call.			
6. If you have a phone number for a member of the family or contact person, give that number also.			
7. Stay with the individual until help arrives. Follow advice or direction offered by the EMS operator.			
8. Document the time of the emergency and anything unusual that you observed.			
9. Discuss the situation with the emergency responders and your immediate supervisor to determine appropriate follow-up.			

Charting:

____

____

____

____

Date of Satisfactory Completion ______________________

Instructor's Signature ______________________

Bedmaking

11

Key Terms Review

Match the key terms in the right column with the definitions in the left column by placing the letter of each correct answer in the space provided.

____ **1.** A bed that is made when the bed is available for a patient admission; covers are pulled all the way to the top of the bed.

____ **2.** Small sheet made of plastic or cotton placed across the middle of the bed to cover and protect the bottom sheet and assist in moving the patient.

____ **3.** Method of arranging bed linens so that the covers and bedspread are folded at the foot of the bed out of the way.

____ **4.** A bed with a patient in it.

____ **5.** Bed made with the top bed linens fan-folded to give patient easy entrance to the bed.

____ **6.** Bed made with the top sheet folded lengthwise and positioned to one side, allowing transfer of the patient from the surgical stretcher to the bed without unnecessary movement.

Terms

A. Closed bed

B. Fan-fold

C. Open (fan-folded) bed

D. Postoperative (surgical) bed

E. Occupied bed

F. Draw sheet

MULTIPLE-CHOICE QUESTIONS

Circle the letter next to the word or statement that best completes the sentence or answers the question.

1. By fan-folding the top of the bed, you make it easier for the patient to
   a. roll out of bed in the morning.
   b. bathe himself.
   c. make his own bed.
   d. get back into the bed.
2. Shaking the bed linen
   a. can be done safely in the hallway.
   b. should not be done because it disturbs the doctors.
   c. should be done daily.
   d. spreads germs and should not be done.
3. When a cotton draw sheet is not available,
   a. you do not need to use one.
   b. reuse the one that was taken off earlier.
   c. use a large sheet that has been folded in half lengthwise. Avoid wrinkles.
   d. use a large sheet that has been folded in half widthwise. Avoid wrinkles.
4. Wrinkles in the sheet indent the skin and
   a. promote good circulation by stimulating the skin.
   b. may be avoided by pulling the sheet tightly to smooth it.
   c. can be removed by the patient lying on it for 2 hours.
   d. will not occur if it is made of cotton fabric.
5. You can save time and energy when making a bed if you
   a. get someone else to do it.
   b. stand either at the head or at the foot of the bed.
   c. make one side of the bed and then quickly crawl across to the other side.
   d. use good body mechanics to make as much of the bed as possible on one side before going to the other side.
6. The ________ side of a bed protector should never touch a patient's skin.
   a. cotton
   b. wet
   c. plastic
   d. white
7. A rubber or plastic bed protector can be used if it is
   a. clean.
   b. covered by a cotton sheet.
   c. dry.
   d. all of the above.
8. Wrinkles in the sheets can
   a. make the patient sleep soundly.
   b. cause skin breakdown.
   c. be ignored.
   d. be removed by shaking them vigorously.
9. Taking extra linen into a patient's unit
   a. is a good idea, because if it is not used it can be put back on the linen cart and used later for someone else.
   b. is a wasteful practice.
   c. makes the patient feel cared for.
   d. is convenient because you will have extra linen if you need it.
10. A patient is highly sensitive to the fibers in the pillow you have given him. You should
    a. offer another pillow from the linen cart.
    b. place a sign on the door noting the patient's allergies.
    c. ask family if there is any way they can provide a pillow from home.
    d. place a pillow protector on the pillow you offered.
11. For each type of bed made,
    a. it is important to always wear gloves.
    b. make sure the bed is always placed in the lowest position when finished.
    c. it is essential to document in the chart how the patient tolerated the procedure.
    d. you should follow the policy and procedure for standard precautions set forth by your facility.

12. A closed bed is
a. used for those residents who may be up for most of the day.
b. the standard way housekeeping leaves a bed once the unit is cleaned.
c. when the top sheet, blanket, and bedspread are near the head of the bed.
d. all of the above.

13. Another name for the fan-folded bed is
a. open.
b. closed.
c. surgical.
d. half made.

14. A recovery bed
a. is made with top linens folded to one side of the bed.
b. can be called a *postsurgical bed.*
c. should be left in the highest position.
d. all of the above.

15. Usually, when making a postoperative bed, no less than ___ blanket(s) is (are) used.
a. one
b. two
c. three
d. four

16. In some cases, a heated blanket is used for a postoperative patient. What is the purpose of a heated blanket?
a. Decrease circulation
b. Maintain body temperature
c. Increase movement
d. Provide privacy for the patient

17. Which of the following is true of the pillow?
a. The case opening should face the door.
b. It should be placed at the headboard for a postoperative bed.
c. It must be removed every time when making an occupied bed.
d. All of the above.

18. What is the purpose of using a towel when making a bed?
a. It provides a barrier between the dirty chair and the fresh linens to reduce bacteria.
b. A towel should be placed under the draw sheet to absorb extra body fluids from the patient.
c. All dirty linens should be placed on top of the towel that has been placed on the floor to prevent contamination.
d. All of the above.

19. What is the purpose of a toe pleat?
a. It gives that extra detail to make the bed look tidy.
b. It allows for some extra room for the patient's feet.
c. Skin breakdown is prevented.
d. All of the above.

20. When you are finished making an occupied bed, the next step you should take is to
a. wash all the linens.
b. get rid of soiled linens and place them in the appropriate container.
c. lower the height of the bed and keep all side rails up.
d. offer a call bell and make sure the patient is comfortable.

21. If the mattress has shifted, you should
a. call a colleague who can help you reposition the mattress when the patient is showering.
b. rely on the help of a colleague to move the mattress when making an occupied bed.
c. not worry about it because you can still tuck the bottom linens under the mattress.
d. use a mechanical lift to move the mattress back into place.

22. What goes on the bed last?
a. Flat sheet or fitted sheet
b. Bedspread
c. Blanket
d. Draw sheet

23. A small sheet that goes in the middle of the bed and is used to help reposition a patient is called a
a. draw sheet.
b. bath blanket.
c. plastic protector.
d. top sheet.

24. When changing a pillowcase, you should
  a. hold the pillow firmly under your arm and pull the case onto the pillow to prevent the pillow from falling to the floor.
  b. tuck the edges inside and place the opening away from the window so the room looks tidy.
  c. turn the pillowcase inside out, grasp the pillow at the center, fit the corners into the case and pull the case down around the pillow.
  d. always use a pillow protector after the case is applied to prevent the spread of bacteria.

25. When is the best time to make a patient's bed?
  a. When evening care is offered to an ambulatory patient.
  b. Before a complete bath is given to a patient in a coma.
  c. When a patient leaves the floor before breakfast to go for an x-ray.
  d. When visitors are in the room and you can ask them to help you.

TRUE OR FALSE QUESTIONS

Determine whether each question is true or false. In the space provided, write "T" for true and "F" for false. If the statement is false, rewrite it on the line provided to make it a true statement.

_____ **1.** Usually, about 18" of linen is left to tuck under the mattress to help secure the sheets.

____

_____ **2.** A draw sheet should be placed approximately 14" from the top of the mattress.

____

_____ **3.** A patient should always be placed in a flat (supine) position when an occupied bed is being made to ensure no wrinkles occur in the linen.

____

_____ **4.** The bed should always be left in the lowest position after making it no matter what type of bed has been made.

____

_____ **5.** You must report to the nurse in charge how the patient tolerated you making the empty bed.

____

_____ **6.** When you are finished with bedmaking, you should ask the patient if he would like the head of the bed raised.

____

_____ **7.** A well-made bed can promote the appearance of the room.

____

_____ **8.** The type of bed you make depends on the needs of the patient.

____

_____ **9.** Hold linens close to your body so they do not fall to the ground.

____

_____ **10.** When gathering supplies, place them in a stack with the item you will use first on top.

____

EXERCISE 11-1

Objective: To apply what you have learned about the different methods of bedmaking.

Directions: Choose terms from the word list to label the four methods of bedmaking in Figure 11-1.

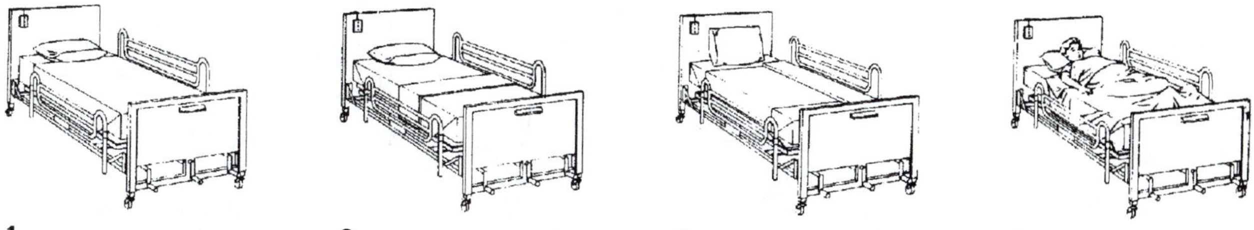

1. ____________ **2.** ____________ **3.** ____________ **4.** ____________

Figure 11-1

Word List

Occupied	Surgical (Postoperative) (Postsurgical)	Open	Closed

EXERCISE 11-2

Directions: Use the word list provided in Exercise 11-1 and write the number of the correct method of bedmaking you should use when reviewing the following practice description exercise.

Practice Description

_____ **1.** Mrs. O'Shea will be returning from surgery in the next 2 hours.

_____ **2.** You have finished giving Mr. Garcia a complete bath. He has had a stroke and is too weak to get out of bed.

_____ **3.** Mrs. Chang is being ambulated in the hallway, so you decide to make her bed now.

_____ **4.** Your patient has been discharged, the room and bed have been cleaned, and your immediate supervisor asks you to make the bed.

EXERCISE 11-3

Directions: Using the pictures provided, place them in the order that makes the most sense when making a closed bed.

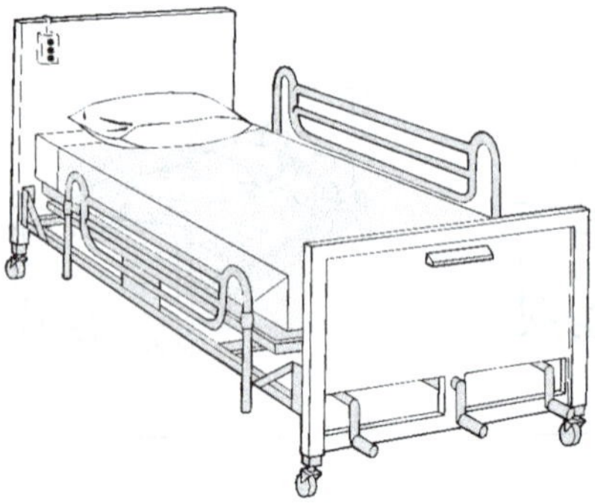

____

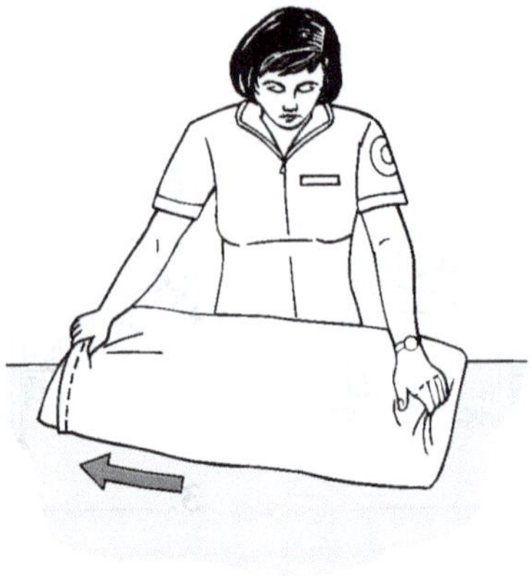

____

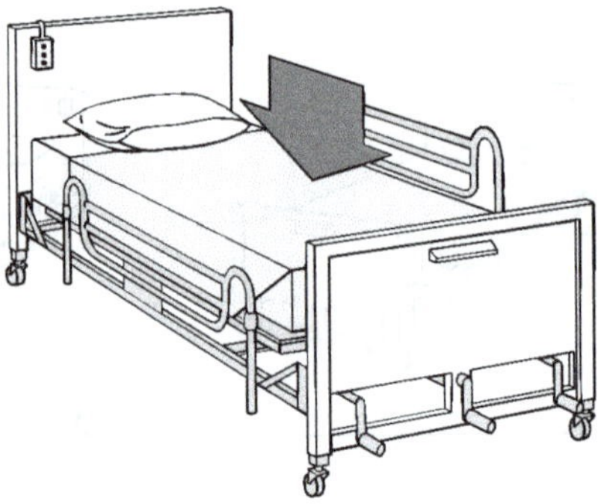

____

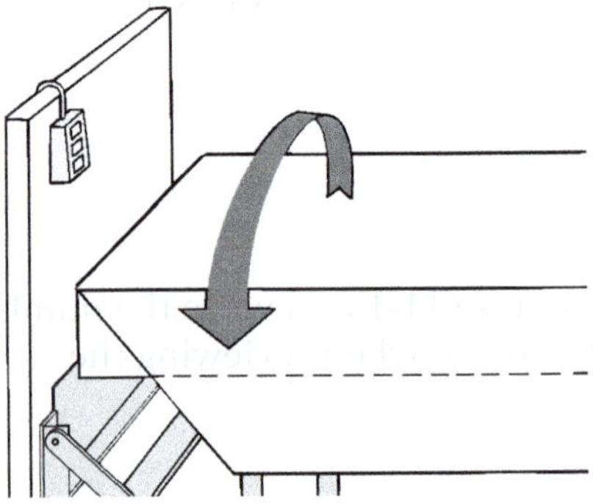

____

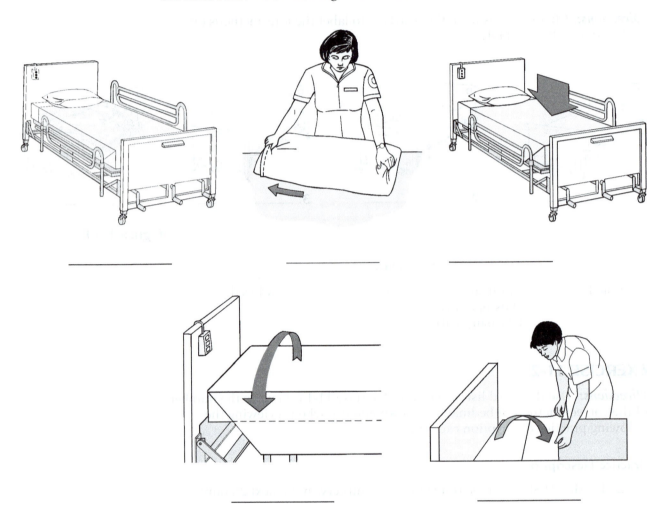

____

THE NURSING ASSISTANT IN ACTION

1. You are in the process of completing the last few steps of making an occupied bed when you realize your patient has soiled himself and the bed linens are completely wet. What should you do?

____

____

____

____

2. You have the patient's bed rails up and the bed in the highest position when making an occupied bed. Half the bed is stripped of linen when you realize you did not get enough supplies. What should you do?

3. You pass by a patient's room where a colleague is making a bed. You notice dirty linen on the floor. What should you do?

4. A patient who is ambulatory refuses to get out of bed after breakfast so you can make his bed. What should you do?

5. A new patient is being admitted to your unit. The room has not yet been cleaned by housekeeping and the old bed linen is still on the bed. What should you do?

LEARNING ACTIVITIES

1. Using your partner, practice making an occupied bed, and then switch. Discuss how it felt to be the patient and offer ideas as to what could make the situation more comfortable. Discuss strengths each person had while the bed was being made.
2. Make a postsurgical bed. Place your partner on a stretcher and pretend she is the patient. Get a second partner to help you practice transferring from the stretcher to the bed and back again. Switch roles. Discuss how it felt to be the patient and offer ideas as to what could make the situation safe and comfortable. Discuss strengths each person had while the transfer occurred.

PROCEDURE CHECKLISTS

PROCEDURE 11-1: MAKING A CLOSED BED

Name: ____________________ Date: ____________________

STEPS	S	U	COMMENTS
1. Assemble your supplies a. Mattress cover (if used) b. Bottom sheet (flat or fitted) c. Cotton or plastic draw sheets (if used) d. Top sheet e. Blanket f. Bedspread g. Pillowcase h. Pillow i. Pillow protector (if used) j. Towel (to use as a barrier) k. Linen hamper			
2. Place a chair near the bed.			
3. Wash your hands.			
4. Open the towel and place as a barrier on the seat of the chair.			
5. Place the pillow on the chair.			
6. Stack the bed linen on the chair in the order you will use them: first things to be used on top, last things to be used on bottom.			
7. Lower rails to the down position on the bed.			
8. Remove any dirty linens and place in the soiled linen hamper, being careful to avoid contact with your uniform.			
9. Adjust the bed to the highest horizontal position for comfort while you work.			
10. Push the mattress to the head of the bed.			
11. Place a fitted sheet on the bed and carefully unfold it.			
12. Anchor the sheet under all four corners of the bed mattress by standing and working on one side of the bed until that side is finished before going to the opposite side. Proceed to step 17. If using an unfitted sheet, follow steps 13–16.			
13. Fold the bottom sheet lengthwise and place it on the bed.			

14. Open the sheet. It should now hang evenly the same distance over each side of the bed.			
15. There should be 18 inches of the sheet to tuck smoothly and tightly under the head of the mattress.			
16. To make a mitered corner a. Pick up the edge of the sheet at the side of the bed 12 inches from the head of the mattress. b. Place the triangle (folded corner) on top of the mattress. c. Tuck the hanging portion of the sheet under the mattress. d. While you hold the fold at the edge of the mattress, bring the triangle down over the side of the mattress. e. Tuck the sheet under the mattress from head to foot.			
17. Fold in half and place the draw sheet 14" down from the head of the bed. Tuck it in. Straighten each piece of linen as you tuck it in.			
18. Fold the top sheet lengthwise and place it on the bed. a. Place the center fold on the center of the bed from the head to the foot. b. Put the large hem at the head of the bed, even with the top edge of the mattress. c. Open the sheet, with the rough edge of the hem up, fan-folding half to the center of the bed. d. Tuck the sheet under tightly at the foot of the bed. e. Make a mitered corner at the foot of the bed. f. Do not tuck in sides.			
19. Fold the blanket lengthwise and place on the bed. a. Place the center fold of the blanket in the center of the bed from head to foot. b. Place the upper hem 6'' from the top edge of the mattress. c. Open the blanket. d. Tuck it under the foot tightly. e. Make a mitered corner at the foot of the bed. f. Do not tuck in sides.			

20. Fold the bedspread lengthwise and place it on the bed. a. Place the center fold in the center of the bed from the head to the foot. b. Place the upper hem even with the head edge of the mattress. c. Keep the rough edge down. d. Open the spread. e. Tuck it under at the foot of the bed tightly. f. Make a mitered corner at the foot of the bed. g. Do not tuck in sides.			
21. Go to the other side of the bed. Start with the bottom sheet. a. Pull the sheet tight to get rid of the wrinkles. b. Miter the top corner. c. Pull the draw sheet tight and tuck it in. d. Straighten out the top sheet, making a mitered corner at the foot of the bed. e. Miter the corner of the blanket. f. Miter the corner of the bedspread.			
22. To make the cuff a. Fold the top hem of the spread under the top hem of the blanket. b. Fold the top hem of the sheet back over the edge of the spread and the blanket to form a cuff. The hemmed side of the sheet must be on the underside so that it does not come in contact with the patient.			
23. To put the pillowcase on a pillow a. Hold the pillowcase at the center of the end seam. b. With your hand outside the case, turn the case back over your hand. c. Grasp the pillow through the case at the center of one end of the pillow. d. Fit the corner of the pillow into the seamless corner of the case. e. Bring the case down over the pillow. f. Fold the extra material from the side seam under the pillow. g. Place the pillow on the bed with the open end away from the door.			

24. Adjust the bed to its lowest horizontal position.			
25. Bag and dispose of soiled linen in the laundry hamper.			
26. Wash your hands.			
27. Report to your supervisor that you made the closed, empty bed.			

Charting:

____

____

____

____

Date of Satisfactory Completion ______________________

Instructor's Signature ______________________

PROCEDURE 11-2: MAKING AN OPEN (FAN-FOLDED) BED

Name: ____________________ Date: ____________________

STEPS	S	U	COMMENTS
1. Assemble your supplies for making the closed bed. a. Mattress cover (if used) b. Bottom sheet c. Cotton and plastic draw sheets d. Top sheets e. Blanket f. Bedspread g. Pillowcase e. Pillow f. Pillow protector (if used)			
2. Wash your hands and make the closed bed.			
3. Grasp the cuff of the bedding in both hands.			
4. Fan-fold to the foot of the bed.			
5. Fold the bedding back on itself toward the head of the bed. The edge of the cuff must meet the fold.			
6. Smooth the hanging sheets on each side neatly into the folds you have made.			
7. Wash your hands.			

Charting:

____

____

____

____

Date of Satisfactory Completion ____________________

Instructor's Signature ____________________

PROCEDURE 11-3: MAKING A POSTOPERATIVE (POSTSURGICAL) BED

Name: ____________________ Date: ____________________

STEPS	S	U	COMMENTS
1. Assemble your supplies for making a closed bed with the addition of at least two additional blankets a. Mattress cover (if used) b. Bottom sheet c. Cotton and plastic draw sheets d. Top sheet e. Blankets (3) f. Bedspread g. Pillowcase h. Pillow i. Pillow protector (if used)			
2. Wash your hands.			
3. Adjust the bed to the highest horizontal, comfortable working position. Lock the bed in place. Strip all used linen from the bed and place in a laundry bag.			
4. Make the bottom part of the bed. Follow instructions for making a closed bed.			
5. Spread one bath blanket across the bed, on top of the draw sheet and bottom sheet. The bottom end of the bath blanket or blanket should be even with the foot of the mattress. Tuck the edge under the mattress on your side of the bed.			
6. Go to the other side of the bed. Tuck the blanket or bath blanket under the mattress.			
7. Spread the second blanket or bath blanket across the bed. The upper edge should be about 6'' from the head of the bed. This blanket gives the patient extra warmth.			
8. Put the top sheet, the regular blanket, and the spread on the bed. Do this the same way as when making the closed bed, but do not tuck them in at the foot of the bed. Instead, all the bedding at the foot end should be folded back on the bed so the folded edge is even with the foot of the mattress.			
9. Make the cuff the same as for the open bed, except you fold the blanket over the cuff.			
10. Go to the side of the bed where the stretcher will be in place.			

11. Grasp the top bedding at the side with both hands. Fold the bedding across the bed so the folded edge is even with the far side of the mattress. Again, fold the bedding to the edge so it is twice folded onto itself.			
12. Put the pillow into the pillowcase. Put the pillow upright against the headboard. Place it so as to protect the patient from hitting his or her head on the headboard during the transfer from the stretcher.			
13. Move the bedside table, chair, and any other furniture out of the way to make room for the stretcher.			
14. Remove everything from the bedside table except a box of tissues and an emesis basin.			
15. Bring an IV pole into the room and place near the head of the bed.			
16. Position the surgical bed to match stretcher height.			
17. Wash your hands.			
18. Report to your supervisor that the postoperative (postsurgical) bed has been made.			

Charting:

____

____

____

____

Date of Satisfactory Completion ____________________

Instructor's Signature ____________________

PROCEDURE 11-4: MAKING AN OCCUPIED BED

Name: ____________________ Date: ____________________

STEPS	S	U	COMMENTS
1. Assemble your supplies in the order in which they will be used, and place on a chair near the bed. a. Two large sheets b. Draw sheet c. Disposable or reusable bed protectors d. One bath or regular blanket e. Pillowcase f. One blanket (depending on room temperature) g. One bedspread h. One plastic laundry bag			
2. Identify the patient by checking the ID bracelet.			
3. Inform the patient that you are going to make the bed.			
4. Provide privacy and comfort for the patient.			
5. Wash your hands and put on gloves.			
6. Lower the backrest and knee rest until the bed is flat, if that is allowed. Raise the bed to a comfortable working height and lock in place. Keep side rails up to provide safety for the patient. Raise the bed to a comfortable working height and lock in place.			
7. Loosen all the sheets around the entire bed.			
8. Take the bedspread and blanket off the bed and fold them over the back of the chair, leaving the patient covered with the top sheet.			
9. Cover the patient with the bath blanket by placing it over the top sheet. Ask the patient to hold the blanket, if he is able to do so. Some patients may not be able to hold the blanket; therefore, it is acceptable to place the blanket under the shoulders to help hold the blanket in place. Remove the top sheet under the bath blanket.			
10. Be sure the mattress is in its proper position touching the headboard. If you must move the mattress, ask for assistance.			
11. Raise the side rail on the opposite side from where you will be working and lock it in place.			
12. Assist the patient with turning on her side toward the side rail, facing away from you.			

13. Adjust the pillow for the patient according to instructions. If the patient cannot sit up, lock arms with her and raise her to remove the pillow, if permitted.			
14. Fold the draw sheet toward the patient and tuck it against her back.			
15. Raise the plastic or disposable draw sheet over the blanket and the patient, if it is clean. If it is soiled, also fold it toward the patient.			
16. Fold the bottom sheet toward the patient and tuck it against her back. This strips your side of the bed down to the mattress.			
17. Take the large clean sheet and fold it in half lengthwise. Do not let the sheet touch the floor or your clothing.			
18. Place the sheet on the bed, still folded, with the fold running along the middle of the mattress. The small hem end of the sheet should be even with the foot edge of the mattress. Fold the top half of the sheet toward the patient. Tuck the folds against her back.			
19. Miter the corner at the head of the mattress. Tuck in the clean bottom sheet from the head to the foot of the mattress.			
20. Pull the plastic draw sheet toward you, over the clean bottom sheet, and tuck in.			
21. Place the clean cotton draw sheet over the plastic sheet, folded in half. Fold the top half toward the patient, tucking the folds under her back, as you did with the bottom sheet. Tuck the draw sheet under the mattress.			
22. Raise the bedside rail on your side of the bed and lock it in place.			
23. Go to the opposite side of the bed.			
24. Lower the bedside rail. Assist the patient with rolling over the "lump" onto the clean sheets, away from you. Be careful not to let the patient become entangled in the sheets as she turns.			
25. Remove the old bottom sheet and cotton draw sheet from the bed by rolling dirty sheets from headboard to footboard and place in linen bag or hamper. Pull the fresh bottom sheet toward the edge of the bed. Tuck it under the mattress at the head of the bed and make a mitered corner. Then tuck the bottom sheet under the mattress from the head to the foot, pulling firmly to remove any wrinkles.			
26. Pull the plastic draw sheet and clean cotton draw sheet toward you.			

27. Then, one at a time, tuck the draw sheets under the mattress along the side.			
28. Be sure to pull all the sheets tight as you tuck them in, removing all wrinkles.			
29. Assist the patient with turning on her back.			
30. Change the pillowcase and place the pillow under the patient's head.			
31. Spread the clean top sheet over the bath blanket with the wide hem to the top. The middle of the sheet should run along the middle of the bed. The wide hem should be even with the head edge of the mattress. Remove the bath blanket, moving toward the foot of the bed, without exposing the patient.			
32. Tuck the clean top sheet under the mattress at the foot of the bed. Be sure to leave enough room for the patient to move her feet freely by gathering the linens and making a 2" to 4" horizontal toe pleat across the foot of the bed. Miter the corners of the sheet.			
33. Spread the blanket over the top sheet. Be sure the middle of the blanket runs along the middle of the bed. The blanket should be high enough to cover the patient's shoulders.			
34. Tuck the blanket in at the foot of the bed. Make a mitered corner with the blanket.			
35. Place the spread on the bed in the same way. Make a mitered corner with the spread.			
36. Go to the other side of the bed, and pull the top sheet, blanket, and spread over and straighten them. Remove the bath blanket. Turn the top covers back and miter the top sheet, then the blanket, then the spread. Be sure the top covers are loose enough for the patient to move her feet.			
37. To make the cuff a. Fold the top hem edge of the spread over and under the top hem of the blanket. b. Fold the top hem of the top sheet back over the edge of the spread and blanket to form a cuff. The rough edge of the hem of the sheet must be turned down so the patient does not come into contact with it.			
38. Raise the backrest and knee rest to suit the patient, if allowed.			
39. Make the patient comfortable and replace the call light.			
40. Lower the bed to a position of safety for the patient.			

41. Raise the side rails when ordered or indicated.			
42. Bag and dispose of used linen in the laundry hamper.			
43. Tidy up the patient's room.			
44. Dispose of gloves and wash your hands.			
45. Report to your supervisor • That you made the occupied bed • How the patient tolerated the procedure • Any unusual observations			

Charting:

____

____

____

____

Date of Satisfactory Completion ____________________

Instructor's Signature ____________________

12

Admitting, Transferring, and Discharging a Patient

Key Terms Review

Match the key terms in the right column with the definitions in the left column by placing the letter of each correct answer in the space provided.

_____ **1.** The process that covers the period of time from when the patient enters the institution door to the time the patient is settled.

_____ **2.** The official procedure for helping patients to leave the health care institution, including how to care for themselves at home.

_____ **3.** Moving a hospital patient from one room, unit, or facility to another.

_____ **4.** Gathering facts to identify needs and problems.

_____ **5.** Determining whether a plan has been effective.

_____ **6.** Deciding what to do and how to do it.

_____ **7.** Carrying out or accomplishing a given plan.

_____ **8.** A written plan stating the nursing priorities, the patient goals, or expected outcomes, and the nursing orders or actions to be taken.

_____ **9.** Verbal or written information passed from one caregiver to another, giving information about a patient, to ensure continuity of care.

Terms

A. Spiritual
B. Sociocultural
C. Psychological
D. Physiological
E. Holistic
F. Assessing
G. Planning
H. Evaluating
I. Implementing
J. Plan of care
K. Report
L. Admission
M. Transfer
N. Discharge

_____10. An approach that includes the four aspects of a whole person; physiological, psychological, sociocultural, and spiritual.

_____11. Referring to a person's biological responses to alterations in the body's structures and functions.

_____12. Referring to a person's cognitive and emotional responses to the self and surrounding environment.

_____13. Referring to a person's interpersonal responses to socialization practices in the family and community.

_____14. Referring to a person's response to inspirational forces.

MULTIPLE-CHOICE QUESTIONS

Circle the letter next to the word or statement that best completes the sentence or answers the question.

1. At the time of admission, the nursing assistant is very important to the patient because
   a. the patient may be frightened and uncomfortable.
   b. the patient may be in pain.
   c. the patient may be seriously ill.
   d. all of the above.

2. The nursing assistant, by being _____________ and _____________, makes the patient's admission process easier.
   a. irate, hasty
   b. slow, disorganized
   c. confused, sleepy
   d. pleasant, courteous

3. The nursing assistant should address the adult patient
   a. with his first name to be informal and friendly.
   b. with his initials only.
   c. as "Grandma" or "Grandpa" to make them feel part of the health care family.
   d. as Mr., Miss, or Ms. and the patient's last name.

4. When admitting a patient, the nursing assistant should keep in mind
   a. the reason for the patient's admission.
   b. the remaining work to be done with other patients.
   c. the tasks the nurse has asked the nursing assistant to do for this patient.
   d. a and c.

5. An important tool for 24-hour communication for the health care team is the
   a. care strategy log.
   b. physician's log.
   c. nursing care plan.
   d. Internet.

6. The nursing care plan helps the team deliver
   a. the mail.
   b. continuous and consistent care.
   c. floral bouquets.
   d. uncoordinated care.

7. The registered nurse _____________ the care plan on admission.
   a. finishes
   b. begins
   c. rejects
   d. approves

8. The registered nurse reevaluates the plan of care each day to reflect
   a. the sun.
   b. the changing needs of the team.
   c. the staffing limits.
   d. the changing needs of the patient.

9. It is important that the nursing assistant review the plan of care each day to
   a. see what information on the plan has changed.
   b. make suggestions, as a way to contribute to the plan.
   c. identify goals the patient is achieving.
   d. all of the above.

10. The plan of care influences how the nursing assistant
   a. organizes his work.
   b. plans his work.
   c. observes and reports the patient's activities.
   d. all of the above.

11. The nursing assistant is responsible for
   a. gathering data objectively.
   b. reporting data after returning from break or before leaving for the day.
   c. calling the doctor when something is not right.
   d. telling other colleagues about the patient's diagnosis.

12. The patient must be identified by _______________ before preparing to transfer him.
   a. asking the family or visitors who he is
   b. asking him if he is the one to be transferred
   c. checking the identification bracelet
   d. calling the doctor

13. The nursing assistant should be aware that some patients will be _______________ that they must be transferred to another facility or even to another unit.
   a. scared
   b. upset
   c. anxious
   d. all of the above

14. The nursing assistant can give the patient emotional support after transferring him by
   a. reassuring him that his family will find him eventually.
   b. telling him he shouldn't worry so much because he could be moved again tomorrow.
   c. telling him about other patients that were transferred today.
   d. reassuring him that his family and visitors will be given the new room number.

15. A common way to transfer the patient is
   a. on a wheelchair scale.
   b. on a draw sheet.
   c. on a stretcher or in a wheelchair.
   d. by allowing the patient to walk to the new unit.

16. After the transfer, the nursing assistant should
   a. report the time of the transfer to the supervisor.
   b. keep all the patient's belongings on the old unit until the patient needs them.
   c. keep the patient's medications locked in a drawer in the new room.
   d. take a break.

17. If the patient is discharged to another health care facility,
   a. the patient may require a caregiver or nurse to accompany her.
   b. the nursing assistant will not be involved in this kind of transfer.
   c. an ambulance is never used.
   d. there will be no special instructions from the nurse.

18. Teaching patients how to care for themselves at home is the responsibility of
   a. the nursing assistant only.
   b. the nurse only.
   c. the entire nursing team.
   d. the person who chooses to take on that responsibility.

19. The patient's family must be included in the discharge education process because
   a. it's nice to be included.
   b. the family may be the primary caregivers at home.
   c. they want to be included.
   d. they are paying the bill.

20. The best approach to discharge teaching is the
  a. partial approach.
  b. complete approach.
  c. holistic approach.
  d. discharge approach.

21. The discharge instructions include
  a. detailed housekeeping instructions.
  b. detailed travel arrangements.
  c. details on diet, activity, and medications.
  d. information on how to discharge a patient.

22. Explanation of care in the home environment could include
  a. maps on how to get from place to place.
  b. coupons they can use when food shopping.
  c. steps to take to plan a vacation.
  d. information on how to eliminate hazards in the home.

23. It is the nursing assistant's responsibility to read and understand the institution's policies and procedures for ________ of the patient.
  a. admission
  b. discharge
  c. transfer
  d. all of the above

24. When admitting a teenager to a new unit, a nursing assistant should
  a. keep the privacy curtain open when they are changing.
  b. speak to only their parents about their care and the tasks she performs.
  c. include the teen when instructions about care is being offered.
  d. not orient the teen to how the TV, radio, or other electronic equipment work because teens know all about these things.

25. When discharge occurs, the nursing assistant should
  a. allow the patient to walk from his room to the car.
  b. buckle the patient into his car, noting who came to take him home.
  c. pay the bill for the patient.
  d. give the patient a kiss and a hug and wish him well.

TRUE OR FALSE QUESTIONS

Determine whether each question is true or false. In the space provided, write "T" for true and "F" for false. If the statement is false, rewrite it on the line provided to make it a true statement.

_____ **1.** It is not a good idea to introduce yourself to a patient being admitted, even if he is in a lot of pain.

____

_____ **2.** If it is possible, allow the parents to stay with a child during admission to a health care facility.

____

_____ **3.** The nursing assistant is a representative of the institution.

____

_____ **4.** The registered nurse identifies patient problems and nursing diagnoses.

____

_____ **5.** Nowadays, patients tend to have shorter stays in the hospital and tend to go home faster to recover.

____

_____ **6.** The nursing assistant should ask the patient if he has the written discharge information before wheeling him off the floor.

____

_____ **7.** A patient is discharged when he no longer requires or benefits from the services a facility offers.

____

_____ **8.** The patient care plan is a very important tool to providing quality care.

____

_____ **9.** A transfer may occur because the patient's condition may have worsened.

____

_____ **10.** In most situations, families will transfer their loved ones to another facility.

____

FILL-IN-THE-BLANK QUESTIONS

Provide the meaning of the following abbreviations.

1. ADL _______________________________

2. NPO _______________________________

3. ID _______________________________

4. RN _______________________________

5. EMS _______________________________

6. DRGs _______________________________

EXERCISE 12-1

In the top row of the following sample care plan form, identify the information provided as the Nursing Diagnosis, Evaluation, Patient Goal, Nursing Intervention, or Assessment.

NURSING CARE PLAN

S: "I am so afraid of falling in my room." O: Pt demonstrates difficulty using his walker and carries it around the facility.	Knowledge deficit with use of walker will be determined by the registered nurse.	The pt will understand the correct steps of how to use his walker.	Follows PT/OT goals when ambulation with walker occurs.	Pt verbalizes and demonstrates understanding of how to use his walker. No falls occurred × 6 wks.

EXERCISE 12-2

Select the letter of the word or phrase that best answers each question. Write the correct letter(s) on the blank line next to the question.

a. Admitting

b. Transfer to another unit in the same facility

c. Transfer to another facility

d. Discharge home

____**1.** When is it appropriate to gather a washbasin, bedpan, and urinal and place it in the patient's room?

____**2.** When is it appropriate to orient the patient to his surroundings?

____**3.** When do you report to the nursing staff the patient has arrived?

____**4.** When should a wheelchair be used?

____**5.** When does a copy of the chart accompany the patient?

____**6.** When should unusual issues be reported to your supervisor?

____**7.** When should the nursing assistant strip the bed?

THE NURSING ASSISTANT IN ACTION

1. The patient insists that he is done with his treatment and that the hospital can do nothing more for him. He packs his bags, calls his wife, and tells you he is leaving. There are no discharge orders from the physician. What should you do?

____

____

____

____

2. A husband tells you he will help his wife by assisting her to walk to the unit she is to be transferred to in another part of the facility. What should you do?

____

____

____

____

3. On admission, the family hands you a shoebox that contains about 30 bottles of medication the patient takes each day. What should you do?

____

____

____

____

4. You are assigned to help admit a 6-year-old to your unit. Her mother is holding her in her arms. Both look very anxious and scared. What should you do?

____

____

____

____

5. A teenager has been discharged from your unit and tells you, "I don't need that wheelchair. I can walk to the door outside where my mom plans to meet me. I can carry all this stuff myself. You do not have to come with me." What should you do?

____

____

____

____

LEARNING ACTIVITIES

1. Create a checklist you can use each time you admit, transfer, or discharge a patient so you do not forget your assigned duties.
2. Practice with a friend the steps you should take when admitting a patient to your unit. Remember to bring in all the equipment you might need to set the room up correctly and to bring equipment you need to gather data. Remember to orient the patient to the new surroundings while maintaining a friendly demeanor. After the role-playing is finished, ask your friend what you could have done to help the patient feel more comfortable and aware of his surroundings.

PROCEDURE CHECKLISTS

PROCEDURE 12-1: ADMITTING THE PATIENT

Name: ______________________ Date: ______________________

STEPS	S	U	COMMENTS
1. Assemble equipment a. Admission checklist b. Urine specimen container and laboratory requisition slip (if used) c. Institution gown or pajamas (per policy) d. Clothing list e. Portable scale f. Blood pressure cuff and stethoscope g. Admission pack (contents vary) h. Thermometer i. Bedpan or urinal, emesis basin, and washbasin.			
2. Wash your hands.			
3. Fan-fold the bed covers down to the foot of the bed to open the bed.			
4. Place the hospital gown or pajamas at the foot of the bed.			
5. Put the bedpan, urinal, emesis basin, washbasin, and admission pack in the proper place in the bedside table drawer or stand. The bedpan, urinal, or other toileting equipment is generally kept in the bathroom.			
6. When the patient arrives on the floor, introduce yourself to the patient and visitors. Be friendly and address the patient by name. Be sure to tell the patient your job title.			
7. Escort the patient to his room.			
8. Politely ask the visitors to leave the room while you complete the admission process, if this is policy.			
9. Close the door and maintain privacy.			
10. Ask the patient to change into the gown or pajamas. Assist the patient if needed.			
11. Weigh the patient before assisting him into the bed or chair.			
12. Assist the patient into bed, or chair if bedrest is not ordered.			
13. Raise the side rails of the bed as necessary.			
14. Complete the admission checklist.			

15. Assist the patient with storing personal belongings. Any valuables should be given to family or locked in the facility safe, per institutional policy.			
16. Ask your supervisor if the patient is NPO or is allowed drinking water. If water is allowed, fill the ice pitcher.			
17. Instruct the patient in the use of the call bell. Attach the call bell to the bed where the patient can reach it. Demonstrate how the intercom works.			
18. Explain the facility policies about a. Radios b. Television c. Newspapers d. Mail e. Meals f. Visitors			
19. Make sure the patient is comfortable, and that the lighting and temperature are sufficient.			
20. Adjust the bed to a comfortable position, as allowed.			
21. Open the curtains, if the patient prefers.			
22. Raise the side rails if ordered and if appropriate for the patient.			
23. Wash your hands.			
24. Report to your supervisor a. That you completed the admission. b. That the patient is in bed or in a chair. c. That you have completed the admission checklist. d. The position of the side rails and bed. e. How the patient tolerated the procedure. f. Any unusual observations.			

Charting:

____

____

____

____

Date of Satisfactory Completion ______________

Instructor's Signature ______________

PROCEDURE 12-2: TRANSFERRING THE PATIENT

Name: ______________________ Date: ______________________

STEPS	S	U	COMMENTS
1. Assemble equipment appropriate to the needs of the patient a. Bag(s) for patient belongings b. Wheelchair c. Stretcher d. Cart e. Patient's chart (or copies of pertinent information in the patient's chart, according to the institution's transfer policy and procedure).			
2. Check to be sure the new unit is ready to receive the patient.			
3. Wash your hands.			
4. Identify the patient by checking the ID bracelet.			
5. Ask visitors to step out of the room, if this is policy.			
6. Tell the patient that he or she is being transferred to another room, unit, or facility. The patient should be given detailed instructions before the transfer procedure begins.			
7. Collect the patient's personal belongings, chart, and equipment.			
8. If the patient is being transferred within the facility to a new unit, transfer the patient a. The patient may be moved from one room to another in his own bed, on a stretcher, or in a wheelchair. b. Provide the patient with both physical and emotional support. c. Follow safety precautions when wheeling the patient to the new unit. d. Make the patient comfortable in the new unit. e. Introduce the patient to nursing staff and hand the chart to the caregiver accepting the patient. f. Arrange the room and assist the patient in putting away belongings. g. Place the bed in a position of safety (bedrails up or down, as per policy) and comfort for the patient. h. Open the curtains, if the patient would like them open. i. Place the call bell within easy reach of the patient.			

9. Report to the nurse manager or RN in the new nursing unit that the patient has arrived.			
10. Return to your own unit; if a cart is being used to transport patient belongings, transport the patient's belongings to the new room.			
11. If the patient is being transferred to another facility, greet the transport service when they arrive and assist with transferring the patient to a stretcher. a. Ensure the patient has all belongings. b. Give a copy of the patient record to the transport service or EMS personnel. c. Inform family or visitors that the patient is about to be transferred. d. Notify the supervisor or admissions office that the patient is being transferred out of the facility.			
12. Wash your hands.			
13. Report to the nurse manager or RN in the new nursing unit that the patient has arrived.			
14. Return to your own unit; if a cart is being used to transport patient belongings, transport the patient's belongings to the new room.			
15. Strip the bed in the original room and take used equipment to the soiled utility room, per institutional policy.			
16. Wash your hands.			
17. Report to your supervisor a. That the patient was taken to the new unit. b. The time of the transfer. c. The patient's reaction to the transfer. d. Any unusual observations.			

Charting:

____

____

____

____

Date of Satisfactory Completion ____________________

Instructor's Signature ____________________

PROCEDURE 12-3: DISCHARGING THE PATIENT

Name: ____________ Date: ____________

STEPS	S	U	COMMENTS
1. Assemble equipment according to the needs of the patient a. Wheelchair b. Stretcher c. Discharge slip d. Cart			
2. Wash your hands.			
3. Identify the patient by checking the identification bracelet.			
4. Help the patient collect and pack personal belongings.			
5. Be sure all valuables and medications are returned to the patient.			
6. Help the patient get dressed, if necessary.			
7. Check that the written instructions are given to the patient by your supervisor, such as a. Doctor's orders to follow at home b. Prescriptions c. Follow-up schedule of appointments with the doctor or clinic			
8. Assist the patient into the wheelchair.			
9. Obtain the discharge slip (if used) from your supervisor.			
10. Take the patient to the business office or discharge desk. Facility policy may allow family to perform this step. Follow policy and procedures set forth by your employer.			
11. Wheel the patient to the discharge and patient pick-up waiting area.			
12. When the patient's transportation arrives, wheel him to a waiting car.			
13. Help the patient out of the wheelchair and into the car.			
14. Secure the seatbelt in place.			
15. Say goodbye to the patient.			
16. Take the wheelchair back to the floor.			

17. Strip the linen from the bed, unless housekeeping does this in your institution. Place the linens in the soiled linen hamper.			
18. Notify housekeeping of the discharge and that the unit is ready to be cleaned.			
19. Wash your hands.			
20. Inform your supervisor that the patient was discharged, and report a. The time of discharge. b. The type of transport used to take the patient to his car. c. Who accompanied the patient at discharge. d. The patient was given a copy of discharge instructions. e. The patient's reaction to the discharge. f. That housekeeping has been notified that the unit is ready to be cleaned. g. Any unusual observations.			

Charting:

____

____

____

____

Date of Satisfactory Completion ____________________

Instructor's Signature ____________________

The Human Body

13

Key Terms Review

Match the key terms in the right column with the definitions in the left column by placing the letter of each correct answer in the space provided.

_____ **1.** The study of the structure of an organism.

_____ **2.** The study of the functions of the body dealing with the physical and chemical processes of cells, tissues, and organs of living organisms.

_____ **3.** The basic unit of living matter.

_____ **4.** A group of cells of the same type.

_____ **5.** A part of the body made of several types of tissue grouped together to perform a certain function. Examples are the heart, stomach, and lungs.

_____ **6.** A group of organs acting together to carry out one or more body functions.

_____ **7.** Located in the front; opposite of posterior.

_____ **8.** Refers to the back or to the back part of an organ.

_____ **9.** The lower portion of the body.

_____ **10.** Located in the back or toward the rear; opposite of anterior.

_____ **11.** The upper portion of the body.

_____ **12.** On the abdominal, anterior, or front side of the body.

Terms

A. Inferior
B. Superior
C. Ventral
D. Posterior
E. Dorsal
F. Anterior
G. Anatomy
H. Physiology
I. System
J. Organ
K. Tissue
L. Cell
M. Nerve tissue
N. Epithelial tissue
O. Muscle tissue
P. Connective tissue
Q. Cardiac muscle tissue
R. Blood and lymph tissue

_____ **13.** Tissue composed of singular cells that move within a fluid to every part of the body. It circulates nutrients, oxygen, and antibodies and removes waste products.

_____ **14.** Involuntary muscle tissue found only in the heart.

_____ **15.** Tissue that connects, supports, covers, lines, pads, or protects other body structures.

_____ **16.** Tissue that lines, protects, secretes, absorbs, and receives sensations.

_____ **17.** Tissue that ensures movement; it is capable of stretching and contracting.

_____ **18.** Tissue that carries nervous impulses between the brain, the spinal cord, and all parts of the body.

MULTIPLE-CHOICE QUESTIONS

Circle the letter next to the word or statement that best completes the sentence or answers the question.

1. The body systems cannot work by themselves and
- a. are dependent on each other.
- b. so must get help from tissues.
- c. are independent of each other.
- d. let you know by complaining often.

2. The digestive system takes in and
- a. absorbs nutrients at night.
- b. absorbs daylight.
- c. absorbs nutrients as waste.
- d. absorbs nutrients and eliminates wastes.

3. An example of the integumentary system is
- a. the kidney.
- b. the heart.
- c. the brain.
- d. the skin.

4. An organ of the respiratory system is the
- a. larynx.
- b. spleen.
- c. pancreas.
- d. thymus.

5. The front side of a person is referred to as the
- a. anterior side.
- b. posterior side.
- c. the frontal lobe.
- d. first side.

6. The human back side, containing the spine, is called the
- a. anterior or upper side.
- b. posterior or under side.
- c. posterior or weak side.
- d. posterior or dorsal side.

7. Cells
- a. can grow and repair themselves.
- b. need oxygen to break food down.
- c. need water to transport substances.
- d. all of the above.

8. The purpose of the cell membrane is to
- a. create a boundary so all of the cytoplasm can pass out of a cell.
- b. contain all of the heredity activity inside the entire cell.
- c. copy a new cell exactly.
- d. allow some substances to pass in and out of the cell.

9. Tissues
- a. are groups of cells working together to perform certain functions.
- b. come together to form organs.

c. divide to make identical copies of themselves.
d. only a and b.

10. Glands, skin, and intestines are made of ________ tissue.
a. nerve
b. epithelial
c. thin
d. porous

11. The only place in the body where cardiac tissue is located is the
a. heart.
b. muscle in the arms and legs.
c. nervous system.
d. intestines.

12. Which organ can be found in the abdominal cavity?
a. Brain
b. Stomach
c. Deltoid muscle in the upper arm
d. Heart

13. The purpose of the peritoneum is to
a. protect organs from rubbing and keep them in place.
b. allow fluids to flow through vessels smoothly.
c. carry messages from the brain and spinal cord.
d. form organs from many different tissue types.

14. If the heart is superior to the intestines, then it is located
a. underneath the intestines.
b. behind the intestines.
c. above the intestines.
d. in front of the intestines.

15. The purpose of the skeletal system is to
a. allow messages from the brain to get to all parts of the body.
b. make sure movement can occur in all muscles.
c. move fluids like blood and gastric juices within the body.
d. protect vital organs like the brain and the organs in the thoracic cavity.

16. Ligaments and tendons are part of which system?
a. Cardiac
b. Gastrointestinal
c. Skeletal
d. Muscular

17. Which organs can be classified in either the endocrine or reproductive systems?
a. Heart and lungs
b. Testes and ovaries
c. Pancreas and intestines
d. Thyroid and parathyroid glands

18. The main function of the respiratory system is to
a. push fluids through vessels so cells can get the food necessary to survive.
b. supply oxygen to the body and release carbon dioxide as waste.
c. take in nutrients.
d. all of the above.

19. Which is an example of a body system that helps eliminate waste?
a. Excretory system
b. Gastrointestinal system
c. Respiratory system
d. All of the above

20. Chromosomes
a. can be found in the nucleus of a cell.
b. are contained in the RNA.
c. contain all the hereditary information needed.
d. only a and c.

21. The lungs and heart are found in the
a. dorsal cavity.
b. thoracic cavity.
c. abdominal cavity.
d. posterior cavity.

22. An organ in the urinary system is the
a. ascending colon.
b. urethra.
c. anus.
d. alveoli.

23. What other organ (besides the heart and blood vessels) can be found in the cardiac system?

a. Spleen
b. Duodenum
c. Pancreas
d. Gallbladder

24. The teeth are usually classified as an organ in which system?

a. Skeletal
b. Gastrointestinal
c. Urinary
d. Muscular

25. A wound is noted below the kneecap; therefore, the wound is located _____ to the kneecap.

a. inferiorly
b. anteriorly
c. posteriorly
d. dorsally

TRUE OR FALSE QUESTIONS

Determine whether each question is true or false. In the space provided, write "T" for true and "F" for false. If the statement is false, rewrite it on the line provided to make it a true statement.

_____ **1.** The urinary system controls activities of the body.

____

_____ **2.** Groups of cells of the same type that work together to perform a particular function are called *tissues.*

____

_____ **3.** Organs that work together to perform similar tasks make up body systems.

____

_____ **4.** The ovaries are part of the female reproductive system.

____

_____ **5.** The larynx is classified as an organ in the gastrointestinal system.

____

_____ **6.** One function of the reproductive system is to allow species to reproduce.

____

_____ **7.** Female and male reproductive organs can be found in the abdominal cavity.

____

_____ **8.** DNA is contained in the cytoplasm of the cell.

____

_____ **9.** RNA is responsible for making protein.

____

_____ **10.** Striated muscle tissue is found in arm and leg muscles and can be controlled voluntarily.

____

FILL-IN-THE-BLANK QUESTIONS

Provide the meaning of the following abbreviations.

1. GI _______________

2. DNA _______________

3. RNA _______________

EXERCISE 13-1

Objective: To apply understanding of how the body cells, tissues, organs, and systems relate to each other.

Directions: Label the diagram in Figure 13-1 with the correct words from the word list. Place the words in the order of their complexity.

Word List

Organs	Cells	Systems	Tissues

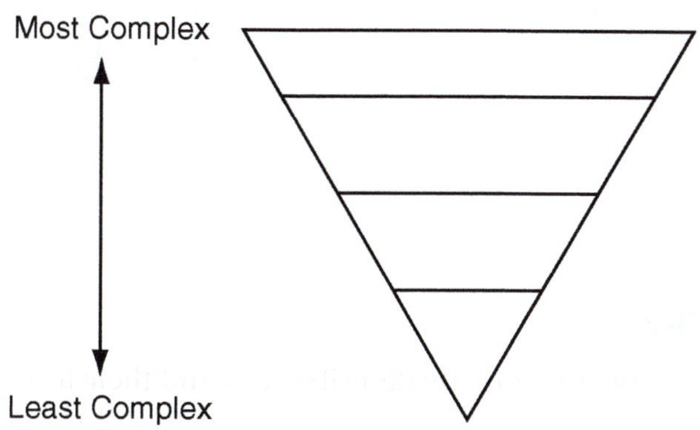

FIGURE 13-1

EXERCISE 13-2

Objective: To recognize and be able to correctly spell the names of various organs of the human body.

Directions: Label the diagrams in Figure 13-2 with the correct words from the following word list.

Word List

Heart	Lung	Kidney	Large intestine	Thyroid
Brain	Uterus	Liver	Small intestine	Trachea
Bladder	Stomach	Ovary	Testicles	Skin

FIGURE 13-2

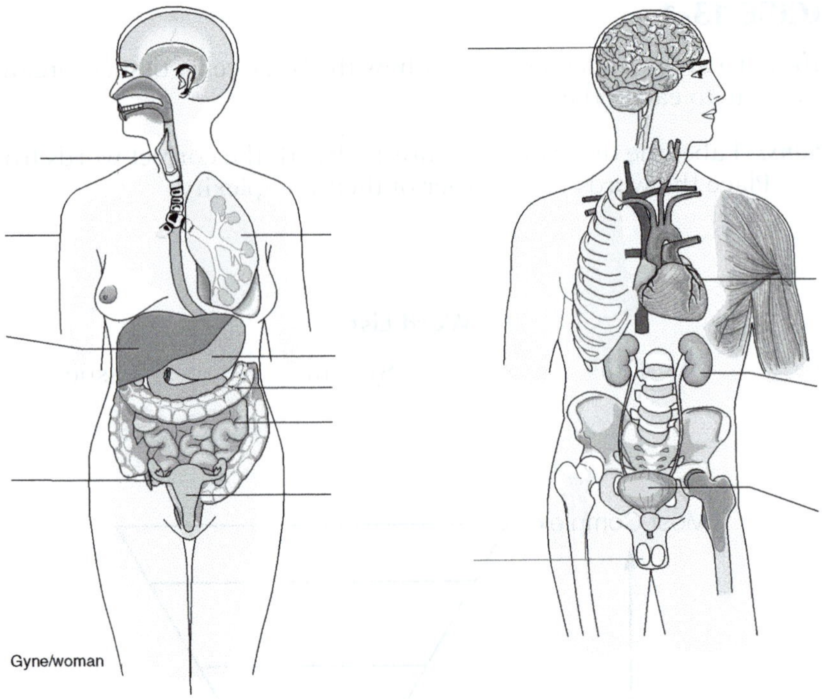

EXERCISE 13-3

Objective: To be able to correctly describe cells and their functions.

Directions: Select the word(s) from the following word list to complete the following sentences.

Word List

building blocks	microscope	existed
living	oxygen	water
reproduce		

1. The cells are the fundamental ________________ of all living matter.
2. Cells can be seen only under the _________.
3. Cells use ______ to transport substances.
4. Most living cells grow and __________ themselves.
5. Cells use _____ to break down food.
6. Cells are the _________ parts of organisms.
7. Cells come from cells that have already ______.

EXERCISE 13-4

Objective: To be able to apply the correct meaning of words used to name tissues of the body.

Directions: Choose the correct word(s) from the following word list to complete the sentences.

Word List

muscle tissue	nerve tissue	connective tissue
epithelial tissue	cardiac muscle tissue	blood and lymph tissue
striated muscle tissue	smooth muscle tissue	tissues

1. Skin, linings of the intestines, and linings of the glands and organs are examples of ______________________.
2. The function of ______________________ is to connect, support, cover or line, and pad or protect the body.
3. ______________________ makes body movement possible.
4. The smooth, involuntary muscles made up of ______________________ keep the heart beating.
5. Muscles that can be moved with a conscious effort are made up of ______________________.
6. ______________________carries impulses to and from the brain, spinal cord, and other parts of the body.
7. The tissue that has single cells and flows through vessels is known as ______________________.
8. The dilation of such structures as the pupil of the eye and blood vessels is made possible by means of ______________________.
9. ______________________are groups of the same type of cells that work together.

THE NURSING ASSISTANT IN ACTION

1. Your supervisor tells you to be careful of the pressure ulcers located dorsally on your patient. What area of the body must you observe frequently and pay close attention to?

____

____

____

____

2. Your supervisor asks you to help her prepare a patient for surgery by shaving the anterior and posterior aspects of his left leg. What part(s) of the leg should you shave?

____

____

____

____

3. A patient complains of pain in his upper chest that is moving down his stomach and into his intestines. Using correct anatomical location and referring to body systems, what should you report to the supervisor?

____

____

____

____

4. You notice a new bruise on the back of the left forearm of a small child for whom you are caring. What words should you use to describe accurately to your supervisor what you noted?

____

____

____

____

5. A male patient is assigned to your care. He is covered from head to toe in body art (tattoos). He has multiple body piercings in his ears, nose, tongue, chest, and penis. What should you do?

____

____

____

____

LEARNING ACTIVITIES

1. Using your own body, locate the organs in the abdominal and thoracic cavities you learned about in this chapter. Using a stethoscope, listen to your heart, lungs, and intestines. What did you hear? Can you use words related to anatomical landmarks and organs to accurately communicate what you observed?
2. Pretend you are preparing a patient for a gastrointestinal test he is about to undergo. He has to drink a certain medicine so the doctors can take pictures of the medicine while it moves through his gastrointestinal system. What do you know about the gastrointestinal system that could help him understand where the medicine he is to drink will travel? If necessary, draw a picture for yourself and label and describe the route from start to finish of the gastrointestinal system. Or, use the Internet to investigate further just how a liquid moves through this system.

Growth and Development

14

Key Terms Review

Match the key terms in the right column with the definitions in the left column by placing the letter of each correct answer in the space provided.

_____ **1.** The physical changes that take place in a person's body over the life span.

_____ **2.** The motor, language, cognitive, and social skills that are gained over the course of the life span.

_____ **3.** Refers to the movement of small muscles, such as those in the hands and fingers.

_____ **4.** Refers to the movement of large muscles, such as those used in walking or in hitting a ball.

_____ **5.** Actual age in years and months.

_____ **6.** The distance around an object or body part, such as the head.

_____ **7.** The mental processes by which knowledge is acquired.

Terms

A. Fine motor

B. Gross motor

C. Growth

D. Development

E. Chronological

F. Cognitive

G. Circumference

MULTIPLE-CHOICE QUESTIONS

Circle the letter next to the word or statement that best completes the sentence or answers the question.

1. Growth and development usually follow
a. growth spurts.
b. each other.
c. stages.
d. death.

2. Growth continues through all the stages of life, but it begins
a. at the beginning of labor.
b. at conception.
c. at birth.
d. with life skills.

3. The gain in weight of infants from birth to 1 year
a. is predictable within parameters.
b. helps the mother feel better.
c. is a sign of problems.
d. is not measurable.

4. One indicator of proper growth is detected by
a. measuring the baby's feet.
b. measuring the mother's feet.
c. measuring the umbilical cord.
d. measuring the circumference of the baby's head periodically.

5. Humans build on skills they developed
a. at a previous stage of development.
b. while sleeping.
c. from observing their parents.
d. through a nursing assistant course.

6. The nursing assistant's ability to relate appropriately to patients is dependent on
a. their awareness of the impact illness can have on patients at each stage of growth and development.
b. the patient's attitude.
c. whether they study this chapter.
d. their immediate supervisor.

7. At the end of the first year, it is normal for an infant to
a. weigh twice as much as when it was born.
b. weigh three times as much as when it was born.
c. gain 4 to 6 pounds each month.
d. have a head circumference more than 20".

8. A woman is pregnant for approximately ____ weeks.
a. 9
b. 44
c. 40
d. 12

9. When comparing an infant to a toddler, it is important to remember that
a. there will be slower growth in the first year of life
b. the height will double in the second year of life.
c. the weight will double in the first year of life.
d. the height and weight will double in the first year of life.

10. When taking care of a 2-year-old, you should remember that
a. only the parent is the customer, because he or she is paying the bill.
b. a 2-year-old will answer your questions correctly.
c. the head circumference is not usually measured unless there is a detected problem.
d. a growth spurt of 1' in a year will occur.

11. When comparing toddlers to preschool-age children, it is normal for
a. the trunk to remain the same length while the legs grow longer for 1- to 2-year-olds.
b. a preschooler to grow 3" each month.
c. the trunk to remain the same length for a preschooler while the legs grow longer.
d. a toddler to grow 3" each month.

12. During the ______ period, there is a rapid growth seen both physically and sexually.
   a. school-age
   b. adolescent
   c. middle to older adult
   d. none of the above

13. During adolescence, girls
   a. may grow at least 1' between ages 12 and 18.
   b. mature 5 years earlier than boys.
   c. gain between 50 and 100 pounds.
   d. have significant visual changes and need glasses.

14. The focus on growth and development in the middle- to older-adult stage is
   a. faster more visual changes.
   b. continual height and weight gain at a progressive rate.
   c. the body's response to injury and illness.
   d. learning how to speak and form sentences.

15. A patient who is 86 years old might need
   a. extra time when dressing and walking.
   b. a support group where he can talk about the loss of his wife and friends.
   c. to rest throughout the day.
   d. all of the above.

16. At what development stage should a child begin to master the skills of dressing/undressing, telling you his full name, and using scissors and eating utensils?
   a. Toddler
   b. Preschool
   c. School age
   d. All of the above.

17. What would you expect is normal skill acquisition for a child who is 11 months old?
   a. The child should have the ability to start to pull herself up using the couch or a table.
   b. The child cries when the parent leaves the room or when a health care provider tries to hold them.
   c. The child should be able to roll over and pull herself into a sitting position.
   d. All of the above.

18. A female child in second grade (approximately 7–8 years old) usually
   a. wants to play with only girls her same age.
   b. can create a drawing where the eyes, nose, mouth, hands, and feet are recognizable.
   c. dresses herself.
   d. all of the above.

19. An example of fine motor development is
   a. being able to jump rope.
   b. buttoning, buckling, and zipping one's own clothing.
   c. balancing and walking.
   d. explaining the differences between an apple and an orange.

20. When caring for a teenager, you should
   a. comment on how nice it was for her friends to bring her games and flowers when they last visited.
   b. stay with her while she dresses to make sure she does not hurt herself.
   c. cut her meat up for her when the meal tray arrives.
   d. monitor and report how much time she spends watching TV and talking on the phone with her friends.

21. A patient had a stroke. An example of mastering gross motor coordination is
   a. learning to eat again using a spoon.
   b. walking with a walker 150'
   c. relearning how to button a shirt.
   d. both a and c.

22. An example of cognitive development is
   a. balancing 8 blocks on top of each other.
   b. understanding that a cancer diagnosis can be fatal.
   c. being able to communicate in full sentences.
   d. hopping on one foot.

23. If a patient weighs 100 kg, then he is _____ pounds.
   a. 2.2
   b. 220
   c. 22
   d. 22.2

24. By the time a child has her first birthday, her head circumference may be approximately
a. 13.5".
b. 18".
c. 16.5".
d. 35 cm.

25. You find it difficult to communicate with a patient who is mentally challenged and much older than you are. You should
a. confide in a colleague and ask her to switch patients with you.
b. ask your supervisor to give care to the patient because you do not understand what this patient is saying and this makes you uncomfortable.
c. check the care plan to see if notes have been made about this patient's preferences and methods of communicating.
d. ask the family for advice.

TRUE OR FALSE QUESTIONS

Determine whether each question is true or false. In the space provided, write "T" for true and "F" for false. If the statement is false, rewrite it on the line provided to make it a true statement.

_____ **1.** *Growth* refers to the measurable physical changes humans experience throughout their lives.

____

_____ **2.** *Development* refers to the accomplishment of and the increase in the ability to use skills that people acquire over their life span.

____

_____ **3.** Injuries such as strokes make it necessary to relearn skills from earlier stages of development.

____

_____ **4.** When people are happy, they often behave at a lower developmental stage than their chronological age indicates.

____

_____ **5.** It is normal behavior for an infant to want to stay with his mother when receiving a shot.

____

_____ **6.** Kilograms (kg) are used when measuring height.

____

_____ **7.** You should check with the policy of the facility in which you work to figure out if you should record and report weight and height using metric measurement tools.

____

_____ **8.** An infant's head circumference at birth should be approximately 13½".

____

_____ **9.** A rule of thumb to determine a child's height in adulthood is to double his height recorded at age 2.

____

_____ **10.** Planning for additional time to help an older patient dress is a good way to decrease anxiety and provide a comfortable pace for the patient.

____

FILL-IN-THE-BLANK QUESTIONS

Provide the meaning of the following abbreviations.

1. kg ____________________
2. cm ____________________
3. in ____________________
4. lb ____________________
5. IV ____________________

EXERCISE 14-1

Objective: To be able to recognize developmental skills and the tasks that illustrate them.

Directions: Place the correct letters next to the matching phrase.

CS—cognitive skill
GMS—gross motor skill
SS—social skill
FMS—fine motor skill
LS—language skill

_____ **1.** A preschool child recognizes colors.
_____ **2.** The school-age child defines words.
_____ **3.** The older adult adjusts to retirement.
_____ **4.** The young adult selects a career.
_____ **5.** The infant vocalizes, squeals, and imitates sounds.
_____ **6.** The toddler throws balls.
_____ **7.** The infant rolls over, pulls to sit, crawls, and stands alone.
_____ **8.** The school-age child draws a man having six parts.
_____ **9.** The infant feeds himself crackers.
_____ **10.** The toddler expresses needs or indicates wants without crying.

EXERCISE 14-2

Objective: To apply what you have learned about nursing assistant behaviors and patient age-specific considerations.

Directions: Match the letter of the developmental stage with the correct age-specific consideration. Select only one answer for each statement.

Developmental Stage

A. Infant: Birth–1 year
B. Toddler: 1–2 year(s)
C. Preschool: 2–5 years
D. School-age: 5–12 years
E. Adolescent: 12–18 years
F. Young adult: 18–40 years
G. Middle adult: 40–65 years
H. Older adult: 65+ years

Age-specific Consideration

_____**1.** Place visually interesting objects where the child can observe them.

_____**2.** Explain procedures in simple words, describing only what the patient will see.

_____**3.** Describe for how long children must undergo a painful procedure.

_____**4.** Keep small objects, which may cause choking, out of child's reach.

_____**5.** Patient may request that a family member be present to provide support in making a health care decision.

_____**6.** Remember that body image is very important at this stage.

_____**7.** Remember that they have many obligations, such as parenthood and the care of their parents.

_____**8.** They are often concerned about how illness will affect their lifelong goals.

EXERCISE 14-3

Objective: To be able to correctly match the chronological stage to the developmental stage of human growth and development.

Directions: From the following word list, select and write the name of the developmental stage next to the matching time period on the age list.

Word

Preschool	Adolescent	Toddler	Older adult
School-age	Young adult	Infant	Middle adult

Age

5–12 years ___________
12–18 years ___________
65+ years ___________
Birth–1 year ___________
1–2 years ___________
18–40 years ___________
2–5 years ___________
40–65 years ___________

THE NURSING ASSISTANT IN ACTION

1. A teenager who was recently diagnosed with bone cancer asks you, "What happens now?" What should you do?

2. You are asked to help distract an infant while a procedure is being performed on this child by a doctor. What should you do?

3. A 90-year-old male client who recently broke his arm is admitted to your unit. He needs help with cutting his food and performing activities of daily living. What should you do?

4. A mother confides in you that her 9-year-old has begun to wet the bed again since being hospitalized. What should you do?

5. A 4-year-old is going for surgery early tomorrow morning and an NPO order has been written. He has a temper tantrum when he asks you for a snack and a drink when he wakes up at 2 AM. What should you do?

LEARNING ACTIVITIES

1. Using what you already learned about growth and development, observe a small child at play. Or, if possible, gain permission from the parent(s) to interact with the child. What social, cognitive, language, and fine and gross motor skills do you think this child has mastered?
2. If possible, find a support group in your community that helps people living with an illness or a loss. Call and gain permission to observe the group at their next meeting. Once the meeting is over, reflect on what physical, cognitive, or social issues members may have talked about, how they support each other, and how they cope with their illness, loss, or grief. What insightful information have you gained, and how can you use this new knowledge when working with patients of similar age and with similar issues?

The Musculoskeletal System and Related Care

15

Key Terms Review

Match the key terms in the right column with the definitions in the left column by placing the letter of each correct answer in the space provided.

_____ **1.** The medical specialty that covers the treatment of broken bones, deformities, or diseases that attack the bones, joints, and muscles.

_____ **2.** A part of the body where two bones come together.

_____ **3.** Tough, white, fibrous cord that connects bone to bone.

_____ **4.** A strong connective tissue cord that attaches a muscle to a bone.

_____ **5.** A tear in the connective cord occurring when the joint is twisted or overstretched; often seen with ankle and knee injuries.

_____ **6.** Break in a bone.

_____ **7.** Chronic condition of inflammation of the joints.

_____ **8.** A degenerative and painful bone disease affecting the spine, hips, finger joints, or knees.

_____ **9.** A mild thinning of the bone mass, resulting when the formation of bone is not enough to offset normal bone loss.

_____ **10.** A chronic disease condition affecting the connective tissue of the body, especially the joints.

Terms

A. Adduction
B. Abduction
C. Atrophy
D. Contracture
E. Extension
F. Flex
G. Flexion
H. Relax
I. Contract
J. Orthopedics
K. Joint
L. Tendon
M. Torn ligament
N. Ligament
O. Fracture
P. Arthritis
Q. Rheumatoid arthritis
R. Osteoarthritis

_____11. Exertion of pull by means of weights or pulleys, often used for realignment of bones or other limb tissues.

_____12. A triangle-shape bar attached to the overbed frame of a traction setup that enables the patient to pull himself up in bed.

_____13. Metal frame device with handgrips and four legs and is open on one side; provides stability and security for the patient who is weak on one side or restricted in the amount of weight she can put on one foot.

_____14. To place in a resting position, in which muscle tension decreases and fibers lengthen.

_____15. Get smaller; shortening the length of muscle, thereby making the angle formed by bones and muscles smaller.

_____16. Wasting away of muscles; decrease in muscle size.

_____17. An abnormal, often permanent, shortening of a muscle; also scar tissue.

_____18. Straightening or lengthening a muscle, thereby making the angle formed by bones and muscles greater.

_____19. To bend; the act of bending a body part.

_____20. Bending of a joint (elbow, wrist, knee).

_____21. Movement of an arm or leg away from the center of the body.

_____22. Movement of an arm or leg toward the center of the body.

S. Osteopenia

T. Walker

U. Traction

V. Trapeze

MULTIPLE-CHOICE QUESTIONS

Circle the letter next to the word or statement that best completes the sentence or answers the question.

1. The healing of broken bones is a gradual process in which ______________ is deposited at the fracture site.
   a. iron
   b. calcium
   c. glue
   d. blood

2. Which of the following is a condition or disease of the bone?
   a. Arthritis
   b. Osteoporosis
   c. Rheumatoid arthritis
   d. All of the above

3. The knee is an example of a ______________ joint.
   a. rapid
   b. stiff
   c. painful
   d. hinge

4. The use of a continuous passive range-of-motion machine (CPM) promotes _____ of the knee joint after total knee replacement surgery.
   a. strength
   b. rigidity
   c. flexibility
   d. tenderness

5. The ______________ connect muscle to bone.
a. tendons
b. ligaments
c. nerves
d. synapses

6. Nursing assistants must be familiar with orthopedic equipment such as
a. splints, nasogastric tubes, and casts.
b. casts, walkers, and thermometers.
c. walkers, casts, and zippers.
d. splints, casts, and walkers.

7. In the past, traction and bed rest were the methods of treatment for fractures, but today the emphasis is on
a. low-fat diets.
b. improved methods of surgery and extended hospital stays.
c. lighter casting materials and early ambulation.
d. shortened hospital stays and low-fat diets.

8. A device that replaces a bone or a joint is called a
a. protrusion.
b. prosthesis.
c. proboscis.
d. partition.

9. Restricted ______________ means that an orthopedic patient needs special skin care.
a. permission
b. mobility
c. diet
d. tolerance

10. A *trapeze* is a device that is suspended from an over-the-bed frame and allows the patient to
a. receive better television reception.
b. summon the nurse.
c. swing forward and backward.
d. move or lift himself more easily.

11. Casts are made of which of the following materials?
a. Gortex
b. Plaster
c. Fiberglass
d. All of the above

12. Casted extremities should be compared to uncasted extremities for
a. changes in length.
b. changes in flexibility.
c. changes in size, color, and warmth.
d. the presence of nodules.

13. An unusual odor coming from a cast could mean that
a. fiber in the diet has been increased.
b. it is ready to be removed.
c. the extremity has healed.
d. a pressure ulcer or infection is developing under the cast.

14. If staining is noted on a cast, this could mean
a. the patient dropped coffee on the cast.
b. there is a fever present.
c. lotion was applied to help alleviate itching.
d. bleeding occurred inside the cast.

15. A nursing assistant checks the fingers on a casted arm to find they are cool and blue. What could this mean?
a. The patient is cold and should be offered a blanket.
b. The patient has a fever and the nurse should give medicine immediately.
c. There is poor circulation to the arm and should be reported.
d. This is normal for a patient with a cast.

16. Performing range of motion and encouraging a patient to exercise
a. prevents permanent lengthening of muscles called contractures.
b. weakens key muscles needed to ambulate.
c. helps maintain tone and flexibility of muscles.
d. can only be done by a physical therapist.

17. Large muscle groups like ones found in the legs and the buttocks should be used
a. only for heavy tasks like walking and running.

b. to prevent back injury to the nursing assistant.
c. when flexing and abducting.
d. to avoid weakening other muscles.

18. The _______ are at lowest risk for developing an infection because they have a rich blood supply that helps protect against infection.
a. muscles
b. bones
c. nerves
d. lungs

19. If a patient is bedridden and is not encouraged to move or does not get range of motion, her muscles can ____ and then permanently ______.
a. strengthen; be toned.
b. lengthen; weaken
c. weaken; contract
d. shorten; lengthen

20. One way to prevent osteoporosis is to
a. speak to a doctor about one's health history, family history, and the possibility of using estrogen medications.
b. to perform weight-bearing exercises regularly
c. eat a calcium-rich diet, including sardines, cottage cheese, and broccoli.
d. all of the above.

21. When assisting a patient with a degenerative disorder such as rheumatoid arthritis the nursing assistant should
a. suggest the patient take a warm bath to help decrease some of the pain and swelling.
b. assist the patient by gently holding their fingers or wrists and pulling them to a standing position and encouraging them to walk.
c. encourage the patient to do lots of exercise to help keep failing joints flexible.
d. encourage them to eat a high-fat, low-carbohydrate diet.

22. If tuberculosis is left untreated, it may lead to
a. osteomyelitis.
b. poliomyelitis.
c. paralysis of the spine.
d. osteoporosis.

23. Placing antiembolism stockings on a patient helps
a. make the muscles more limber.
b. decrease the chance of blood clots forming.
c. keep the feet flexed to prevent footdrop.
d. increase flexibility of the joints.

24. When applying prosthetics or assistive devices, a nursing assistant should
a. check to see if rubber or plastic grips are in place on crutches, canes, and walkers.
b. leave splints on the unaffected side for at least 2 hours.
c. encourage the patient to only use these devices when ambulating at home.
d. leave them at the bedside so they do not get lost.

25. When working with a patient in traction, the nursing assistant should
a. place weights on the floor.
b. never check on the apparatus, as this is the nurse's responsibility.
c. report when cables become loose or come off the pulley.
d. leave the patient if he slips down in the bed.

TRUE OR FALSE QUESTIONS

Determine whether each question is true or false. In the space provided, write "T" for true and "F" for false. If the statement is false, rewrite it on the line provided to make it a true statement.

_____ 1. During each body movement, the skeletal system, the muscular system, the circulatory system, and the reproductive system are all interacting.

____

_____ 2. When assisting a total hip replacement (THR) patient to ambulate, it is important to know how much weight bearing is allowed on the affected leg.

____

_____ 3. Offering a patient with a cast a backscratcher, hanger, or a comb to scratch inside the cast when he is itchy is acceptable practice.

____

_____ 4. One of the benefits of early ambulation is fewer circulatory side effects.

____

_____ 5. Some braces must be worn continually, and some are worn only when the patient is out of bed. Therefore, it is important to check the plan of care or ask your immediate supervisor for instructions if your patient is using a brace.

____

_____ 6. The type of surgery a patient has determines what kind of activity she is allowed to perform.

____

_____ 7. You should change the position of an immobile patient at least every 4 hours.

____

_____ 8. In the past, casts were made only out of plaster, a heavy material. Now casts are more often made of plastic or fiberglass. These modern casts are lighter, allowing the patient to move more easily.

____

_____ 9. Casts can become too tight after they are applied, causing the skin on either side of the cast edge to become blue or pale in color or hot to the touch.

____

_____ 10. Any complaint of pain around, under, or near the cast must be reported immediately to the nurse or your immediate supervisor.

____

FILL-IN-THE-BLANK QUESTIONS

Provide the meaning of the following abbreviations.

1. CPM ____

2. THR ____

EXERCISE 15-1

Objective: To recognize and be able to spell correctly the parts of the musculoskeletal system.

Directions: Label the diagram in Figure 15-1 with the correct words from the following word list.

Word List

Muscles

Tibialis anterior	Gastrocnemius	Sartorius
Rectus abdominus	Quadriceps femoris	Deltoid
Pectoralis major	Sternocleidomastoid	Biceps
Tensor facia latae	Peroneus longus	
Abdominal muscles	Intercostals	

Bones

Humerus	Fibula	Clavicle	Metacarpals
Metatarsals	Scapula	Tibia	Ribs
Vertebrae	Maxilla	Radius	Femur
Sternum	Frontal bone	Pelvic bone	Mandible
Cervical vertebrae	Patella	Ulna	
Parietal		Phalanges	

FIGURE 15-1

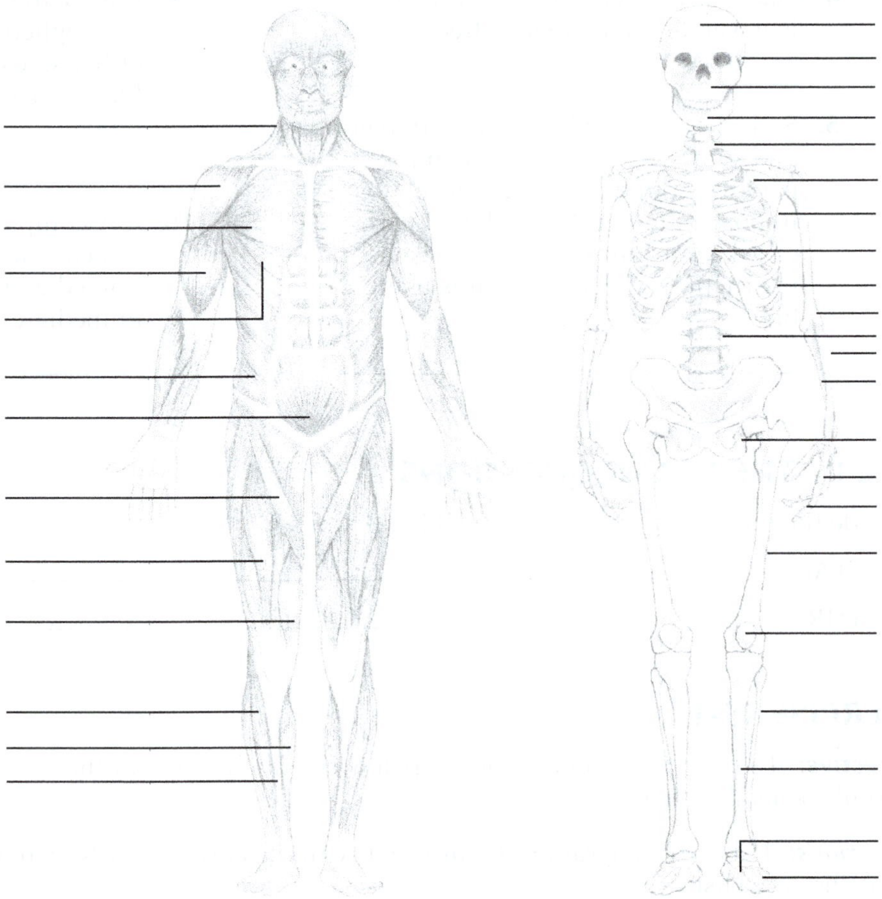

EXERCISE 15-2

Objective: To be able to name the category to which bones belong.

Directions: Draw a line to connect the bone with the correct category.

Category	Bone
Long bones	Vertebrae
Short bones	Ribs
Irregular bones	Phalanges
Flat bones	Femurs

EXERCISE 15-3

Objective: To identify correctly the types of joints of the human body.

Directions: Circle the words in the following word list that identify the major types of joints of the human body.

Shoulder	Metatarsals	Mandible
Femur	Wrist	Scapula
Radius	Ankle	Tibia
Hip	Ball-and-socket	Pivot
Hinge	Knee	
Irregular joints of the spine	Elbow	

EXERCISE 15-4

Objective: To recall common diseases and disorders of the orthopedic patient.

Directions: Complete the sentences with the correct words from the Word List below.

Sprain	Bone	Simple fracture
Joint dislocation	Compound	Guillain-Barré tuberculosis
Muscular dystrophy	Arthritis	Spinal cord
Poliomyelitis	Trauma to spinal cord	Atrophy
Contracture		

1. An injury in which ligaments are partially torn is a(n) ______________.
2. A fracture of a bone with no bone sticking out through the skin is called a(n) ______________________.
3. __________ can be a disease of the bone; usually affects the lungs.
4. _________________ is known as a joint disease.
5. A(n) ______________ ______________ is the pulling out (displacement) of a bone end that forms part of a joint.
6. ____________________ can result in damage to the _________________ ____________________, causing paralysis of some area of the body.
7. A nervous system disease is the ________________ syndrome.

8. ____________ is a disease that is not often seen because of the use of preventive vaccines in babies and young children.
9. A disorder that can occur when muscles are immobile for several weeks or months is __________ ____________________.
10. A(n) __________________ fracture is when the ______________ is broken and there is an external wound or bone protruding through the skin.
11. Wasting away of muscles is called ___________________.
12. A(n) ___________________ is the abnormal shortening of a muscle.

THE NURSING ASSISTANT IN ACTION

1. A patient is admitted to your unit from the Emergency Room with casts to both arms and one leg. What cast-care measures should you use to ensure the cast dries and that the patient is comfortable and healing correctly?

____

____

____

____

2. The patient you are caring for who had a total hip replacement has been ordered to be on bedrest and an abductor wedge is in place. He rings the call bell and tells you he needs to use the bedpan. What should you do?

____

____

____

____

3. The nurse asks you to help Mr. Jones out of the bed and to a wheelchair so he can go for some tests. He cannot bear weight because he had a total hip replacement. What should you do to get him ready for transport to take him to his tests?

____

____

____

____

4. You are asked to assist a patient who had total knee replacement out of bed and into a chair in her room. What measures should you take to assure comfort and care is maintained for this patient?

____

____

____

____

5. A patient with rheumatoid arthritis complains of pain in his shoulders, elbows, ankles, knees, and hips. What should you do to help alleviate some of his pain?

____

____

____

____

LEARNING ACTIVITIES

1. Using the Internet, find video clips of arthroscopic surgery and an arthroplasty being performed. Become familiar with what the differences are in order to understand what actually occurs to patients who undergo these procedures.

2. Make flashcards of key bones and muscles identified in the textbook from the figures provided. Using a partner, place the cards on this person in the correct place. Check your work for accuracy with the textbook pictures to assure you are correct.

16

The Integumentary System and Related Care

Key Terms Review

Match the key terms in the right column with the definitions in the left column by placing the letter of each correct answer in the space provided.

_____ **1.** The body system that includes the skin, hair, nails, and sweat and oil glands. It provides the first line of defense against infection, maintains body temperature, provides fluids, and eliminates wastes.

_____ **2.** The inner layer of the skin.

_____ **3.** The outer layer or surface of the skin.

_____ **4.** The body area between the thighs (external genitalia and rectal area).

_____ **5.** Thin, fragile, less elastic skin frequently associated with aging.

_____ **6.** Places where bones are close to the surface of the skin.

_____ **7.** Unable to control urine or feces.

_____ **8.** Very overweight.

_____ **9.** An abnormality, either benign or cancerous, of the tissues of the body, such as a wound, sore, rash, boil, tumor, or growth.

_____ **10.** Injuries that result from the skin remaining in place on top of a surface while the underlying structures, such as the bone, slide downward.

Terms

A. Epidermis
B. Dermis
C. Integumentary system
D. Obese
E. Incontinent
F. Pressure ulcers
G. Lesion
H. Shear injuries
I. Friction injuries
J. Skin shear
K. Perineum
L. Bony prominences
M. Atrophic skin

_____**11.** Injuries resulting from the patient's skin sliding against hard surfaces or sheets when pulled up in bed.

_____**12.** An internal force caused when surfaces slide across each other, causing a twisting and tearing of the underlying blood vessels; it can lead to tissue ischemia and localized tissue death.

_____**13.** Bedsores; areas of the skin that become broken and painful; caused by continuous pressure on a body part and usually occur when a patient is kept in one position for a long period of time.

MULTIPLE-CHOICE QUESTIONS

Circle the letter next to the word or statement that best completes the sentence or answers the question.

1. The _____ are part of the integumentary system.
   a. lungs
   b. intestines
   c. nails
   d. fingers and toes

2. ____________ is responsible for the color of the skin.
   a. Dermis
   b. Epidermis
   c. Toner
   d. Pigment

3. The primary function of the skin is to
   a. cover and protect underlying body structures from injury and invasion by microorganisms.
   b. provide an area for exchange of oxygen.
   c. help regulate cardiac output.
   d. eliminate wastes through the urine.

4. Serious health problems can cause ________ in the skin.
   a. changes
   b. improvement
   c. illumination
   d. healthy growth

5. Fungus is caused by ________ organisms.
   a. animal-like
   b. plant-like
   c. child-like
   d. solar-like

6. Chickenpox viruses can cause another painful skin disease called
   a. athlete's foot.
   b. *pediculisis pedis*.
   c. shingles.
   d. psoriasis.

7. As people age, the skin
   a. becomes more elastic.
   b. flakes away.
   c. grows thicker and tougher.
   d. becomes less elastic and more fragile.

8. Loss of fat cells in the skin can make a person feel ________ even when room temperatures feel warm to others.
   a. thinner
   b. warmer
   c. cold
   d. sweaty

9. Decreased __________ caused by prolonged pressure in an area can lead to pressure ulcers.
   a. digestion
   b. circulation
   c. exercise
   d. posture

10. In addition to prolonged pressure, another reason pressure ulcers form is from
   a. dry skin.
   b. clean skin.

c. wound drainage.
d. body lotion applied in a circular motion after the bath.

11. Which patient is at high risk for developing a pressure ulcer?
a. A woman who has a high fever and is in a coma
b. The man who can ambulate himself to and from the bathroom
c. The patient with left-side weakness who refuses to eat, drink, and get out of bed
d. Both a and c

12. The best place to check for signs of pressure is
a. the top of the thigh.
b. the forearm.
c. the great toe.
d. the sacrum.

13. Which of the following is a type of pressure ulcer that is the most difficult to heal?
a. Stage I
b. Stage II
c. Stage III
d. Stage IV

14. Friction/shear injuries can occur if
a. the side rails are too high.
b. the patient ambulates often.
c. the gown is not tied tightly.
d. the head of the bed is elevated too high.

15. To prevent friction/shear injuries,
a. use a restraint on active patients.
b. restrict bed movement.
c. use a draw sheet to pull patients up in bed and for turning them.
d. leave the patient on the bedpan for more than 20 minutes.

16. The feet must be kept in good alignment to prevent a serious deformity called
a. alignment disorder.
b. athlete's foot.
c. chin drop.
d. foot drop.

17. Do not place an incontinent patient
a. directly on the plastic side of the bed protector.
b. directly on an incontinent pad.
c. on a clean dry sheet.
d. a chair with an incontinence product.

18. The patient's position should be changed
a. at least every 2 hours.
b. once a shift.
c. when he or she becomes incontinent.
d. during the day only.

19. If the patient's toenails must be trimmed, the nursing assistant should
a. trim them immediately.
b. soak them before trimming them.
c. notify the nurse.
d. call the doctor.

20. In order to provide all the care a patient needs within a limited timeframe, you must
a. stop when tired.
b. arrive earlier or work later than assigned.
c. skip some of the work.
d. plan the day efficiently

21. The integumentary system helps regulate body temperature
a. by allowing heat to escape through a process called *vasodilation.*
b. through perspiration.
c. by conserving heat during vasoconstriction.
d. all of the above.

22. If a patient is very obese, ______ may be noticed under skin folds.
a. maceration
b. infestation
c. body lice
d. scaling

23. Providing good skin care
a. protects wounds and tissue from further injury.
b. prevents infection from occurring.
c. means offering incontinence care as soon as an episode occurs.
d. all of the above.

24. When using cornstarch or powder on a patient, the nursing assistant should
  a. rub either product into the skin as you would lotion.
  b. always use these products with someone who has oxygen.
  c. never wash it off as it creates a barrier to prevent pressure ulcers.
  d. check the policy of your facility to make sure you can use these products.

25. Which device can prevent foot drop?
  a. High-top sneakers
  b. Trochanter rolls
  c. Egg crate
  d. Foam rings

TRUE OR FALSE QUESTIONS

Determine whether each question is true or false. In the space provided, write "T" for true and "F" for false. If the statement is false, rewrite it on the line provided to make it a true statement.

_____ **1.** People who are in shock have skin that is paler than usual.

____

_____ **2.** In some pressure ulcers, the skin damage below the surface can be greater than what is noticeable on the surface of the skin.

____

_____ **3.** The nursing assistant should report the first signs (redness) of a pressure ulcer formation to the immediate supervisor.

____

_____ **4.** To prevent pressure between the legs when positioning the patient, use pillows.

____

_____ **5.** A patient using an egg crate mattress will not develop a pressure ulcer.

____

_____ **6.** When providing foot care, a nursing assistant should always soak patients' feet for approximately 5 minutes before washing with soap and water.

____

_____ **7.** Lotion should be applied between toes to prevent scaling from occurring.

____

_____ **8.** If pressure ulcers are not cared for properly, amputation or even death may occur.

____

_____ **9.** During stage III, bone, nerve, and muscle can be exposed.

____

_____ **10.** When aging occurs, increased oil from sweat glands occurs, making more baths necessary.

____

EXERCISE 16-1

Objective: To recognize and correctly spell the structures of the skin.

Directions: Label the diagram in Figure 16-1 with the correct words from the following word list.

Word List

Sweat gland	Epidermis	Hair
Sebaceous gland	Dermis	Fat
Pores	Blood vessel	Nerve

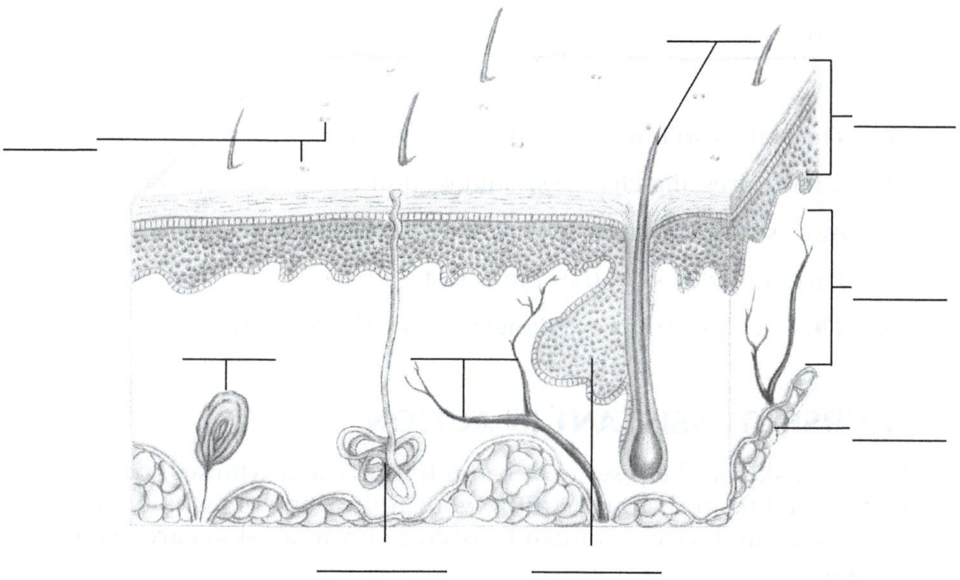

FIGURE 16-1

EXERCISE 16-2

Objective: To identify important protective devices for the skin.

Directions: Read the following riddles carefully before writing the correct answer on the blank line.

1. This device helps to elevate an extremity off the bed. What is it?____________

   (*Hint:* An alternative meaning goes well with coffee in the morning.)

2. This item is used to keep blankets off the legs and feet. What is it?____________

   (*Hint:* An alternative meaning is a small bed for a baby.)

3. This device prevents a serious deformity to the foot. What is it?______________

   (*Hint:* An alternative meaning is something you would want to wear in the snow or rain.)

EXERCISE 16-3

Select from the following list of ulcer stages the letter that best answers each statement. Write the correct letter(s) on the blank line next to the question. You may need to use more than one stage for each statement.

a. Stage I

b. Stage II

c. Stage III

d. Stage IV

_____ **1.** The skin is still intact but may be reddened.

_____ **2.** A daily dressing change should be done.

_____ **3.** At this stage(s), surgery may be required

_____ **4.** Partial thickness of the skin is lost.

_____ **5.** This stage(s) can prove dangerous for the patient.

THE NURSING ASSISTANT IN ACTION

1. You are asked to help set up a room for a patient who will be transferred from the burn unit to your unit. Knowing what you do about special devices that can be used to promote skin care, what should you do?

____

____

____

____

2. A patient has redness on his heels and elbows. What should you do?

____

____

____

____

3. You notice a frail, thin 90-year-old patient has slipped down in bed. What should you do?

____

____

____

____

4. You assist in giving a patient who is rather obese and bedridden a bath. What should you do to promote good skin care?

____

____

____

____

5. While caring for a patient, you notice redness on the patient's ischium and sacrum and some open wounds along her spine. The sheets are bloody and he cries out in pain when you reposition her. What should you do?

____

____

____

____

LEARNING ACTIVITIES

1. Research what types of foods and liquids you should encourage a patient who is at high risk for developing pressure ulcers to eat in order to prevent pressure ulcers from occurring or to help promote healing. Using these food items, create a menu for one day consisting of breakfast, lunch, dinner, and a snack.
2. Ask a fellow student to get into a hospital bed. Have her pretend she cannot move. Reposition her on her back using special devices to prop her arms and heels off the mattress. If available, use mattress devices and bed cradles along with items to decrease the chance that foot drop can occur. Use the bed mechanisms to keep her propped up so she does not slip. Change positions so you are the "patient." Discuss what felt good or bad about the experience, and together figure out other things you could do to make the person more comfortable while promoting skin integrity.

PROCEDURE CHECKLIST

PROCEDURE 16-1: SAFE SKIN CLEANSING FOR THE INCONTINENT PATIENT

Name: ____________________ Date: ____________________

STEPS	S	U	COMMENTS
1. Assemble your equipment a. Disposable gloves b. Tissues or disposable washcloths c. Bedpan d. Incontinent spray or soap e. Towel f. Moisture lotion or barrier g. Corn starch or powder h. Incontinent pad i. Bed sheets			
2. Wash your hands.			
3. Identify the patient by checking the identification bracelet.			
4. Ask visitors to step out of the room, if this is your hospital's policy.			
5. Tell the patient that you are going to wash him.			
6. Provide privacy for the patient.			
7. Raise the bed to a comfortable working position.			
8. Raise the side rail on the far side of the bed.			
9. Put on the disposable gloves.			
10. Using tissue or disposable washcloths, wipe away as much feces and urine as possible. Then wash the area that has urine or feces on it very well, removing all waste material from the skin. Place soiled tissue into the bedpan. If available, use the incontinence sprays to cleanse the skin. These are convenient, help eliminate odors, and the spray can be directed to specific areas.			
11. If there is soap on the skin, rinse well with clean water, changing the water frequently. (Many incontinence sprays do not require rinsing, thus saving time and trauma to the skin. Special cleansing foams do not run and cause less discomfort than cold sprays.)			
12. Pat the skin dry to prevent injury or pain from rubbing. If the skin is red and macerated, use soft tissues to blot the skin dry.			

13. Apply a moisture lotion or barrier to the *perineum* (area between and around rectum and urinary opening) of any patient with incontinence.			
14. Apply cornstarch or powder only where skin surfaces touch other skin surfaces (creases and skin folds). Dust lightly and close to the skin surface to prevent excessive dust particles from floating into the air. The cornstarch or powder should be rubbed into the skin gently. Do not apply powder in areas of open sores or surgical incisions.			
15. Do not put disposable plastic diapers on the patient while still in bed. This holds moisture next to the skin and can cause skin maceration and skin infections.			
16. Place an incontinent pad under the patient. Do not place patient directly on top of a plastic disposable pad. Put a sheet over the disposable plastic pad, between the pad and the patient. Do not use more than two layers of pads under the patient at a time.			
17. Position, cover, and make the patient comfortable.			
18. Lower the bed to a position of safety for the patient.			
19. Replace the side rails to the proper position.			
20. Discard disposable equipment.			
21. Place soiled linen in the laundry bag, and then place the bag into the dirty linen hamper in the utility room.			
22. Remove and discard gloves, then wash your hands.			
23. Check for incontinent episodes every 2 hours. Remake the bed as necessary.			
24. Report to your immediate supervisor • The patient was incontinent of urine or feces. • The patient was washed and the skin is now clean and dry. • The patient's position was changed every 2 hours, and the time of each position change. • Any signs of skin breakdown. • The color, amount, and consistency of the feces and urine you cleaned. • How the patient tolerated the procedure. • Your observations of anything unusual.			

Charting:

____

____

____

____

Date of Satisfactory Completion ______________________

Instructor's Signature ______________________

17

The Circulatory and Respiratory Systems and Related Care

Key Terms Review

Match the key terms in the right column with the definitions in the left column by placing the letter of each correct answer in the space provided.

_____ **1.** Blood vessels that carry blood from parts of the body back to the heart.

_____ **2.** Blood vessels that carry oxygenated blood away from the heart.

_____ **3.** The smallest blood vessel in the body.

_____ **4.** A four-chambered, hollow, muscular organ that lies in the chest cavity and pumps the blood through the lungs and into all parts of the body.

_____ **5.** Relating to the heart.

_____ **6.** The continuous movement of blood through the heart and blood vessels to all parts of the body.

_____ **7.** The heart, blood vessels, blood, and all organs that pump and carry blood and other fluids throughout the body.

_____ **8.** The liquid portion of the blood.

_____ **9.** The force of the blood pushing against the walls of the blood vessels.

_____ **10.** A blood clot.

_____ **11.** A lack of red blood cells.

_____ **12.** A blood clot in the brain.

Terms

A. Respiratory system
B. Pulmonary
C. Aspiration
D. Tuberculosis (TB)
E. Heart
F. Cardiac
G. Circulatory system
H. Circulation
I. Veins
J. Arteries
K. Capillaries
L. Plasma
M. Blood pressure
N. Anemia
O. Thrombus
P. Pulmonary embolism
Q. Cerebral embolism
R. Cyanosis
S. Orthostatic (postural) hypotension
T. Edema

_____ **13.** A blood clot in the lung.

_____ **14.** A bluish discoloration of the skin and mucous membranes caused by a lack of oxygen in the blood.

_____ **15.** Abnormal swelling of a part of the body caused by fluid collecting in that area; usually the swelling is in the ankles, legs, hands, or abdomen.

_____ **16.** A drop in blood pressure that occurs when a person changes positions from lying down to sitting or standing.

_____ **17.** Relating to the lungs.

_____ **18.** The group of body organs that carries on the body function of respiration; the system brings oxygen into the body and eliminates carbon dioxide.

_____ **19.** The inhalation of oral or gastric contents into the lungs.

_____ **20.** A highly infectious disease that usually affects the lungs.

MULTIPLE-CHOICE QUESTIONS

Circle the letter next to the word or statement that best completes the sentence or answers the question.

1. The _________ blood cells fight infection.
  a. red
  b. white
  c. plasma
  d. new

2. The heart is located in the chest cavity,
  a. pointing slightly to the patient's left.
  b. hanging low in the abdomen.
  c. pointing slightly to the patient's right.
  d. behind the large intestine.

3. Myocardial tissue is supplied with blood via the
  a. superior and inferior vena cavae.
  b. coronary arteries.
  c. right ventricle.
  d. pulmonary veins.

4. A pulmonary embolism is a blood clot that lodges in the
  a. feet.
  b. heart.
  c. brain.
  d. lungs.

5. A pulmonary embolism causes chest pain, difficulty in breathing, and
  a. is not serious.
  b. is treated with bed rest.
  c. is life threatening.
  d. requires removal of the lung.

6. One reason older adults tire easily is because
  a. they are lazy.
  b. they do not get enough sleep.
  c. the brain has become smaller.
  d. the heart has reduced output because of weaker heart muscle.

7. The respiratory system's function is to allow
  a. urine to leave the blood.
  b. oxygen to move from the air outside the body into the blood.
  c. urine to enter the kidneys.
  d. blood to enter the brain.

8. If the epiglottis is not functioning, then _________________ may occur in the lungs.
  a. stomatitis
  b. epiglottitis

c. aspiration
d. hypertension

9. *Chronic obstructive pulmonary disease (COPD)* refers to a group of respiratory disorders, including asthma, bronchitis, and
a. epiglottitis.
b. anemia.
c. emphysema.
d. tuberculosis.

10. A patient with COPD has difficulty
a. swimming.
b. running.
c. breathing.
d. all of the above.

11. A person with obstructed breathing may mouth-breathe and require
a. more frequent mouth care.
b. more back rubs.
c. more steaming showers.
d. more sleep.

12. The circulatory and respiratory systems
a. are separate, and one is not affected by the other.
b. are the same system.
c. can take the place of the endocrine system.
d. work closely together and a condition that affects one system may affect the other system.

13. After surgery, patients are encouraged to cough and deep breathe to
a. give them exercise.
b. keep them oriented.
c. expand the alveolar sacs and promote the exchange of oxygen.
d. improve their coughing skills.

14. Tuberculosis is transmitted by which of the following?
a. Coughing
b. Sneezing
c. Speaking
d. All of the above

15. As a nursing assistant, which of the following observations should she report immediately to the nurse?
a. The patient is tired after walking in the hall.
b. The patient is short of breath in bed.
c. The patient is tired of TV.
d. The patient is hungry for a snack.

16. The left side of the heart
a. pumps blood to all body cells to deliver oxygen, nutrients, and hormones.
b. delivers carbon dioxide to the lungs to remove this waste from the blood stream.
c. receives the superior and inferior vena cavae into the atrium.
d. is a weak muscle and needs help from the respiratory system to do its job correctly.

17. A *pulse* is
a. felt when the heart rests during diastole.
b. found in different locations in the body where major arteries lie close to the skin's surface.
c. recorded using a blood pressure cuff and a stethoscope.
d. measured and recorded using mm/Hg.

18. Besides feeling weak, fatigued, and short of breath, a person who is anemic
a. can have warm, moist skin and cheeks that are rosy.
b. may complain of dizziness and feeling faint.
c. will need cool compresses placed to increase vasodilation and promote blood flow.
d. clots easily and therefore should be watched for increased chance of bleeding.

19. When caring for a patient living with peripheral vascular disease, it is important to
a. encourage the use of a space heater placed near his feet at night to keep his body warm.
b. cut his toenails frequently so infection does not start.

c. elevate his feet when he sits to reduce edema that may accumulate in his feet, ankles, and lower legs.
d. all of the above.

20. The most comfortable area to place a pulse oximeter on a patient is his
a. nose when wearing an oxygen mask.
b. forehead
c. toe when he is out of bed.
d. finger.

21. If a pulse oximeter reading ________, the nursing assistant should report this finding immediately to your supervisor.
a. goes below 90%
b. stays at 98%
c. fluctuates between 95% and 100%
d. is 140/90 mm/Hg

22. When caring for a patient who has tuberculosis, the nursing assistant should
a. have visitors wear a mask when entering the room.
b. leave the door open to the patient's room to decrease the feeling of social isolation.
c. wear a mask in the hallway when transporting this patient for testing.
d. place a fan in his room to vent the air into the hallway of the facility.

23. A patient has an incentive spirometer at his bedside. He should
a. be taught how to inhale deeply and hold his breath.
b. cough into the machine 10 times each hour.
c. close his lips around the tubing when exhaling slowly into the machine.
d. be awakened in the middle of the night to practice coughing frequently.

24. When oxygen is ordered, the nursing assistant should
a. check the order and administer 2 liters per minute using a mask or nasal cannula.
b. set up the tubing, oxygen equipment, and mask and then tell your supervisor this task is complete.
c. encourage the patient to wear her mask even if she has skin breakdown.
d. lubricate the tubing with petroleum jelly.

25. When the left valve in the heart becomes weakened, this is called
a. peripheral vascular disease.
b. mitral valve prolapse.
c. tricuspid valve disorder.
d. hypertension.

TRUE OR FALSE QUESTIONS

Determine whether each question is true or false. In the space provided, write "T" for true and "F" for false. If the statement is false, rewrite it on the line provided to make it a true statement.

_____ **1.** Because we need oxygen to live, it is necessary to keep the respiratory system pathway (trachea, larynx, bronchi, and lungs) open and functioning.

____

_____ **2.** In the lungs, the oxygen molecules get exchanged for carbon dioxide in the alveolar sacs.

____

_____ 3. The incidence of tuberculosis (TB) has been decreasing in recent years.

____

_____ 4. High blood pressure can be caused from a diet high in fats.

____

_____ 5. Patients who have diseases or limiting conditions of the circulatory or respiratory system often find activities of daily living (ADLs) difficult to perform.

____

_____ 6. The lungs bring carbon dioxide into the body during inhalation and release oxygen from the body during exhalation.

____

_____ 7. The immune system stops bleeding by initiating a clotting response, thereby allowing healing to occur.

____

_____ 8. Platelets contain red blood cells and white blood cells.

____

_____ 9. It is not unusual for edema to occur in the feet and ankles in a patient who has congestive heart failure.

____

_____ 10. When bathing patients with circulatory disorders, rub lotion vigorously to promote tissue perfusion and reduce edema.

____

FILL-IN-THE-BLANK QUESTIONS

Provide the meaning of the following abbreviations.

1. TB _______________
2. mL _______________
3. O_2 _______________
4. CO_2 _______________
5. MI _______________
6. CHF _______________
7. CVA _______________
8. COPD _______________
9. SpO_2 _______________
10. ID _______________
11. HR _______________
12. IS _______________

EXERCISE 17-1

Objective: To recognize and be able to correctly spell the names of various parts of the circulatory system.

Directions: Label the diagram in Figure 17-1 with the correct words from the following word list.

Word List

Pulmonary capillaries	Pulmonary veins	Aorta (artery)
Pulmonary arteries	Systemic capillaries	Venule
Arteriole	Capillaries	Vena cavae (veins)

FIGURE 17-1

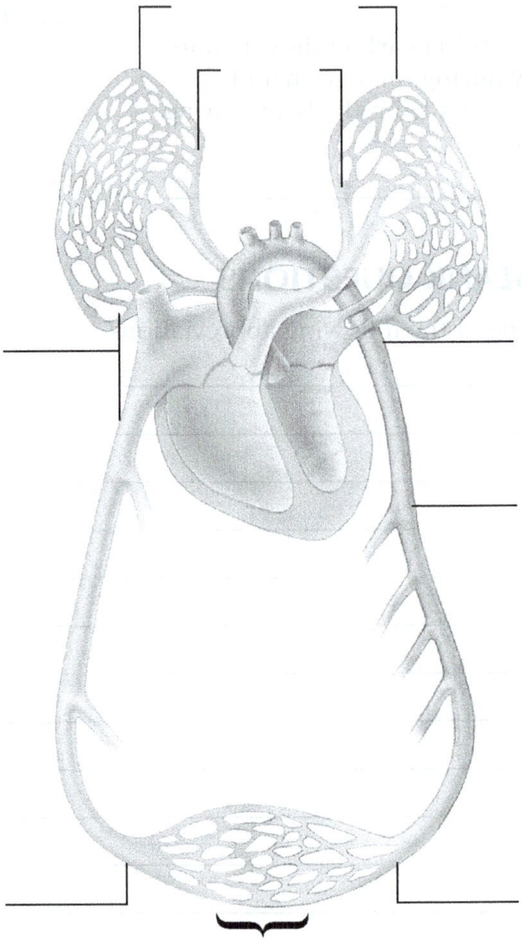

EXERCISE 17-2

Objective: To recognize and be able to correctly spell the names of various parts of the heart.

Directions: Label the diagram in Figure 17-2 with the correct words from the following word list.

Word List

Superior vena cava
Pulmonary artery
Inferior vena cava
Myocardium (muscle)
Aorta
Left atrium
Right atrium
Pulmonary veins
Left ventricle
Right ventricle
Pulmonary artery
Epicardium (outer covering)
Pulmonary veins

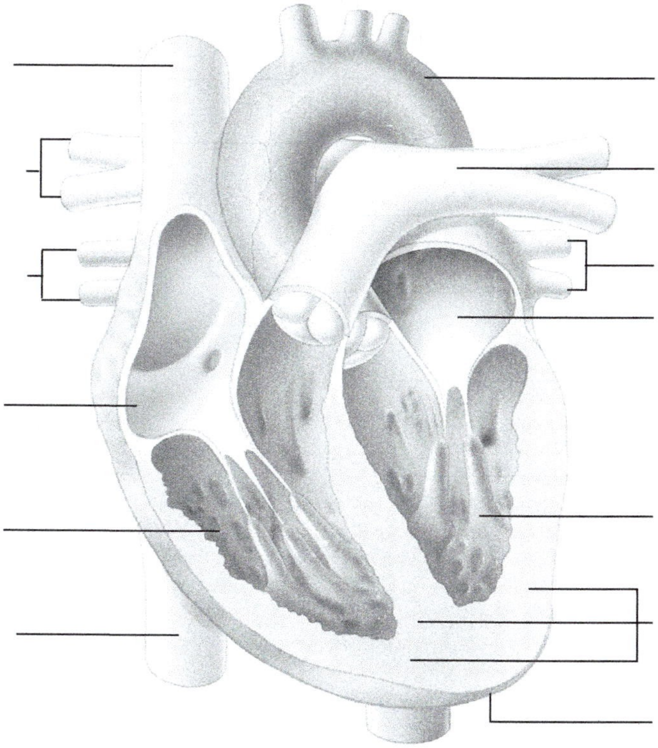

FIGURE 17-2

EXERCISE 17-3

Objective: To recognize and be able to correctly spell the names of various parts of the system of arteries.

Directions: Label the diagram in Figure 17-3 with the correct words from the following word list.

Word List

Right common carotid	Innominate artery	Aortic arch
Pulmonary artery	Right subclavian artery	Common iliac
Descending aorta	Left subclavian artery	Femoral Artery
Left common carotid	Right and left coronary arteries	Ascending aorta

FIGURE 17-3

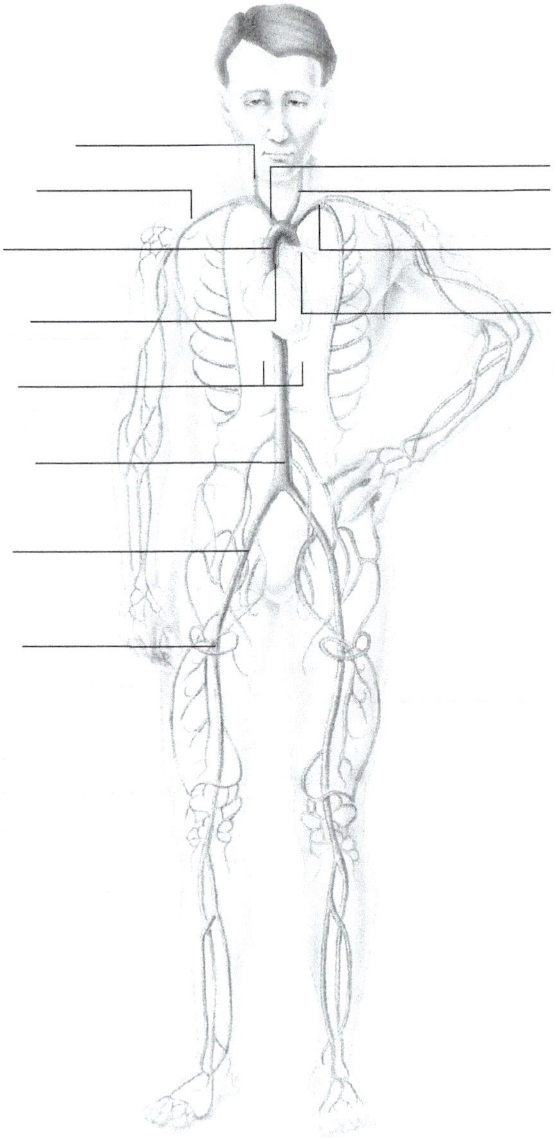

EXERCISE 17-4

Objective: To recognize and be able to correctly spell the names of various parts of the system of veins.

Directions: Label the diagram in Figure 17-4 with the correct words from the following word list.

Word List

Internal jugular vein	External jugular vein	Femoral vein
Iliac vein	Inferior vena cava	Innominate vein
Subclavian vein	Superior vena cava	

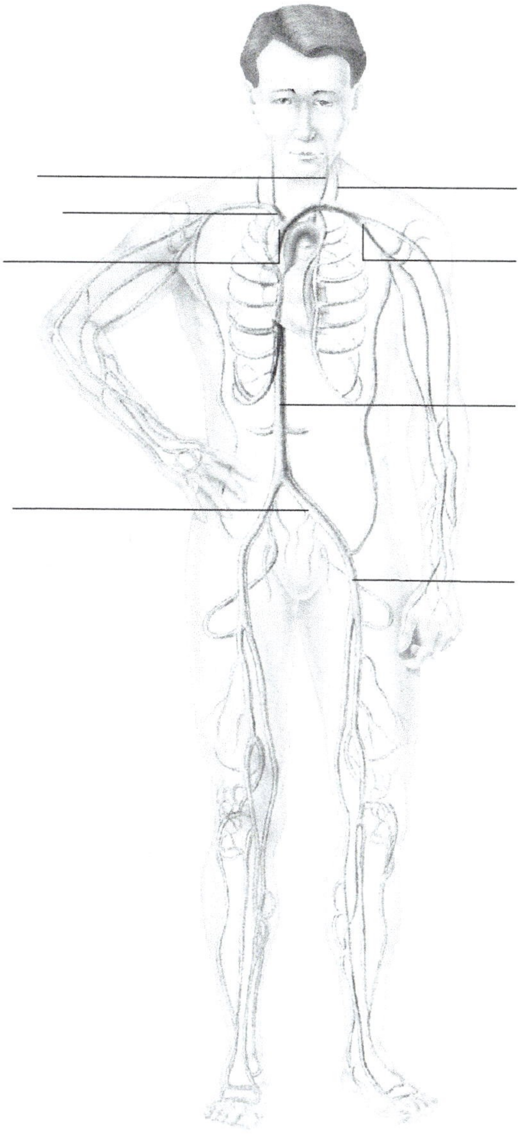

FIGURE 17-4

EXERCISE 17-5

Objective: To recognize and be able to correctly spell the names of various parts of the respiratory system.

Directions: Label the diagram in Figure 17-5 with the correct words from the following word list.

Word List

Left main bronchus	Frontal sinus	Diaphragm	Adenoids	Trachea
Right main bronchus	Pleural space	Bronchiole	Epiglottis	Larynx
Pulmonary artery	Capillaries	Esophagus	Pharynx	Mucus
Pulmonary vein	Nasal cavity	Oral cavity	Tongue	Ribs
Alveolus (air sac)	Bronchial cilia	Pleura	Tonsils	Cells

FIGURE 17-5

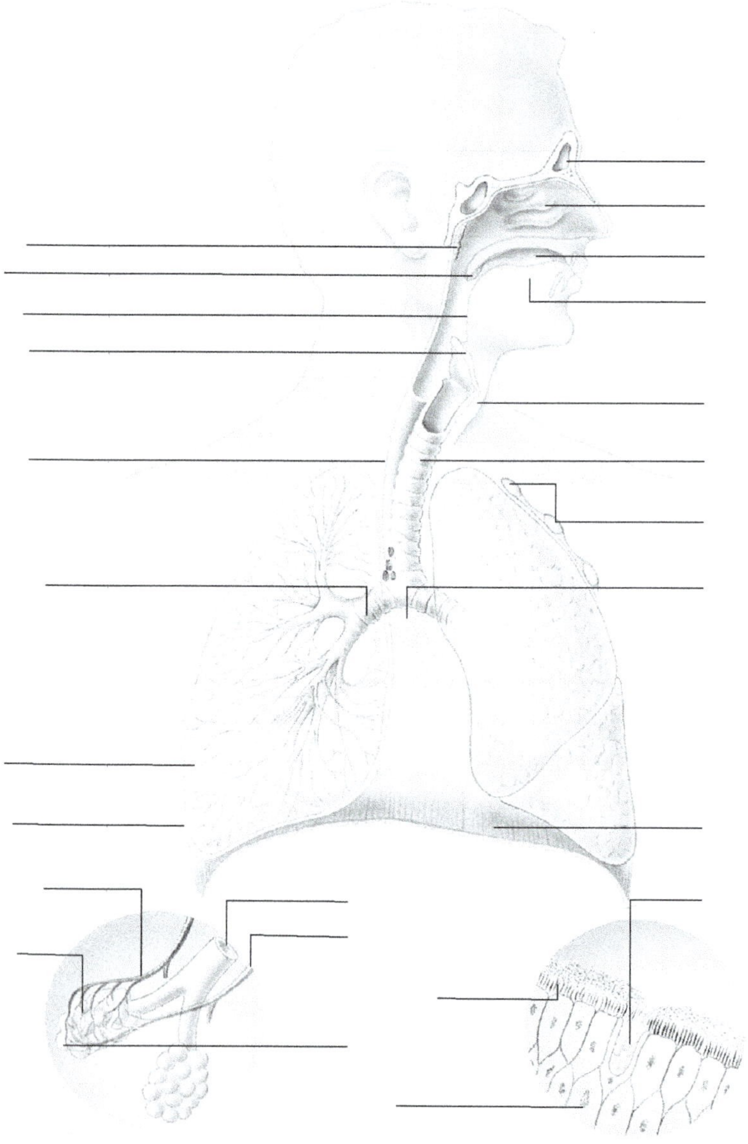

THE NURSING ASSISTANT IN ACTION

1. A postsurgical patient will be transferred to your unit and will need oxygen. Your supervisor asks you to get the room ready. What should you do?

2. A female patient who is on seizure precautions and who had cardiac surgery must have her blood pressure taken and a pulse oximeter machine placed on her finger. What should you do?

3. A patient living with peripheral vascular disease is being discharged from your unit. She is wearing knee-high hose. What information should you give her to promote good circulation?

4. You enter a room where a patient who is on oxygen via a mask is being visited by family. It is his birthday and they want to light candles on a cake they brought in for him. What should you do?

5. A patient has been given an incentive spirometer to use. You come into his room and find he is not using it correctly. What should you do?

LEARNING ACTIVITIES

1. Listen to your chest with a stethoscope to find your apical pulse. Count for 1 full minute to determine how many beats per minute your heart contracts. Each "lub/dub" is considered one beat. Now see if you can feel your carotid, radial, and dorsalis pedis pulses. Count for 1 full minute and record the beats per minute at each pulse point. Were the numbers the same in each spot? Why or why not? Discuss your findings with your peers and instructor.
2. Find a pulse point like the radial pulse or carotid pulse on your body. While sitting, count how many beats per minute you felt at that pulse area. Write that number on a piece of paper. Now count again while standing, while lying down, and after running in place for 1 full minute. Record and compare your findings each after each position. What were your findings? Why do you think there were similarities and differences? Why did this occur? Discuss your findings with your peers and instructor.

PROCEDURE CHECKLISTS

PROCEDURE 17-1: USING A PULSE OXIMETER TO MEASURE OXYGEN IN THE BLOOD

Name: ____________________ Date: ____________________

STEPS	S	U	COMMENTS
1. Assemble equipment a. Pulse Oximeter b. Gloves c. Fingernail polish remover			
2. Identify the patient by checking the ID bracelet.			
3. Wash your hands and put on gloves.			
4. Provide privacy and comfort for the patient.			
5. Explain to the patient that you are going to assess the amount of oxygen in her blood.			
6. Raise the rails on the opposite side of the bed.			
7. Raise the bed to a comfortable working height.			
8. Select a good sensor site a. Generally a finger is selected (although the toe, earlobe, nose, or forehead may also be used, depending on the sensor attachment). b. Do not use a finger site if the person has fake fingernails on. c. If using a finger site, remember that the blood pressure cuff on the same arm may affect the reading. Use the opposite side. d. Shaking, tremors, shivering, or seizures may affect the reading. In these circumstances, use a different sensor site such as the forehead.			
9. Remove fingernail polish from fingernail if a finger site is selected for this procedure.			
10. Attach pulse oximetry sensor to the selected site. Make sure the sensor is in good contact with the skin.			
11. Turn on the pulse oximeter.			
12. Check the patient's pulse (apical or radial) with the pulse on the display. The pulses should be identical. If not, notify your supervisor.			
13. Observe the oxygen saturation (SpO_2) and heart rate indicator findings displayed on the electronic screen.			
14. Discard gloves and wash your hands.			

15. Report and record SpO_2 and pulse rate measurements accurately.			
16. Report your findings to your supervisor.			

Charting:

____

____

____

____

Date of Satisfactory Completion ____________________

Instructor's Signature ____________________

PROCEDURE 17-2: ASSISTING WITH COUGHING AND DEEP-BREATHING EXERCISES

Name: ______________________ Date: ______________________

STEPS	S	U	COMMENTS
1. Assemble equipment a. Incentive spirometer b. Pillow c. Tissues d. Gloves			
2. Identify the patient by checking the ID bracelet.			
3. Inform the patient that you are going to assist him with deep-breathing and coughing exercises.			
4. Wash your hands.			
5. Put on gloves.			
6. Provide for privacy and assist patient to a sitting or semi-Fowler's position, if permitted.			
7. Instruct the patient to a. Breathe out normally. b. Clasp his hands over his abdomen i. Take a deep breath in until he feels his abdomen push out and he can't inhale any more. Have the patient hold his breath for 3 seconds and then exhale slowly; or, if the patient has an incentive spirometer, instruct him to seal his lips tightly around the mouthpiece and breathe in as slowly and deeply as possible through his mouth. Note the highest level the indicator reaches. When the patient can't inhale any further, have the patient hold his breath for 3 seconds then move the incentive spirometer away from his mouth to exhale slowly. c. Rest a few seconds. d. Repeat deep breathing three to four times. e. Cough one to two times. Instruct the patient to hold a pillow across his abdomen to "splint" while coughing to decrease any discomfort. f. Use a tissue to collect any respiratory mucus brought up during coughing. g. Relax and breathe normally. h. Repeat deep-breathing and cough exercises 10 times every hour while awake.			

8. Discard any tissues used in the proper receptacle.			
9. Place the incentive spirometer within the patient's reach on the bedside or overbed table.			
10. Discard gloves and wash your hands.			
11. Report to your supervisor			
• That you assisted the patient with deep-breathing and coughing exercises. • How the patient tolerated the procedure. • Any unusual observations.			

Charting: ______________________________

____

____

____

____

Date of Satisfactory Completion ______________

Instructor's Signature ______________

PROCEDURE 17-3: PREPARING FOR OXYGEN ADMINISTRATION

Name: ____________________ Date: ____________________

STEPS	S	U	COMMENTS
1. Assemble equipment a. Oxygen (wall unit) or portable oxygen tank b. Oxygen connection tubing i. Nasal cannula ii. Face mask c. Flowmeter d. Humidifier (if ordered) e. Water (if using a humidifier)			
2. Identify the patient by checking the ID bracelet.			
3. Wash your hands.			
4. Provide privacy and comfort for the patient.			
5. Explain to the patient that you are going to set up for oxygen administration.			
6. Turn the flowmeter to the OFF position.			
7. Attach the oxygen flowmeter to the wall outlet.			
8. Fill the humidifier (if ordered) with water.			
9. Attach the humidifier to the bottom of the flowmeter.			
10. Attach the oxygen device and connection tubing to the humidifier.			
11. Replace the cap on the water and store the bottled distilled water according to agency policy.			
12. Place oxygen tubing packaging and other waste products in the appropriate receptacle.			
13. Wash your hands.			
14. Notify your supervisor that you are set up for oxygen administration.			

Charting:

____

____

____

____

Date of Satisfactory Completion ____________________

Instructor's Signature ____________________

Measuring Vital Signs

18

Key Terms Review

Match the key terms in the right column with the definitions in the left column by placing the letter of each correct answer in the space provided.

_____ **1.** Measurements reflecting the patient's physical well-being and condition.

_____ **2.** An instrument used for measuring temperature.

_____ **3.** A system for measuring temperature in which the temperature of water at boiling is 212 degrees and at freezing, it is 32 degrees.

_____ **4.** A system for measurement of temperature using a scale divided into 100 units or degrees; in this system, the freezing temperature of water is 0 degrees and water boils at 100 degrees.

_____ **5.** Under the arm.

_____ **6.** Pertaining to the rectum.

_____ **7.** The mouth.

_____ **8.** The rhythmic expansion and contraction of the arteries caused by the beating of the heart.

_____ **9.** A difference between the apical heart rate and the pulse rate.

_____ **10.** A measurement of heart beats counted by listening to the heart directly over the apex on the patient's chest.

_____ **11.** A heart rate of less than 60 beats per minute.

Terms

A. Vital signs
B. Pulse
C. Apical pulse
D. Radial pulse
E. Rhythm
F. Bradycardia
G. Tachycardia
H. Pulse deficit
I. Thermometer
J. Oral
K. Rectal
L. Axillary
M. Fahrenheit
N. Centigrade
O. Exhaling
P. Inhaling
Q. Abdominal respiration
R. Shallow respirations
S. Labored respirations

_____12. A heart rate of more than 100 beats per minute.

_____13. A pulse felt at the radial artery in the wrist.

_____14. Describes the regularity of pulse beats.

_____15. Air going out of the lungs; breathing out.

_____16. Air going into the lungs, breathing in.

_____17. The depth of respirations changes and the rate is not steady.

_____18. Respirations that are difficult for the patient and require extra work.

_____19. Breathing with only the upper part of the lungs.

_____20. Breathing in which the patient is using mostly the abdominal muscles.

_____21. The absence of respirations; not breathing.

_____22. Abnormal respirations.

_____23. Abnormal sounds made with breathing.

_____24. One kind of irregular breathing. At first, the breathing is slow and shallow; then the respiration becomes faster and deeper until it reaches a peak. The respiration then slows down and becomes shallow again. The breathing may then stop completely and the pattern begins again. May be caused by certain cerebral (brain), cardiac (heart), or pulmonary (lung) diseases or conditions.

_____25. A measure of the force of blood against the walls of the arteries as blood is pumped by the heart.

_____26. A device used to measure blood pressure.

_____27. An instrument that allows one to listen to sounds within the body.

_____28. The force with which blood is pumped when the heart muscle is contracting.

_____29. Measurement of the force of blood against the arterial walls when the heart is at rest.

_____30. Dial-type blood pressure equipment.

_____31. Blood pressure that is higher than normal. In an adult, it is a systolic pressure of 140 mmHg or higher or a diastolic pressure of 90 mmHg or higher.

_____32. Blood pressure that is lower than normal. In an adult, it is a systolic pressure of 90 mmHg or lower or a diastolic pressure of 60 mmHg or lower.

T. Irregular respirations

U. Apnea

V. Dyspnea

W. Stertorous respiration

X. Cheyne-Stokes respirations

Y. Blood pressure

Z. Stethoscope

AA. Sphygmomanometer

BB. Systolic blood pressure

CC. Diastolic blood pressure

DD. Hypertension

EE. Hypotension

FF. Aneroid sphygmomanometer

MULTIPLE-CHOICE QUESTIONS

Circle the letter next to the word or statement that best completes the sentence or answers the question.

1. To be sure the patient will not know that you are watching his breathing, you should
   a. count respirations while taking his blood pressure.
   b. hold the patient's wrist just as if you were taking his pulse.
   c. distract him by talking about the weather.
   d. take his temperature first.
2. What should a nursing assistant do if she cannot clearly see the chest rise and fall?
   a. Fold the patient's arm across his chest to feel his breathing as she holds his wrist.
   b. Place her hand on the patient's chin to feel his breathing.
   c. Use a disposable thermometer to distract the patient.
   d. Place her hand on his shoulder and count respirations.
3. If you count the chest rising 15 times in 1 full minute, you should report
   a. 30 respirations per minute.
   b. 15 respirations per minute.
   c. 7 respirations per minute.
   d. 60 respirations per minute.
4. If you count 9 respirations in 30 seconds, you should report
   a. 27 respirations per minute.
   b. 9 respirations per minute.
   c. 18 respirations per minute.
   d. 36 respirations per minute.
5. If you count a radial pulse as 72 beats in 1 full minute, you should report
   a. 72 respirations per minute.
   b. 288 beats per minute.
   c. 72 beats per minute.
   d. 36 beats per minute
6. Measuring the force of the blood flowing through the arteries means you are
   a. measuring a patient's temperature.
   b. counting a patient's respirations.
   c. measuring a patient's blood pressure.
   d. assessing a patient's vital signs.
7. "mm" is the abbreviation for
   a. mercury.
   b. centimeters.
   c. millimeters.
   d. cubic centimeters.
8. "Hg" is the abbreviation for
   a. mercury.
   b. centimeters.
   c. millimeters.
   d. diastolic.
9. When a patient's blood pressure is higher than the normal range for his age and condition, it is referred to as
   a. hypotension.
   b. hypertension.
   c. high diastolic pressure.
   d. low blood pressure.
10. When a patient's blood pressure is lower than the normal range for her age and condition, it is referred to as
    a. hypotension
    b. hypertension.
    c. low systolic pressure.
    d. high blood pressure.
11. Which blood pressure should be reported as high?
    a. When the systolic pressure is 110
    b. When the diastolic pressure is 80
    c. 160/95
    d. 90/60
12. Which blood pressure should be reported as low?
    a. When the systolic pressure is 126
    b. When the diastolic pressure is 90
    c. 160/95
    d. 80/50

13. When using a sphygmomanometer, the nursing assistant

a. must use the correct-size cuff based on the size of the patient's arm.

b. must wait 5–10 minutes after the patient eats or drinks anything hot or cold.

c. count respirations.

d. watch a television monitor.

14. When using the aneroid dial sphygmomanometer, the nursing assistant

a. watches a television monitor.

b. watches a pointer on a dial.

c. counts respirations.

d. watches a digital display.

15. When taking a patient's blood pressure, the nursing assistant listens to how the brachial pulse sounds in the brachial artery in the patient's arm and at the same time

a. pumps air into the cuff and recording the beats per minute per minute at the radial pulse site.

b. watches the aneroid dial to take a reading while slowly releasing air from the cuff.

c. counts the pulse for a 30 seconds and then multiplying the results by 2 to record the accurate beats per minute.

d. watches the clock for a full minute.

16. When recording blood pressure you should write it $\frac{120}{80}$ or $^{120}/_{80}$. The top number is the

a. systolic pressure.

b. diastolic pressure.

c. blood pressure.

d. millimeters of mercury.

17. The bottom number of a recorded blood pressure is the

a. systolic pressure.

b. diastolic pressure.

c. blood pressure.

d. millimeters of mercury.

18. The amount of heat in a body that is a balance between the amount of heat produced and the amount of heat lost is called

a. metabolism

b. body temperature

c. Fahrenheit

d. Centigrade

19. The difference between the apical and radial pulse is the

a. apical heart rate.

b. apical radial rate.

c. pulse deficit.

d. beats per minute.

20. Vital signs

a. are important because they help establish a baseline of information that is normal for the patient.

b. help detect changes in the body.

c. may detect a life-threatening disease or disorder.

d. all of the above.

21. The nursing assistant first takes a rectal temperature on an infant. The infant begins to cry. Then the nursing assistant takes the infant's pulse and respirations. The nursing assistant should expect that

a. the pulse and respirations may be lower than normal.

b. the pulse and respirations may be higher than normal.

c. the infant's crying will stop when she leaves the room.

d. the recordings are accurate.

22. Which site is the most invasive site to use when measuring body temperature?

a. Oral

b. Tympanic

c. Axillary

d. Rectal

23. When a patient complains of pain, it is important to initially

a. ask the nurse to give the patient medication immediately and encourage the patient to sleep to help decrease the pain.

b. get the patient up and moving because it is probably related to constipation.

c. ask the patient to point to the area the pain exists, ask when it started and to describe the pain.

d. offer the patient a pillow and encourage her to hold it to her chest when she coughs because the pain is probably related to her recent surgery.

24. The nursing assistant records an adult patient's TPR as: T = 98.8°F (O); P = 80; R = 32. Which vital sign(s) should he report to his supervisor as being abnormal?

a. The temperature and the respirations
b. The pulse and the respirations.
c. The respirations
d. Nothing, because all vital signs are within normal ranges.

25. The nursing assistant obtains vital signs on a postsurgical patient shortly after he comes from surgery. Which set of vital sign(s) should the nursing assistant report to the nurse as being abnormal?

a. T = 102.8°F (R); P = 90, irreg and weak; R = 30, labored; BP = 98/60.
b. T = 99.8°F (R); P = 80, reg and strong; R = 26; BP = 128/82.
c. T = 98.6°F (O); P = 76, reg and bounding; R = 20; BP = 120/80.
d. T = 97.8°F (O); P = 65, reg and bounding; R = 18; BP = 118/78.

TRUE OR FALSE QUESTIONS

Determine whether each question is true or false. In the space provided, write "T" for true and "F" for false. If the statement is false, rewrite it on the line provided to make it a true statement.

_____ **1.** Pain, height, weight, and abdominal girth can be considered vital signs.

____

_____ **2.** Drinking hot coffee can change a patient's vital signs.

____

_____ **3.** When obtaining a rectal temperature, change the probe to the blue probe, clean the probe before and after use, and insert without lubricant.

____

_____ **4.** The best way to take a combative patient's temperature is rectally to ensure they do not bite the thermometer.

____

_____ **5.** If capillary refill time is recorded as 4 seconds in the left foot, then this may indicate circulatory problems and should be reported.

____

_____ **6.** Using the "Face Scale" is appropriate to assess pain in an 8-year-old.

____

_____ **7.** The nursing assistant must use alcohol wipes when obtaining a rectal, oral, tympanic, or axillary temperature.

____

_____ **8.** When measuring abdominal girth, be sure to place the measuring tape around the back of the person and connect the tape at the breastbone to ensure accurate size is obtained.

____

_____ **9.** When obtaining a height on a patient who cannot get out of bed, the nursing assistant should place a mark on the sheets at the top of the patient's head and another at her heel, then measure with a measuring tape between the two points.

____

_____ **10.** When weighing a bedbound patient, weigh them at the same time each day, wearing the same type of clothing (if possible), and report to the nurse any casts or colostomy bags.

____

FILL-IN-THE-BLANK QUESTIONS

Provide the meaning of the following abbreviations.

1. mm ______
2. Hg ______
3. TPR ______
4. BP ______
5. C ______
6. F ______
7. O ______
8. R ______
9. A ______
10. T ______
11. TA ______
12. ID ______
13. NIBP ______
14. SpO_2 ______
15. OPQRST ______
16. IBW ______
17. BMI ______
18. lb ______
19. kg ______
20. IV ______
21. cm ______

EXERCISE 18-1

Objective: To identify the common areas of the body where a pulse can be measured.

Directions: Label the diagram in Figure 18-1 with the correct words from the following word list.

Word List

Femoral pulse	Temporal pulse	Apical pulse
Popliteal pulse	Radial pulse	Brachial pulse
Pedal pulse	Carotid pulse	

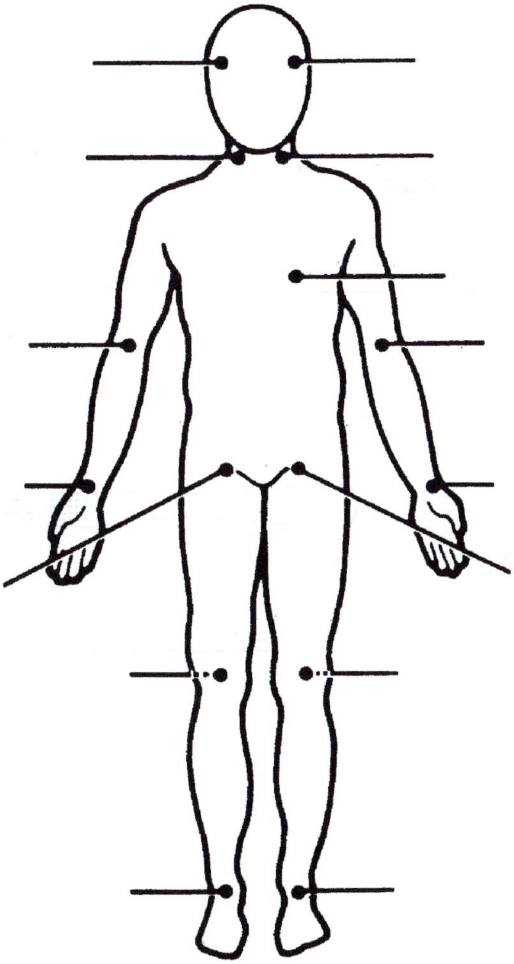

FIGURE 18-1

EXERCISE 18-2

Objective: To recognize the names of equipment commonly used to measure vital signs.

Directions: Label the pictures in Figure 18-2 with the number of the correctly matching name from the following word list.

Word List

1. Electronic oral/rectal thermometer
2. Electronic ear thermometer
3. Disposable thermometer
4. Diaphragm stethoscope
5. Aneroid sphygmomanometer

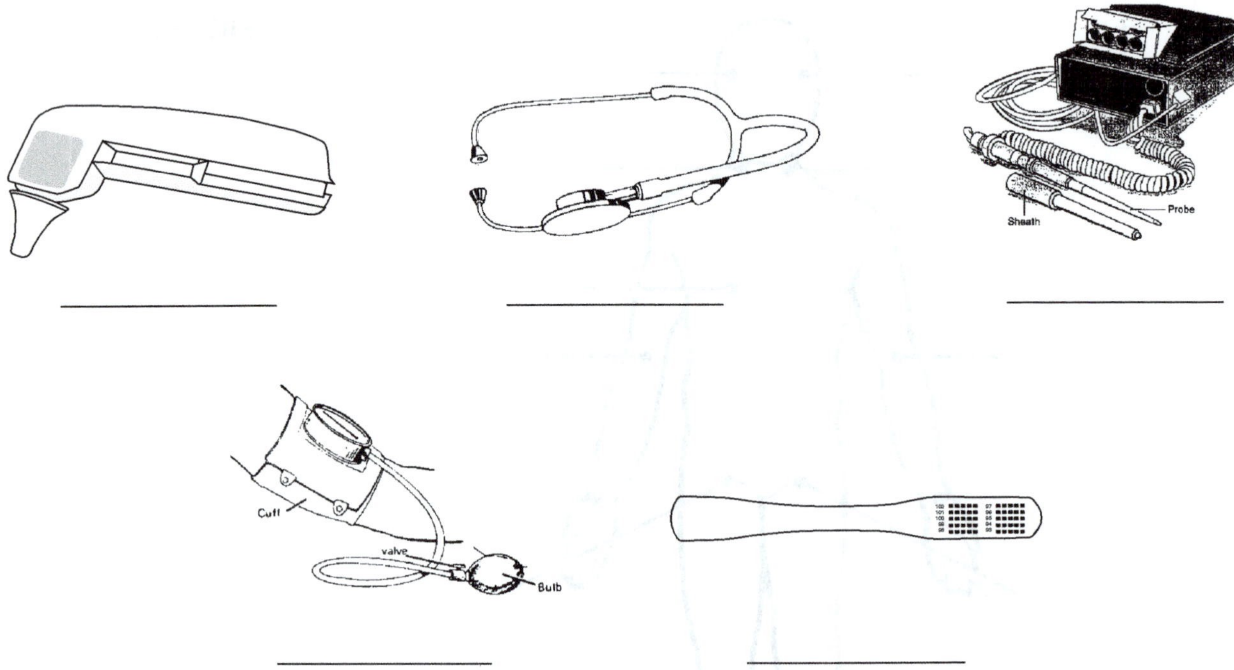

FIGURE 18-2

EXERCISE 18-3

Objective: To identify the correct technique for feeling the radial pulse.

Directions: Look carefully at Figure 18-3. Circle the letter next to the picture that shows the correct technique for feeling the radial pulse.

FIGURE 18-3

A.

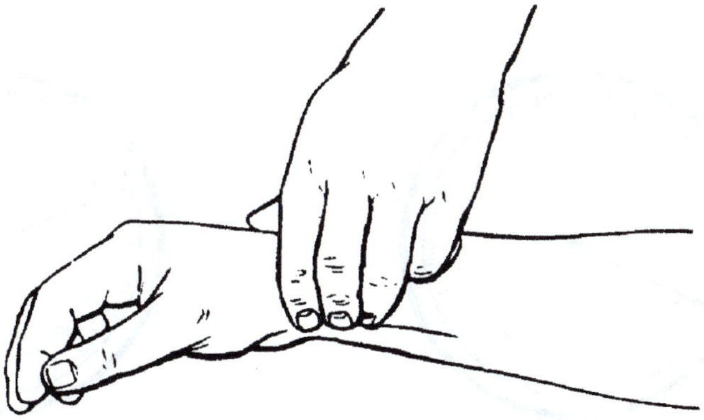

B.

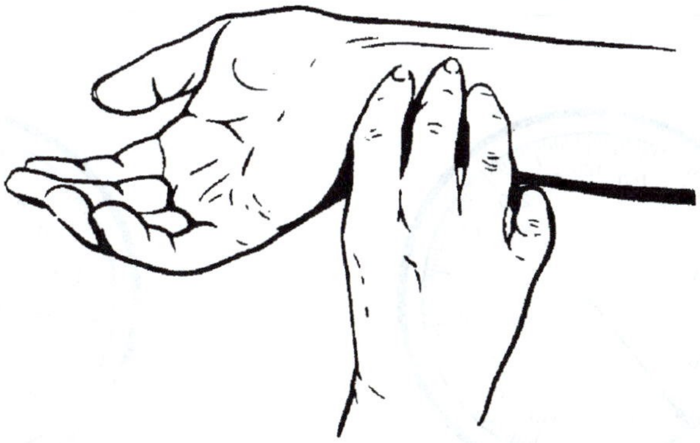

C.

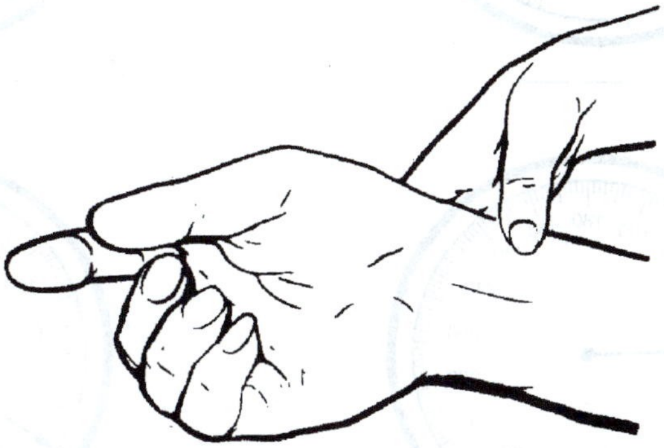

EXERCISE 18-4

Objective: To demonstrate your ability to read an aneroid dial sphygmomanometer correctly.

Directions: Read the gauges in Figure 18-4 and write the correct answer on the blank line next to each gauge.

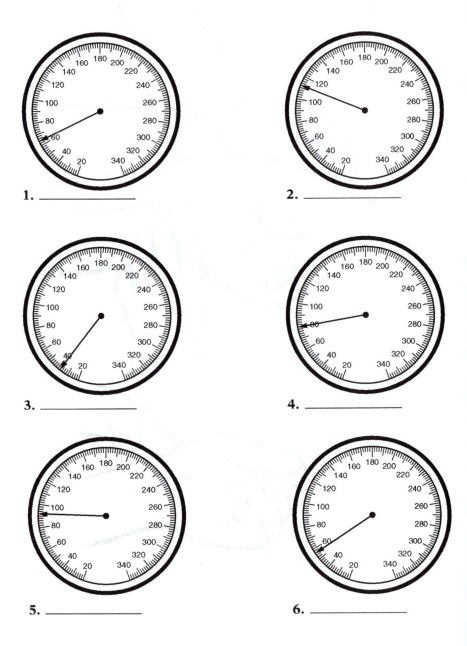

FIGURE 18-4

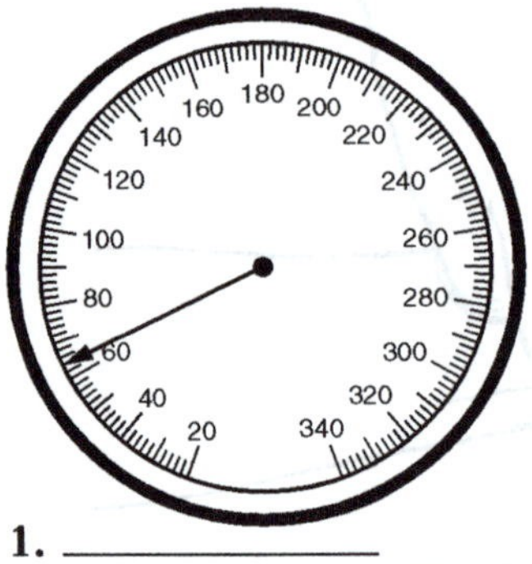

1. ________________

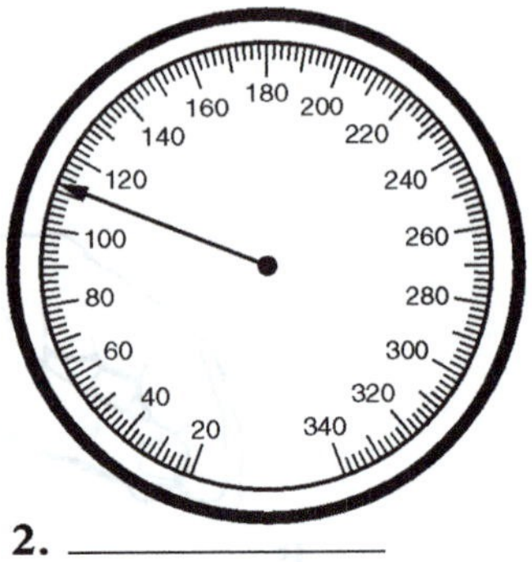

2. ________________

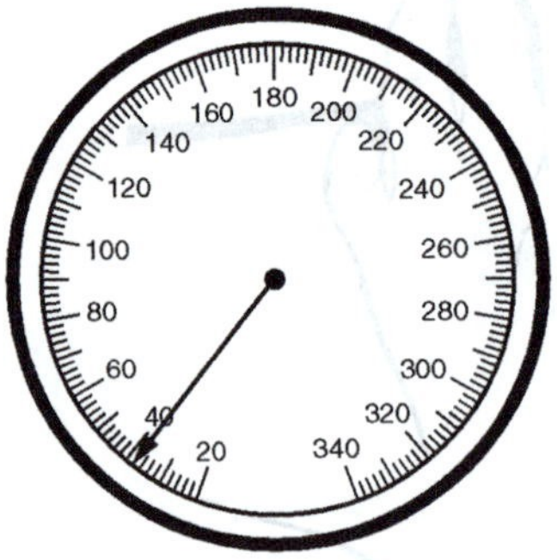

3. ________________

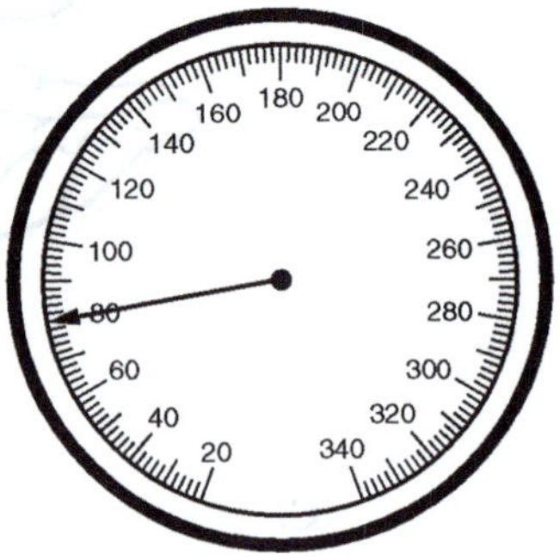

4. ________________

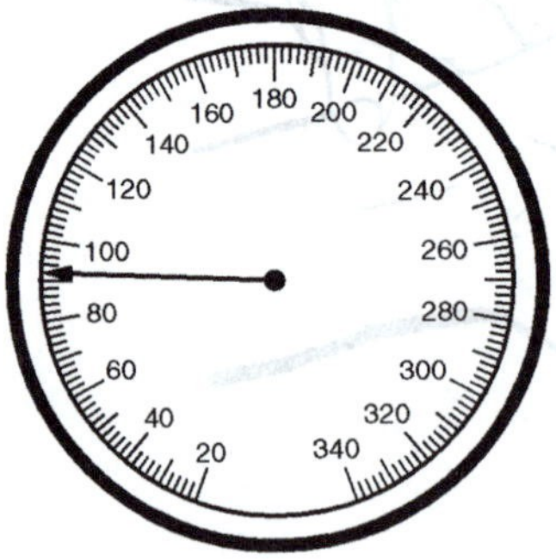

5. ________________

6. ________________

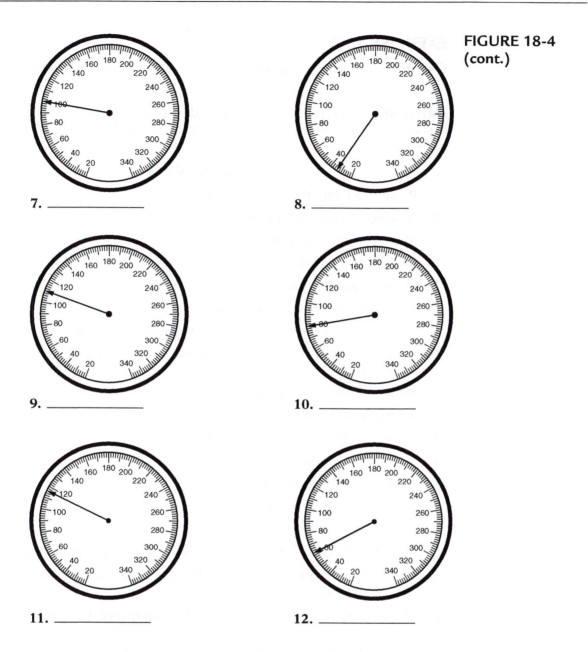

FIGURE 18-4 (cont.)

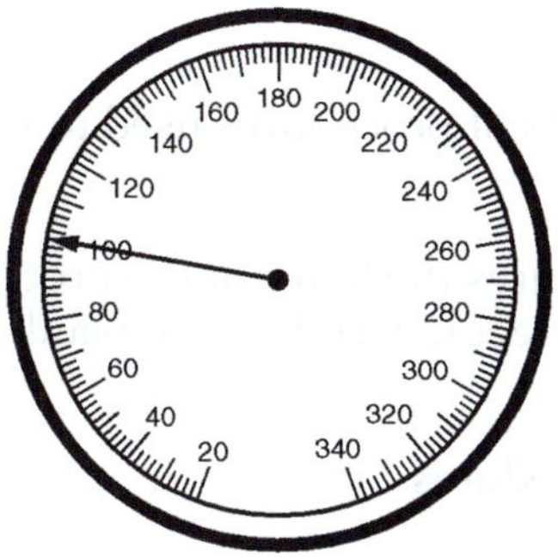

7. ______________

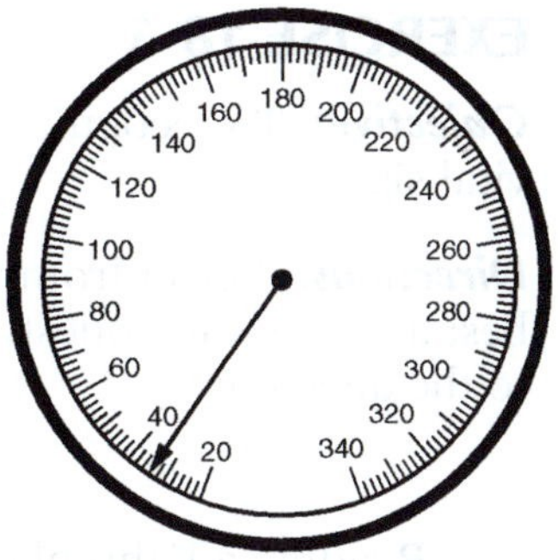

8. ______________

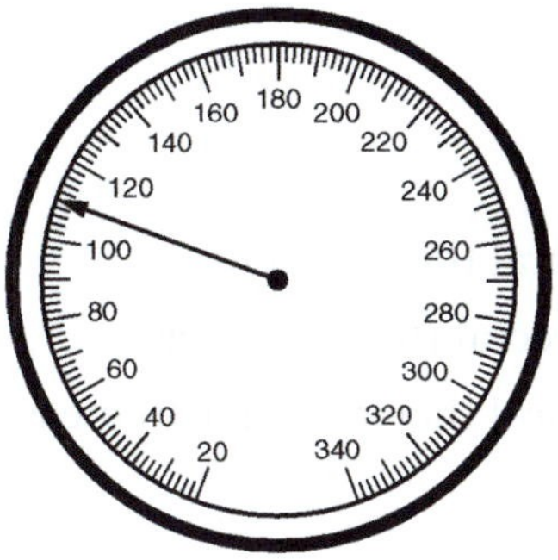

9. ______________

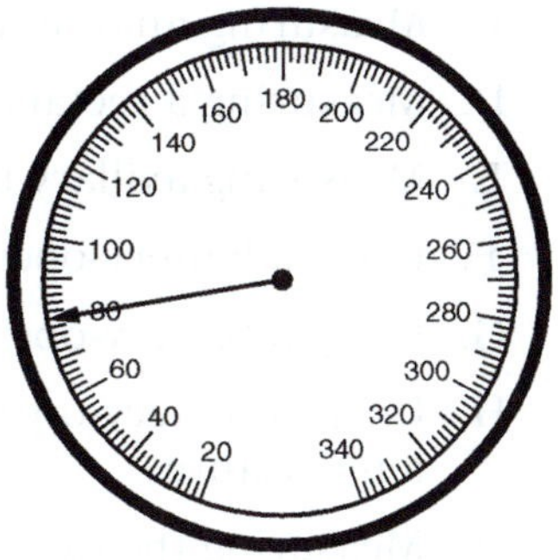

10. ______________

11. ______________

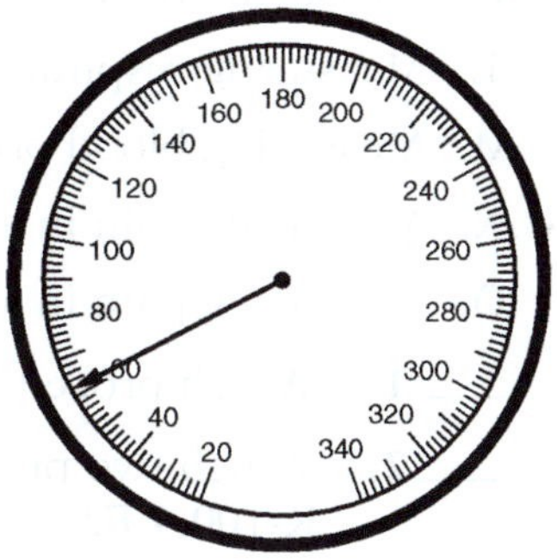

12. ______________

EXERCISE 18-5

Objective: To recognize important aspects of procedures used to measure vital signs.

Directions: Select from the list of procedures the letter of the procedure that best answers each question. Write the correct letter(s) on the blank line next to the question.

List of Procedures

A. Reading a Fahrenheit thermometer
B. Reading a centigrade thermometer
C. Measuring an oral temperature
D. Measuring a rectal temperature
E. Measuring axillary temperature
F. Using a battery-operated electronic oral thermometer
G. Using a battery-operated electronic rectal thermometer
H. Using a battery-operated electronic oral thermometer to measure axillary temperature
I. Measuring the radial pulse
J. Measuring the apical pulse
K. Measuring the apical pulse deficit
L. Measuring respirations
M. Measuring blood pressure
N. Measuring pain in a child
O. Measuring pain in an adult

_____**1.** Which procedure requires the use of a sphygmomanometer?

_____**2.** Which two procedures could be used to get a measurement of R-100.4°F?

_____**3.** In which three procedures would you observe the rate, rhythm, and force?

_____**4.** Which three procedures involve the use of a stethoscope?

_____**5.** For which procedure would the normal adult rate be 16–20 times per minute?

_____**6.** Which procedure could involve two nursing assistants working together?

_____**7.** Which procedure involves counting by twos (e.g., 2, 4, 6, 8)?

_____**8.** Which three procedures would you follow if your immediate supervisor asked you to take vital signs?

_____**9.** Which two procedures could you use to measure temperature if the patient is receiving oxygen by cannula, catheter, facemask, or oxygen tent?

_____**10.** Which procedure involves a happy and sad face scale?

_____**11.** Which procedure involves using a 0–10 rating scale?

EXERCISE 18-6

Objective: To recognize important aspects of abnormal respirations.

Directions: Select the letters of the abnormal respiration from the following word list that match the definitions provided. Write the letter next to the matching description.

Word List

A. Stertorous respiration
B. Abdominal respiration
C. Shallow respiration
D. Irregular respiration
E. Cheyne-Stokes respiration

_____**1.** Breathing with only the upper part of the lungs.

_____**2.** Using mostly abdominal muscles for breathing.

_____**3.** A pattern where the breathing is slow and shallow, then faster and deeper to peak, then slow and shallow again. The breathing may stop for several seconds before beginning the pattern again.

_____**4.** Abnormal sounds (e.g., snoring) while breathing.

_____**5.** The depth and rate are not steady.

THE NURSING ASSISTANT IN ACTION

1. Your male patient is from Germany and does not speak English very well. You ask him about his pain level. He says, "I am fine. How are you?" When he moves in bed, you notice he is sweating and is holding his abdominal area where he was stitched. How should you assess his pain correctly and what should you do?

____

____

____

____

2. A 90-year-old woman with dementia was recently admitted to your unit. You are assigned to give her a bed bath. You notice she has severe contractures in both arms and legs and a large pressure ulcer on her buttocks. She cries out in pain throughout the day and especially when you go to turn her. She does not use words but has repetitive speech that makes no sense. How should you assess her pain and offer her care?

____

____

3. A relatively new nursing assistant has been working on your unit for the past 2 weeks. She confides in you that she really does not know how to use the equipment used to take vital signs. She tells you she has been looking at the vital signs on her patients obtained from the other shift and has been changing the numbers slightly when asked to obtain and record her patient's vital signs during her shift. What should you do?

4. You obtain an oral temperature on a patient. His temperature reading is 100.0°F. You feel his skin. It is warm and dry. He is not sweating. He is not complaining of feeling ill. You notice his dinner tray was just cleared. What should you do?

5. A dialysis patient recently arrived to your floor after having her right breast removed because of cancer. She has an AV shunt in her left arm. You must obtain her blood pressure. What should you do?

LEARNING ACTIVITIES

1. Listen to a friend's chest with a stethoscope. What sounds do you hear? Find a friend who will allow you to locate his apical pulse and radial pulse. Try to determine his pulse deficit. Discuss your findings with your peer and instructor.
2. Using a stethoscope and sphygmomanometer, take a friend's blood pressure in the left arm. Wait 3 minutes and try taking the blood pressure while the person is lying down. Wait 3 minutes and then take the blood pressure while standing. What do you notice about the readings you obtained? What do you think the reason for this is? Discuss your findings with your peer and instructor.

PROCEDURE CHECKLISTS

PROCEDURE 18-1: USING A BATTERY-OPERATED ELECTRONIC THERMOMETER

Name: ____________________ Date: ____________________

STEPS	S	U	COMMENTS
1. Assemble equipment a. Disposable plastic probe cover b. Alcohol swabs c. Battery-operated electronic thermometer d. Pen e. Vital sign form used in your institution			
2. Identify the patient by checking the ID bracelet.			
3. Inform the patient that you are going to take his temperature.			
4. Wash your hands.			
5. Provide privacy and comfort for the patient.			
6. Remove the probe from its stored position and clean with an alcohol swab.			
7. Insert the probe into the probe cover or sheath.			
8. Insert the covered probe into the patient's mouth slowly until the tip is at the base under the tongue.			
9. Hold the probe in the patient's mouth.			
10. Wait for the sensor to alarm indicating that a temperature reading has been obtained.			
11. Record the temperature on the vital sign form used in your institution.			
12. Without touching it, discard the used probe cover into the waste receptacle.			
13. Clean the probe with an alcohol swab.			
14. Return the probe to its stored position in the face of the thermometer.			
15. Store the thermometer in its charging stand when it is not in use.			
16. Make the patient comfortable and replace the call light.			
17. Lower the bed to a position of safety.			
18. Raise the side rails when ordered or indicated.			
19. Wash your hands.			

20. Report to your supervisor • The temperature was taken • Any abnormal or unusual findings			
21. Record temperature measurement on patient flow sheet.			

Charting:

____

____

____

____

Date of Satisfactory Completion ____________________

Instructor's Signature ____________________

PROCEDURE 18-2: USING A TYMPANIC (EAR) THERMOMETER

Name: ____________________ Date: ____________________

STEPS	S	U	COMMENTS
1. Assemble your equipment a. Disposable plastic tympanic cover b. Battery-operated tympanic thermometer c. Vital sign form used in your institution d. Pen			
2. Identify the patient by checking the ID bracelet.			
3. Inform the patient that you are going to take her temperature.			
4. Wash your hands.			
5. Provide privacy and comfort for the patient.			
6. Remove the thermometer from its stored position. Insert the cone-shape end of the thermometer into a disposable tympanic cover and attach.			
7. Position the patient's head so one ear is directly in front of you.			
8. For an adult or child, pull the outer ear up and back to open the ear canal. For an infant, pull the ear straight back.			
9. Gently insert the tympanic thermometer into the patient's ear. Use a slow, slight rocking motion, as needed, to insert the probe as far as possible and seal the ear canal.			
10. Watch and wait until the sensor sounds indicating that a temperature measurement has been obtained.			
11. Read and record the digitally displayed temperature on the vital sign form used in your institution.			
12. Without touching it, eject and discard the used probe cover immediately into the waste receptacle.			
13. Store the thermometer in its charging stand whenever it is not in use.			
14. Make the patient comfortable and replace the call light.			
15. Lower the bed to a position of safety.			
16. Raise the side rails when ordered or appropriate for patient safety.			
17. Wash your hands.			

18. Report to your supervisor • That you obtained a tympanic temperature • Any abnormal or unusual observations			

Charting:

____

____

____

____

Date of Satisfactory Completion ____________________

Instructor's Signature ____________________

PROCEDURE 18-3: USING A BATTERY-OPERATED ELECTRONIC RECTAL THERMOMETER

Name: ____________________ Date: ____________________

STEPS	S	U	COMMENTS
1. Assemble your equipment a. Disposable thermometer probe cover b. Battery-operated electronic thermometer with red, rectal probe attachment c. Lubricant (water-soluble) d. Alcohol swabs e. Vital signs form used in your institution			
2. Identify the patient by checking the ID bracelet.			
3. Inform the patient that you are going to take his temperature.			
4. Wash your hands and put on gloves.			
5. Provide privacy for the patient.			
6. Raise the rails on the opposite side of the bed.			
7. Raise the bed to a comfortable working height.			
8. Assist the patient to a side-lying position.			
9. Check to be sure the rectal probe connector is in the appropriate receptacle on the base of the thermometer.			
10. Remove the probe from its stored position, and clean it with an alcohol swab.			
11. Insert the probe into a probe cover or sheath. Lubricate the tip of the probe cover.			
12. Insert the covered probe slowly and gently through the patient's anus into the rectum ½".			
13. Wait for the alarm indicating that a temperature reading has been obtained, then remove the probe from the rectum.			
14. Dispose of the probe in the waste receptacle.			
15. Discard your gloves and wash your hands.			
16. Clean the probe with an alcohol swab.			
17. Return the probe to its stored position in the thermometer.			
18. Record the temperature on the vital signs form.			
19. Store the thermometer in its charging stand whenever it's not in use.			

20. Make the patient comfortable and place the call light within easy reach.			
21. Set the bed to a position of safety.			
22. Raise the side rails when ordered, indicated, and appropriate for patient safety.			
23. Wash your hands.			
24. Report to your supervisor • That you took a rectal temperature on the patient • How the patient tolerated the procedure • Any unusual or abnormal observations			

Charting:

____

____

____

____

Date of Satisfactory Completion ____________________

Instructor's Signature ____________________

PROCEDURE 18-4: USING AN ELECTRONIC THERMOMETER TO MEASURE AXILLARY TEMPERATURE

Name: ______________________ Date: ______________________

STEPS	S	U	COMMENTS
1. Assemble your equipment a. Plastic probe cover b. Battery-operated electronic thermometer with oral attachment probe c. Vital sign form used in your institution d. Pen			
2. Identify the patient by checking the ID bracelet.			
3. Inform the patient that you are going to take her temperature.			
4. Wash your hands.			
5. Provide privacy and comfort for the patient.			
6. Remove the probe from its stored position. Insert it into a probe cover.			
7. Put the covered probe in the center of the patient's armpit, or axilla.			
8. Put the patient's arm across her chest. Hold the probe in place.			
9. Wait until the sensor alarms indicating a temperature reading has been obtained. Remove the probe from the patient's axilla.			
10. Discard the used probe cover in a waste receptacle.			
11. Return the probe to its stored position.			
12. Record the temperature on the vital sign form.			
13. Wash your hands.			
14. Store the thermometer in its charging stand when it is not in use.			
15. Make the patient comfortable and replace the call light.			
16. Lower the bed to a position of safety.			
17. Raise the side rails when ordered or indicated.			

18. Report to your supervisor • That you obtained an axillary temperature measurement • Any abnormal or unusual observations			

Charting:

____

____

____

____

Date of Satisfactory Completion ____________________

Instructor's Signature ____________________

PROCEDURE 18-5: MEASURING THE RADIAL PULSE

Name: ______________________ Date: ______________________

STEPS	S	U	COMMENTS
1. Assemble your equipment a. Watch with a second hand b. Vital sign form used in your institution c. Pen			
2. Identify the patient by checking the ID bracelet.			
3. Inform the patient that you are going to take his pulse.			
4. Wash your hands.			
5. Provide privacy and comfort for the patient.			
6. Place the patient is a seated or lying position.			
7. The patient's hand and arm should be well supported and resting comfortably below the heart.			
8. Find the pulse by placing the middle three fingers on the palm side of the patient's wrist in a line with his thumb directly next to the wrist bone. Press very lightly until you feel the beat. (Do not feel with your thumb, as your thumb has its own pulse, and you may count your pulse instead of the patient's.) When you have found the pulse, note the rate, rhythm, and force.			
9. Look at the position of your second hand on your watch. Start counting the pulse beats that you feel until the second hand comes back to the same number on the clock. a. Method A: Count the pulse beats for 1 full minute and report the full minute. Always use this method if the patient's pulse is irregular. b. Method B: Count for 30 seconds, until the second hand on the watch is opposite its position where you started. Then multiply the number of beats by 2, and record that number. For example, if you count 30 beats for 30 seconds, the count for 1 full minute is 60. Use this method only if the patient is known to have a regular heart rate.			
10. Record the pulse count on the vital sign form used in your institution.			
11. Make the patient comfortable and replace the call light.			
12. Lower the bed to a position of safety.			

13. Raise the side rails when ordered or indicated.			
14. Report to your supervisor • That you took the patient's pulse. • Any pulse rate over 100 or under 60, or any irregular pulse rhythm • Any unusual observations			

Charting:

____

____

____

____

Date of Satisfactory Completion ________________

Instructor's Signature ________________

PROCEDURE 18-6: MEASURING THE APICAL PULSE

Name: ____________________ Date: ____________________

STEPS	S	U	COMMENTS
1. Assemble your equipment a. Stethoscope and antiseptic wipe b. Watch with a second hand c. Vital sign form in your institution. d. Pen			
2. Identify the patient by checking the ID bracelet.			
3. Inform the patient that you are going to take her apical pulse.			
4. Wash your hands.			
5. Provide privacy and comfort for the patient.			
6. Clean the earpieces and diaphragm on the stethoscope with an antiseptic wipe. Put the earpieces in your ears. Warm the diaphragm of the stethoscope by holding it tightly for a few seconds.			
7. Uncover the left side of the patient's chest. Avoid overexposing the patient.			
8. Locate the apex of the patient's heart under the patient's left breast, located at the fifth intercostal space and to the left of the sternum. Place the diaphragm of the stethoscope on the patient's skin and listen for heart sounds.			
9. Count the heart sounds for 1 full minute.			
10. Write the full minute count on the vital signs sheet.			
11. Cover and make the patient comfortable.			
12. Replace the call light.			
13. Lower the bed to a position of safety.			
14. Raise the side rails if ordered or indicated.			
15. Clean the earpieces of the stethoscope with antiseptic wipes. Return equipment to its proper place.			
16. Wash your hands.			

17. Report to your supervisor • That you took the patient's apical pulse • The apical pulse rate • Any unusual or abnormal observations			

Charting:

____

____

____

____

Date of Satisfactory Completion ____________________

Instructor's Signature ____________________

PROCEDURE 18-7: MEASURING THE APICAL PULSE DEFICIT (ADVANCED PROCEDURE)

Name: ______________________ Date: ______________________

STEPS	S	U	COMMENTS
1. Assemble your equipment a. Stethoscope and antiseptic wipe b. Watch with a second hand c. Vital sign form in your institution d. Pen			
2. Identify the patient by checking the ID bracelet.			
3. Inform the patient that you are going to take his pulse.			
4. Wash your hands.			
5. Provide privacy and comfort for the patient.			
6. There are two methods of taking the apical pulse deficit a. Method A: Two nursing assistants do this procedure together at the same time. One counts the radial pulse and the other counts the apical pulse for 1 full minute. The difference between the two pulses is known as the *apical pulse deficit*. This is the most accurate method. b. Method B: The nursing assistant first takes the apical pulse, then the radial pulse. The difference between the two pulses is known as the *apical pulse deficit*. However, because the readings are not taken at the same time, this is not quite as accurate as method A.			
7. Count the apical pulse and the radial pulse for 1 full minute and record both figures.			
8. Record the difference between the figures as the pulse deficit.			
9. Make the patient comfortable and replace the call light.			
10. Lower the bed to a position of safety.			
11. Raise the side rails when ordered or indicated.			
12. Clean the equipment and return to its proper place.			
13. Wash your hands.			

14. Report to your supervisor • That you took the patient's apical pulse deficit • The apical pulse rate • The radial pulse rate • The pulse deficit • Any unusual or abnormal observations			

Charting:

____

____

____

____

Date of Satisfactory Completion ______________

Instructor's Signature ______________

PROCEDURE 18-8: MEASURING RESPIRATIONS

Name: ______________________ Date: ______________________

STEPS	S	U	COMMENTS
1. Assemble your equipment a. Watch with a second hand b. Vital sign form used in your institution c. Pen			
2. Identify the patient by checking the ID bracelet.			
3. Wash your hands.			
4. Provide privacy and comfort for the patient.			
5. Hold the patient's wrist as though you were taking a pulse. This way he will not know that you are watching his breathing. Count the respirations, without him knowing it, immediately after counting his pulse rate.			
6. If the patient is a child who is crying or restless, wait until he is quiet before counting respirations. If a child is asleep, count his respirations before he wakes up. Always count a child's pulse and respirations before measuring temperature, as taking a temperature may upset a child, which would elevate pulse and respirations.			
7. One rise and one fall of the patient's chest counts as one respiration.			
8. If you cannot clearly see the chest rise and fall, fold the patient's arms across his chest. You can feel his breathing as you hold his wrist.			
9. Check the position of the second hand on the watch. Count "1" when you see the patient's chest rising as he breathes in. The next time his chest rises, count "2." Continue doing this for 1 full minute. (Many states require a full minute count as a standard of care for elderly persons.) Report the number you count in that minute of respirations.			
10. You may be permitted to count for 30 seconds. Multiply the 30-second count of respirations by 2.			
11. If the patient's breathing rhythm is irregular, count for a full minute. Observe the depth of the breathing while counting respirations.			
12. Write down the number you counted on the vital sign form used by your institution.			
13. Note whether respirations were noisy or labored.			
14. Make the patient comfortable and replace the call light.			

15. Lower the bed to a position of safety.			
16. Raise the side rails when ordered or appropriate for patient safety.			
17. Wash your hands.			
18. Report to your supervisor • The rate of the patient's respirations • Whether the respirations were noisy or labored • Whether the respirations were irregular • The amount of time they were measured • If the respirations were less than 12 or more than 28 per minute • Any abnormal or unusual observations			

Charting:

____

____

____

____

Date of Satisfactory Completion ______________

Instructor's Signature ______________

PROCEDURE 18-9: MEASURING BLOOD PRESSURE USING A SPHYGMOMANOMETER

Name: ____________________ Date: ____________________

STEPS	S	U	COMMENTS
1. Assemble your equipment a. Sphygmomanometer (blood pressure cuff) b. Stethoscope c. Antiseptic wipes d. Vital sign form used in your institution e. Pen			
2. Identify the patient by checking the ID bracelet.			
3. Tell the patient that you are going to measure his blood pressure.			
4. Wash your hands.			
5. Provide privacy and comfort for the patient.			
6. Raise the rails on the opposite side of the bed.			
7. Raise the bed to a comfortable working height.			
8. Wipe the earpieces and diaphragm of the stethoscope with antiseptic swabs.			
9. Have the patient resting quietly. He should be either lying down or sitting up in a chair.			
10. If you are using the mercury apparatus, the measuring scale should be level with your eyes.			
11. The patient's arm should be bare up to the shoulder, or the patient's sleeve should be well above the elbow without limiting or constricting circulation.			
12. The patient's arm from the elbow down should be resting, palm up to the ceiling, fully extended on the bed or the arm of a chair.			
13. Leave the area clear where you will place the bell or diaphragm of the stethoscope.			
14. Unroll the blood pressure cuff and loosen the valve on the bulb. Make sure all air is out of the cuff.			
15. Snugly and smoothly, wrap the cuff around the patient's arm ½" to 1" above the elbow. (Do not wrap it so tightly that the patient is uncomfortable from the pressure.) You may need to use a different size cuff for a patient with very small or very large arms.			
16. Be sure the sphygmomanometer is in position so you can read the numbers easily.			
17. Put the earpieces of the stethoscope into your ears.			

18. With your fingertips, find the patient's brachial pulse at the inner aspect of the arm above the elbow (brachial artery). This is where you will place the diaphragm of the stethoscope. The diaphragm should be held firmly against the skin, but should not touch the cuff.			
19. Tighten the thumbscrew of the valve to close it by turning it clockwise. (Be careful not to turn it too tightly. If you do, you will have trouble releasing it.)			
20. Hold the stethoscope in place. Inflate the cuff quickly. When the radial pulse is no longer felt, inflate the cuff an additional 30 mmHg.			
21. Open the valve counterclockwise. This allows the air to escape. Let air out slowly until the sound of the pulse comes back. A few seconds must go by without sounds. If you do hear sounds immediately, you must deflate the cuff and reinflate the cuff to a higher pressure.			
22. Listen for blood pressure sounds. Note the number the pointer passes as you hear the first sound. This is the systolic pressure. Continue releasing the air from the cuff. When you hear the last beat, note the number. This is the diastolic pressure.			
23. Deflate the cuff completely and remove it from the patient's arm.			
24. Record your reading on the vital sign form.			
25. After using the blood pressure cuff, roll it up over the sphygmomanometer and replace it in the case.			
26. Wipe the earpieces and diaphragm of the stethoscope again with an antiseptic swab.			
27. Make the patient comfortable and replace the call light.			
28. Lower the bed to a position of safety.			
29. Raise the side rails if ordered or indicated.			
30. Wash your hands.			
31. Report to your supervisor • That you measured the patient's blood pressure • The time that you measured the blood pressure • Any unusual or abnormal observations			

Charting:

____

____

____

____

Date of Satisfactory Completion ______________

Instructor's Signature ______________

PROCEDURE 18-10: MEASURING HEIGHT OF A PATIENT IN BED

Name: ______________________ Date: ______________________

STEPS	S	U	COMMENTS
1. Assemble your equipment a. Measuring tape b. Vital sign form used in your institution c. Pen			
2. Identify the patient by checking the ID bracelet.			
3. Inform the patient that you are going to measure her height.			
4. Wash your hands.			
5. Provide privacy and comfort for the patient.			
6. Raise the rails on the opposite side of the bed.			
7. Raise the bed to a comfortable working height.			
8. Lower the bed rail nearest to you.			
9. Have the patient lie on her back as straight as possible with limbs straight.			
10. Make certain the bottom sheet is pulled taut without wrinkles.			
11. With the patient on her back, ask her to stretch as much as possible.			
12. Place a mark on the bottom sheet at the top of the patient's head and at the bottom of the patient's heel.			
13. Measure between these two marks.			
14. Record the patient's height (in centimeters or inches) on the vital sign form used in your institution.			
15. Make the patient comfortable and replace the call light.			
16. Lower the bed to a position of safety.			
17. Raise the side rails when ordered or indicated.			

18. Report to your supervisor • That you measured the patient's height • Any unusual observations			

Charting:

____

____

____

____

Date of Satisfactory Completion ____________________

Instructor's Signature ____________________

PROCEDURE 18-11: MEASURING THE WEIGHT OF A PATIENT IN BED

Name: ____________________ Date: ____________________

STEPS	S	U	COMMENTS
1. Assemble your equipment a. Bed scale b. Pen			
2. Identify the patient by checking the ID bracelet.			
3. Inform the patient that you are going to measure his weight using a bed scale.			
4. For safety reasons, always obtain assistance from another nursing assistant before operating the bed scale.			
5. Wash your hands.			
6. Provide privacy and comfort for the patient.			
7. Raise the rails on the opposite side of the bed.			
8. Raise the bed to a comfortable working height.			
9. Lower the bed rail nearest to you.			
10. Place a protective plastic covering over the bed scale sling.			
11. Balance the scale with the sling attached.			
12. Assist the patient to roll to his far side, facing away from you.			
13. Slide the bed scale sling lengthwise next to the patient and under the patient's head.			
14. Assist the patient to roll to his side closest to you and facing you.			
15. Pull the bed scale sling under the patient and assist the patient to roll on his back, centered over the bed scale sling.			
16. Center the bed scale over the bed and carefully lower the circular weighing arms of the scale over the patient and attach them securely to the sling bars.			
17. Instruct the patient to keep his arms next to his side while being weighed.			
18. Lock the hydraulic mechanism.			
19. Reassure the patient.			
20. Pump the hand of the bed scale with long, slow strokes to raise the patient a few inches off the bed. The patient in the sling should hang freely over the bed.			

21. Check to be sure nothing is pulling against the sling, which may affect the weight. Lift patient tubing (e.g., IV, catheter) away from the sling.			
22. Push the operate button and read the patient's weight on the digital display.			
23. Record the patient's weight (lb or kg) on the vital sign form used in your institution.			
24. Press in on the bed scale handle to release the hydraulic and lower the patient back on to the bed.			
25. Release the locks on the bed scale and remove it from the patient.			
26. Assist the patient to roll off the sling by turning the patient side to side and moving the sling out of the way.			
27. Make the patient comfortable and replace the call light.			
28. Lower the bed to a position of safety.			
29. Raise the side rails when ordered or indicated.			
30. Report to your supervisor • That you measured the patient's weight • Any unusual observation			

Charting:

____

____

____

____

Date of Satisfactory Completion ____________________

Instructor's Signature ____________________

PROCEDURE 18-12: MEASURING THE PATIENT'S ABDOMINAL GIRTH

Name: ____________________ Date: ____________________

STEPS	S	U	COMMENTS
1. Assemble your equipment a. Measuring tape b. Marking pen			
2. Identify the patient by checking the ID bracelet.			
3. Inform the patient that you are going to measure his abdominal girth.			
4. Wash your hands.			
5. Provide privacy.			
6. Raise the rails on the opposite side of the bed.			
7. Raise the bed to a comfortable working height.			
8. Lower the bed rail nearest you.			
9. Position the patient in a supine position.			
10. Move aside the gown or any clothing that interferes with the ability to place the measuring tape around the abdomen on the patient's skin.			
11. Measure the girth on the patient in the same location each time.			
12. Slide the measuring tape under the patient's back, bringing tape up to the umbilicus on both sides of the patient. Be certain the tape is lying flat and not twisted under the patient.			
13. Place the measuring tape snugly across the abdomen at the widest part, generally at the level of umbilicus ("belly button").			
14. Take the measurement in centimeters at the end of expiration.			
15. Record the abdominal girth measurement on the vital sign flow sheet.			
16. Make the patient comfortable and replace the call light.			
17. Lower the bed to a position of safety.			
18. Raise the side rails when ordered or indicated.			

19. Report to your supervisor • That you measured the patient's abdominal girth • Any unusual observations			

Charting:

____

____

____

____

Date of Satisfactory Completion ____________________

Instructor's Signature ____________________

19

The Gastrointestinal System and Related Care

Key Terms Review

Match the key terms in the right column with the definitions in the left column by placing the letter of each correct answer in the space provided.

_____ **1.** Consists primarily of the mouth, esophagus, stomach, small intestines, and large intestines.

_____ **2.** Breaking down the food that is eaten into a form that can be used by the body cells; this process is both mechanical and chemical.

_____ **3.** Part of the digestive process in which digestive juices and enzymes break down food into usable parts.

_____ **4.** The secretion of the salivary glands into the mouth; it moistens the food and helps in swallowing; it contains an enzyme (protein) that helps digest starches.

_____ **5.** The first, smaller portion of the bowel, including the duodenum, where most of digestion and food breakdown occurs; also known as the small bowel.

_____ **6.** The first loop of the small intestine.

_____ **7.** Responsible for manufacturing bile and is a storage area for glucose; also is the place where toxins, or poisons, are removed from the blood.

_____ **8.** Organ that produces digestive enzymes responsible for food breakdown in the small intestines; also produces insulin and glucagon hormones.

Terms

A. Small intestine
B. Duodenum
C. Appendicitis
D. Pancreas
E. Liver
F. Bile
G. Sphincter
H. Anus
I. Rectum
J. Large intestine
K. Saliva
L. Digestion
M. Absorption
N. Gastrointestinal (GI) system
O. Diarrhea
P. Constipation
Q. Evacuation
R. Sims' position

_____ 9. Substance manufactured by the liver that helps the food breakdown process.

_____ 10. Inflammation (swelling and irritation) and infection of the appendix, typically with pain in the right lower quadrant; surgery called an *appendectomy* is usually performed to remove the appendix.

_____ 11. Distal colon that absorbs water from stool.

_____ 12. The lowest portion of the large intestine called the *sigmoid* (*S*-shape) colon that stores fecal material and leads to the anus.

_____ 13. Muscular opening that controls elimination of stool from the rectum.

_____ 14. Ring-shaped muscle that surrounds and controls a natural opening in the body, such as the anus.

_____ 15. Uninterrupted, without a stop.

_____ 16. Alternating; stopping and beginning again.

_____ 17. Abnormally frequent discharge of fluid fecal material from the bowel.

_____ 18. Difficult and infrequent defecation with passage of unduly hard and dry fecal material.

_____ 19. Discharge of the contents of the lower bowel through the rectum and anus.

_____ 20. Hard, putty-like fecal material resulting from prolonged retention of stool in the rectum.

_____ 21. Patient positioned on the left side with the right knee bent toward the chest, often called the *enema position*.

_____ 22. Procedure of evacuation or washing out of waste materials (feces or stool) from a person's lower bowel.

_____ 23. Intestinal gas.

_____ 24. A surgically created opening for the discharge of body wastes (urine or feces). The part of the new opening that can be seen is called a *stoma*.

_____ 25. Collecting pouch usually attached to the skin around the stoma with adhesive.

_____ 26. An opening made through the abdomen to the stomach for the purpose of feeding.

_____ 27. Tube inserted into the abdomen for the introduction of fluids.

_____ 28. The actual opening or end of the ureter, or the small or large intestine that can be seen protruding through the abdominal wall. This surgically made opening connects the urinary or intestinal tract with the outside, such as in a urostomy or colostomy.

S. Fecal impaction

T. Enema

U. Flatus

V. Peristalsis

W. Suction

X. Nasogastric tube

Y. Lavage

Z. Gavage

AA. Continuous

BB. Intermittent

CC. Ostomy

DD. Ostomy appliance

EE. Gastrostomy

FF. Gastrostomy tube (GT)

GG. Stoma

HH. Rectal irrigation

II. Retention

_____ **29.** Using negative pressure to remove material, usually fluid.

_____ **30.** The washing out of the stomach through a nasogastric tube, usually with normal saline.

_____ **31.** Feeding through a nasogastric tube.

_____ **32.** A tube placed through one of the patient's nostrils, down the back of the throat, and through the esophagus into the patient's stomach.

_____ **33.** Rhythmic contractions of the muscle walls of the small and large intestines.

_____ **34.** Repeated washing out of the rectum; clean water runs into the rectum, gas (flatus) and water run out of the rectum, as in the Harris flush.

_____ **35.** Occurs when the patient keeps the enema fluid (oil) in the rectum for 20 minutes.

MULTIPLE-CHOICE QUESTIONS

Circle the letter next to the word or statement that best completes the sentence or answers the question.

1. Good nutrition and a functioning ___________ are vital to a patient's health.
a. nexus
b. apex
c. bowel
d. tube

2. A large amount of ___________ is necessary for the chemical breakdown of food.
a. mercury
b. lead
c. water
c. copper

3. The lining of the duodenum is composed of thousands of
a. tilli.
b. silli.
c. billi.
d. villi.

4. As a person ages, what change occurs to the gastrointestinal system?
a. The flow of saliva increases.
b. The number of taste buds increases.
c. Chewing and swallowing are more difficult.
d. Absorption of vitamins and minerals increases.

5. _________ is a disease/disorder of the gastrointestinal system.
a. Myocardial infarction
b. Asthma
c. Cholecystitis
d. A urinary tract infection

6. ________ are growths on the lining of the intestines that can become cancerous if not treated.
a. Jauntoids
b. Rectoids
c. Polyps
d. All of the above

7. For removing fluids from a patient's body, the degree of suction most commonly used is
a. high.
b. low.

c. intermittent.
d. b and c.

8. Before giving fluid through the NG tube, listen with a stethoscope over the stomach while inserting air into the tube. The sound of air in the stomach means
a. the tube is not properly placed.
b. the lungs are inflating.
c. the tube is loose.
d. the tube is properly placed in the stomach.

9. If you notice that the formerly greenish fluid in the drainage container connected to the nasogastric tube has suddenly become bright red, what would you do?
a. Empty the container when it is full.
b. Measure and record the amount and color of the drainage.
c. Notify your immediate supervisor at once.
d. Tell the patient at once.

10. When administering a tube feeding, the formula
a. must be chilled and shaken thoroughly.
b. is given when it has reached boiling.
c. should be room temperature.
d. must be 98.6° F.

11. If the patient does not have a functioning GI tract, he may be able to receive a venous feeding called
a. total parenteral nutrition (TPN).
b. total food nutrition (TFN).
c. fast-food nutrition (FFN).
d. venous food nutrition (VFN).

12. If a patient has diarrhea, it is important to note the amount of ________ output, because it may indicate dehydration.
a. blood
b. work
c. lavage
d. urine

13. A device used to relieve flatus is
a. high bulk foods.
b. a rectal connector.
c. a rectal tube with connected bag.
d. a bowel bag.

14. A nursing assistant never
a. inserts a rectal tube.
b. administers a medicated rectal suppository.
c. is asked to place a non-medicated rectal suppository.
d. gives a back rub.

15. If a colon is diseased, a surgical procedure ____________ may be performed.
a. to create a stoma
b. to staple stomach
c. called a *hysterectomy*
d. all of the above

16. _____ and _____ are two diseases commonly treated with a stoma.
a. AIDS; pneumocystic disease
b. Diabetes; hypertension
c. Inflammatory bowel disease (IBD); Crohn's disease
d. Diaphoresis; vertigo

17. The nursing assistant should immediately report
a. bleeding around the stoma.
b. feces coming from the stoma.
c. odor coming from the stoma.
d. bleeding from the stoma that doesn't stop.

18. What psychological changes might you expect to note in a patient with an ostomy?
a. Anxiety
b. Depression
c. Being quiet and withdrawn
d. All of the above.

19. If the patient is able, the best time to empty an ostomy bag is when the patient is
a. on the toilet.
b. in bed.
c. has visitors.
d. sleeping.

20. The nursing assistant should place the patient in which position when a tube feeding occurs to prevent aspiration?
   a. Supine
   b. Sims'
   c. Semi-Fowler's or Fowler's
   d. Prone

21. Why is it important to encourage a BRAT diet when diarrhea occurs?
   a. The bananas and rice help to restore nutrients lost when diarrhea occurs and slow down the loss of fluids.
   b. The applesauce helps to thicken the stool.
   c. The tea restores lost fluids.
   d. All of the above.

22. What food(s) on the patient's food tray should the nursing assistant encourage the patient to eat if he is experiencing constipation?
   a. Chocolate pudding and the banana
   b. Grilled cheese sandwich
   c. Warm prune juice and oatmeal with lots of milk stirred into it
   d. Side dish of rice and the tea

23. Which position is used when fecally disimpacting a patient?
   a. Sims'
   b. Supine
   c. Knee–chest
   d. Prone

24. At which temperature should a cleansing enema solution be prepared?
   a. 105° F
   b. 32° C
   c. 98.6° F
   d. Room temperature

25. Which type of enema may be administered approximately 20 minutes after an oil retention enema is given?
   a. Soap suds
   b. Harris flush
   c. Tapwater
   d. Saline

TRUE OR FALSE QUESTIONS

Determine whether each question is true or false. In the space provided, write "T" for true and "F" for false. If the statement is false, rewrite it on the line provided to make it a true statement.

_____ **1.** Varicose veins of the anal canal are called *hemorrhoids*.

____

_____ **2.** When fluids are removed with a gravity nasogastric tube, it is important that the collecting container is higher than the patient's body.

____

_____ **3.** The nursing assistant is responsible for watching the level of the feeding and making sure the formula is being fed as fast as possible into the patient's stomach.

____

_____ **4.** For adults, the NG tube must be flushed with 75 cc of water before and after the feeding or every 8 hours.

____

_____ **5.** The cause of constipation is lack of adequate fluid intake.

____

_____ **6.** A physician's order is necessary to remove a fecal impaction.

____

_____ **7.** Practicing with the patient to empty his ostomy bag helps her develop independence and confidence in her ability to care for it.

____

_____ **8.** The liver makes bile, stores glucose, and removes toxins in our body.

____

_____ **9.** When preparing a saline enema, place 2 teaspoons of salt into 1000 ccs of water.

____

_____ **10.** When performing an enema, it is essential to make sure the person is not cramping, feeling dizzy, or that his heart rate is dropping.

____

FILL-IN-THE-BLANK QUESTIONS

Provide the meaning of the following abbreviations.

1. GI _______________

2. GT _______________

3. *C. diff* _______________

4. NG _______________

5. NPO _______________

6. PEG _______________

7. PEG-J _______________

8. NA _______________

9. TPN _______________

10. BRAT _______________

11. A&D _______________

12. IBD _______________

EXERCISE 19-1

Objective: To recognize and correctly spell words related to the gastrointestinal system and related care.

Directions: Label the diagram in Figure 19-1 with the correct words from the following word list.

Word List

Mouth	Rectum	Pharynx
Appendix	Tongue	Gallbladder
Large intestine	Stomach	Liver
Teeth	Small intestine	Esophagus
Pancreas	Salivary glands	Duodenum

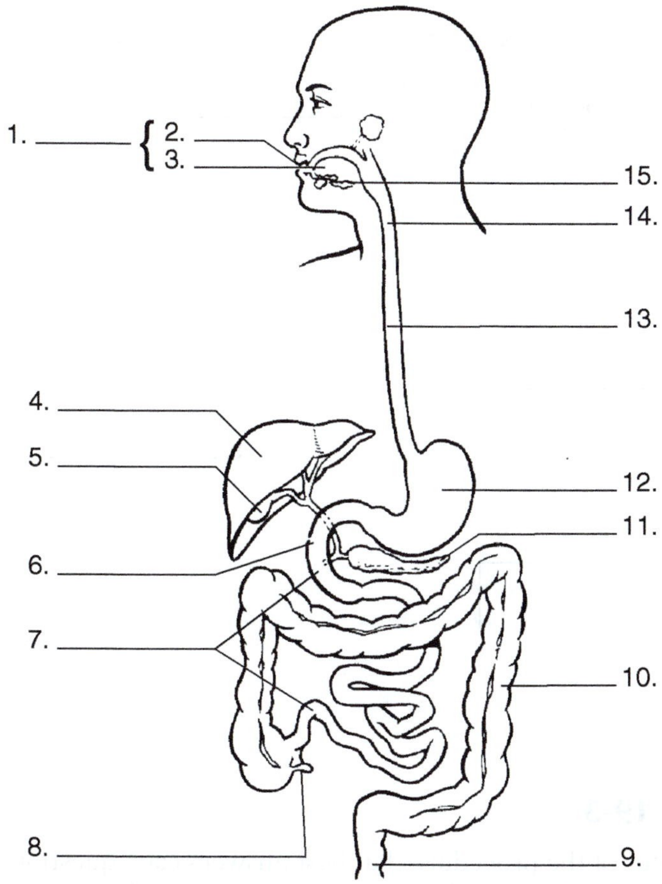

FIGURE 19-1

EXERCISE 19-2

Objective: To recognize and correctly spell words related to tube feedings and stomach lavage.

Directions: Label the diagram in Figure 19-2 with the correct words from the following word list.

Word List

Nostrils (naso)
Esophagus
Stomach (gastric)
Gastric irrigation (lavage)
Nasogastric feeding (gavage)

FIGURE 19-2

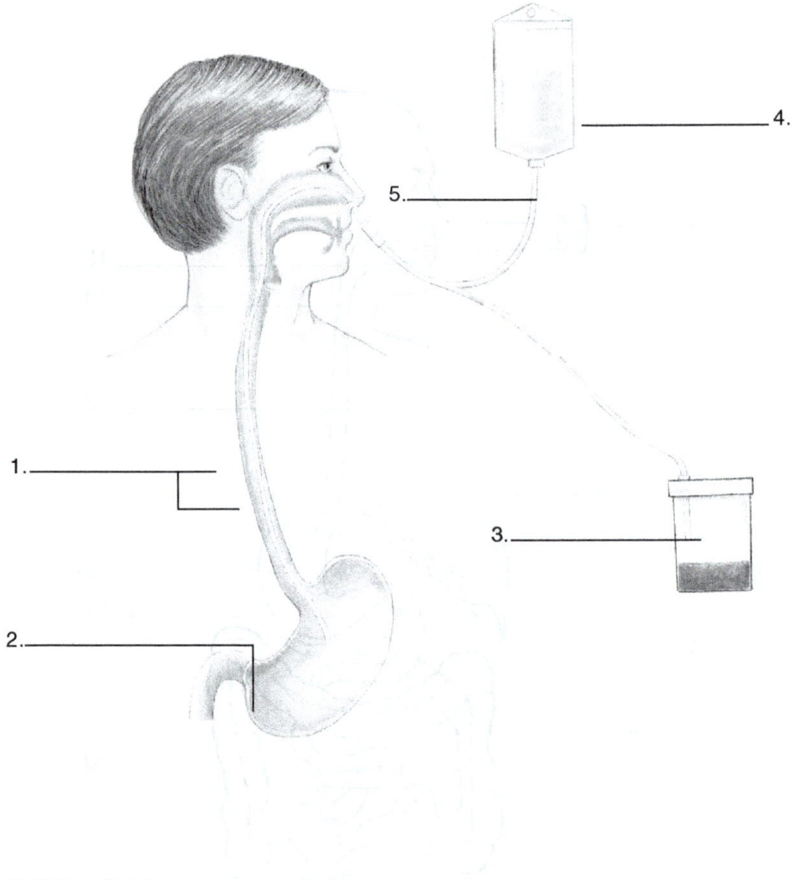

EXERCISE 19-3

Select the letter of the procedure that best answers each question. Write the correct letter(s) on the blank line next to the question. Answers may be used for more than one question.

A. cleansing enema

B. non-medicated suppository

C. Harris flush

D. Removing fecal impaction

_____ 1. Which procedure(s) requires entering at least 2 inches inside the rectum?

_____ 2. In which procedure(s) should the nursing assistant observe for cramping?

_____ 3. Placing a digit (finger) into the rectum occurs in which procedure(s)?

_____ 4. The heart rate can drop during which procedure(s)?

_____ 5. Which procedure(s) helps alleviate constipation?

THE NURSING ASSISTANT IN ACTION

1. You enter a patient's room to find him gagging. There is vomitus all over his sheets. His NG tube feeding is attached. You go to his bedside and notice leaking around his nose. What should you do?

____

____

____

____

2. You are asked by your supervisor to perform GT care. You gather your equipment and enter the room of the patient who has had her GT in place for 1 month already. What should you do?

____

____

____

____

3. You are to remove feces that are impacted in a patient. What should you do, and what safety precautions must you remember?

____

____

____

____

4. You are administering a cleansing enema when the patient tells you his stomach does not feel right and he is cramping badly. In a very loud anxious voice, he says "I cannot hold the enema any longer!" What should you do?

____

____

____

____

5. You take a patient who has a new colostomy into the bathroom to help her bathe. You suggest she use the toilet first. You know now is a good time for her to begin learning how to care for the colostomy. Up to this point, she has refused to do any care for the colostomy herself. What should you do?

____

____

____

____

LEARNING ACTIVITIES

1. If possible, job-shadow an ostomy or wound-care nurse for a day and become familiar with the types of patients for whom she cares, the equipment she uses, and the lessons she teaches. If this is not possible, use the Internet to find out more about the role and responsibilities of this health care provider.

2. If you have the equipment readily available, fit yourself for a colostomy bag. Or, use a resealable plastic food storage bag and tape it to your abdomen. Fill the bag with sticky fluids, cooking oil, or honey and odiferous substances like herbs such as garlic, dried basil, oregano, and cheeses. Wear the colostomy bag for 3 days. Shower with it as well. By the end of the experience, discuss with your instructor what occurred while wearing the colostomy bag. Did anyone you know react differently to you while wearing the colostomy bag? Was there anything you needed to do differently during the 3 days? What clothing helped conceal the bag? How did you sleep? Did your self-esteem and body image change at all? Use what you learned from this experience when providing care to patients who have an ostomy.

PROCEDURE CHECKLISTS

PROCEDURE 19-1: CHECKING FOR FECAL IMPACTION (ADVANCED PROCEDURE)

Name: ____________________ Date: ____________________

STEPS	S	U	COMMENTS
1. Assemble equipment a. Lubricant b. Gloves (two pair) c. Basin of warm water d. Soap e. Protective underpad f. Bedpan and tissue g. Bath blanket h. Towel			
2. Identify the patient by checking the ID bracelet.			
3. Explain the procedure to the patient, emphasizing the need to relax as much as possible.			
4. Ask about any allergies, including iodine-based antiseptics, latex, and adhesive tape.			
5. Ask about any history of slow heart rate or dizziness.			
6. Provide privacy for the patient.			
7. Wash your hands.			
8. Place the protective pad under the patient's buttocks.			
9. Position the patient in the left side-lying, or Sims', position.			
10. Drape the patient with the bath blanket so that only the buttocks are exposed.			
11. Put on gloves.			
12. Liberally lubricate your index finger.			
13. With your nondominant hand, separate the buttocks to expose the anus.			
14. Ask the patient take a deep breath through the mouth. While they are taking the breath, insert your lubricated finger into the anus.			
15. Check for a hard fecal mass, then withdraw your finger. Observe for any signs of rectal bleeding. Discard and put on clean gloves.			
16. Offer the bedpan if needed.			

17. Wash the patient's anal area with soap and water and towel dry.			
18. Remove underpad. Return bedpan to proper place.			
19. Remove and discard gloves and all disposable items used.			
20. Wash your hands.			
21. Document and report the results to your supervisor.			

Charting:

____

____

____

____

Date of Satisfactory Completion ____________________

Instructor's Signature ____________________

PROCEDURE 19-2: REMOVING A FECAL IMPACTION (ADVANCED PROCEDURE)

Name: ____________________ Date: ____________________

STEPS	S	U	COMMENTS
1. Assemble equipment a. Lubricant b. Gloves (two pair) c. Basin of warm water d. Soap e. Protective underpad f. Bedpan and tissue g. Bath blanket h. Towel			
2. Identify the patient by checking the ID bracelet.			
3. Explain the procedure to the patient, emphasizing the need to relax as much as possible.			
4. Ask about any allergies, including iodine-based antiseptics, latex, and adhesive tape.			
5. Ask about any history of slow heart rate or dizziness.			
6. Provide privacy for the patient.			
7. Wash your hands.			
8. Place the protective pad under the patient's buttocks.			
9. Position the patient in the left side-lying, or Sims', position.			
10. Drape the patient with the bath blanket so that only the buttocks are exposed.			
11. Put on gloves. Check and record patient's pulse and rhythm.			
12. Liberally lubricate your finger.			
13. With your nondominant hand, separate the buttocks to expose the anus.			
14. Ask the patient take a deep breath through the mouth. While they are taking the breath, insert your lubricated finger into the anus.			
15. Check for a hard fecal mass, hook your finger around a portion of feces, and then withdraw your finger.			
16. Drop the feces in the bedpan and observe for any signs of rectal bleeding.			

17. Clean your finger with toilet tissue, lubricate it again, and repeat steps 13 through 16 until you no longer feel any feces to remove.			
18. Stop and check the patient's pulse and note how she are tolerating the procedure after each one to two times you repeat steps 13 through 16. If the patient experiences a slowed pulse rate or a change in heart rhythm, call your supervisor or RN to check the patient. Discard and put on clean gloves.			
19. Offer the bedpan if needed.			
20. Wash the patient's anal area with soap and water and towel dry.			
21. Remove underpad. Return bedpan to proper place.			
22. Remove and discard gloves and all disposable items used.			
23. Wash your hands.			
24. Document and report the results to your supervisor.			

Charting:

____

____

____

____

Date of Satisfactory Completion ____________________

Instructor's Signature ____________________

PROCEDURE 19-3: GIVING A CLEANSING ENEMA (ADULT)

Name: ____________________ Date: ____________________

STEPS	S	U	COMMENTS
1. Assemble your equipment a. Disposable enema kit: enema container, tubing, and clamp b. Lubricating jelly c. Graduated pitcher d. Bath thermometer e. Solution as instructed by the registered nurse • *Soapsuds:* 1 package of enema soap, 1000 cc of water, 105° F (40.5° C) • *Saline:* 2 teaspoons salt, 1000 cc of water, 105° F (40.5° C) • *Tapwater:* 1000 cc of water, 105° F (40.5° C) f. Bedpan and cover/bedside commode g. Urinal, if necessary h. Emesis basin i. Toilet tissue j. Disposable bed protector k. Paper towel l. Bath blanket m. Disposable plastic gloves			
2. Wash your hands.			
3. Identify the patient by checking the ID bracelet.			
4. Ask visitors to step out of the room, if this is your hospital's policy.			
5. Tell the patient that you are going to give him an enema while he is in bed.			
6. Provide privacy for the patient.			
7. Cover the patient with a bath blanket. Without exposing the patient, fan-fold the top sheets to the foot of the bed. Have the patient covered only with the bath blanket.			
8. Place the disposable bed protector under the patient's hips and buttocks.			
9. Turn the patient on the left side. Bend the right knee toward the chest (left Sims' position).			

10. Place the bedpan at the foot of the bed within easy reach.			
11. Close the clamp on the enema tubing.			
12. Fill the graduated pitcher with 1000 ccs of water at 105°F (40.5°C).			
13. Pour the water from the graduate into the enema container.			
14. a. If your instructions call for a soapsuds enema, add one package of enema soap to the water in the container. Use the tip of the tubing to mix the solution gently so that no suds form. b. If your instructions call for a saline enema, add 2 teaspoons of salt to the water in the container. c. If your instructions call for a tapwater enema, do not add anything to the water.			
15. Open the clamp on the enema tubing. Let a little of the solution run through the tubing into the bedpan. (This eliminates any air in the tubing, warms the tube, and avoids giving the patient flatus.) Then close the clamp.			
16. Put the lubricating jelly on a piece of toilet tissue. Lubricate the enema tip by rubbing the jelly on it with the tissue, beginning at the end and going up the tube 2" to 4". Be sure the tip is well lubricated and the opening is not plugged.			
17. Expose the patient's buttocks by raising the blanket in a triangle over the anal area. Put on disposable gloves.			
18. Raise the upper buttocks so you can see the anal area.			
19. Gently insert the enema tip 2" to 4" through the anus into the rectum (slow insertion prevents spasm of the sphincter). If you feel resistance or if the patient complains of pain, stop and report this to your immediate supervisor.			
20. Open the clamp and hold the enema container 12" above the anus or 18" above the mattress (the higher the container, the greater the pressure exerted).			
21. Tell the patient to take slow, deep breaths. Explain that this helps relieve any cramps caused by the enema and also helps the patient relax.			
22. When most of the solution has flowed into the patient's rectum, close the clamp. Slowly withdraw the rectal tubing. Wrap it in the paper towel to avoid contamination, and place the tubing into the empty enema container. Encourage the patient to hold the solution for as long as possible.			

23. Help the patient onto the bedpan or commode. If using a bedpan, raise the back of the bed, if allowed. Put the toilet tissue where the patient can reach it easily.			
24. The patient may be allowed to go to the bathroom to expel the enema. If so, assist the patient to the bathroom and stay near the bathroom to assist the patient if needed. Tell the patient not to flush the toilet. This is so the results can be observed.			
25. When the patient is in the bathroom or on the bedpan, make sure the signal cord is within reach. Check on the patient every few minutes.			
26. Dispose of the enema equipment while the patient is on the bedpan.			
27. When observing the results of an enema, look for anything that does not appear normal. Check color, consistency, odor, and amount. a. Report findings to the registered nurse if the stool • Is very hard • Is very soft • Is large in amount • Is small in amount • Is accompanied by flatus (gas) b. Collect a specimen and report to the registered nurse if the stool • Is black (tarlike) • Is streaked with red, white, yellow, or gray • Has a very bad odor • Looks like perked coffee grounds			
28. Empty the bedpan, clean it, and put it in its proper place.			
29. Remove the disposable bed protector and discard.			
30. Remove the bath blanket. At the same time, raise the top sheets to cover the patient.			
31. Wash the patient's hands or have the patient wash his own hands.			
32. Make the patient comfortable.			
33. Lower the bed to a position of safety for the patient.			
34. Raise the side rails where ordered, indicated, and appropriate for patient safety.			
35. Place the call light within easy reach of the patient.			

36. Wash your hands.			
37. Report to your immediate supervisor • That you gave the patient a cleansing enema • The time the enema was given • The type of solution used • The results, color of stool, consistency, flatus (gas) expelled, and unusual material noted • Whether a specimen was obtained • How the patient tolerated the procedure • Your observations of anything unusual			

Charting:

____

____

____

____

Date of Satisfactory Completion ______________________

Instructor's Signature ______________________

PROCEDURE 19-4: GIVING A SMALL-VOLUME, READY-TO-USE CLEANSING ENEMA

Name: ____________________ Date: ____________________

STEPS	S	U	COMMENTS
Note: Always read the package instructions for giving the enema. 1. Assemble your equipment a. Disposable prepackaged enema b. Bedpan and cover/bedside commode c. Urinal (if necessary) d. Disposable bed protector e. Toilet tissue f. Disposable plastic gloves			
2. Wash your hands.			
3. Identify the patient by checking the ID bracelet.			
4. Ask visitors to step out of the room, if this is your hospital's policy.			
5. Tell the patient that you are going to give her an enema while she is in bed.			
6. Provide privacy for the patient. Ask patient if she needs to urinate. If so, provide equipment.			
7. Cover the patient with a bath blanket. Without exposing the patient, fan-fold the top sheets to the foot of the bed. Have the patient covered only with the bath blanket.			
8. Place the disposable bed protector under the patient's hips (buttocks). Warm the enema, if this is the policy of your employing health care institution.			
9. Turn the patient on the left side and bend the right knee toward the chest (left Sims's position).			
10. Place the bedpan at the foot of the bed within easy reach.			
11. Open the enema package. Take out the disposable enema. Remove the cap. Put on disposable plastic gloves.			
12. Expose the patient's buttocks by raising the blanket in a triangle over the anal area.			

13. Raise the buttocks so you can see the anal area.			
14. Gently insert the enema tip, which is prelubricated, 2" through the anus into the rectum.			
15. Squeeze the plastic bottle gently until all the liquid goes into the patient's rectum.			
16. Remove the tube from the patient's anus. Put the empty plastic bottle back in the box. (You will discard it later, in the dirty utility room.) Encourage the patient to hold the solution as long as possible.			
17. Help the patient onto the bedpan. Raise the back of the bed, if allowed. Put the toilet tissue where the patient can reach it easily.			
18. The patient may be allowed to use a bedside commode or go to the bathroom to expel the enema. If so, assist the patient to the bathroom and stay near the bathroom to assist the patient if needed. Tell the patient not to flush the toilet. This is so the results can be observed.			
19. When the patient is in the bathroom or on the bedpan, make sure the signal cord is within reach. Check on the patient every few minutes.			
20. Discard the disposable enema equipment. Return to the patient when she is finished using the bedpan. Check the contents for color of stool, consistency, amount, unusual material, or anything abnormal. If you observe anything unusual, collect a specimen.			
21. Empty the bedpan. Clean it and put it in its proper place.			
22. Remove the disposable bed protector and discard it.			
23. Remove the bath blanket. At the same time, raise the top sheets to cover the patient.			
24. Wash the patient's hands or have the patient wash her own hands.			
25. Make the patient comfortable.			
26. Lower the bed to a position of safety for the patient.			
27. Raise the side rails where ordered, indicated, and appropriate for patient safety.			
28. Place the call light within easy reach of the patient.			
29. Wash your hands.			

30. Report to your immediate supervisor • That you gave the patient a cleansing enema • The time the enema was given, the results, color of stool, consistency, flatus expelled, and any unusual material noted • How the patient tolerated the procedure • Your observations of anything unusual			

Charting:

____

____

____

____

Date of Satisfactory Completion ____________________

Instructor's Signature ____________________

PROCEDURE 19-5: GIVING A READY-TO-USE OIL-RETENTION ENEMA

Name: ______________ Date: ______________

STEPS	S	U	COMMENTS
Note: Always read the package instructions for giving the enema. 1. Assemble your equipment a. Disposable, ready-to-use enema kit b. Bedpan and cover/bedside commode c. Urinal, if necessary d. Disposable bed protector e. Equipment for soapsuds enema if ordered by the physician; give 20 minutes after oil retention enema. f. Toilet tissue g. Disposable gloves			
2. Wash your hands.			
3. Identify the patient by checking the ID bracelet.			
4. Ask visitors to step out of the room, if this is your hospital's policy.			
5. Tell the patient that you are going to give him an oil-retention enema while he is in bed.			
6. Provide privacy for the patient. Ask patient if she needs to urinate. If so, provide equipment.			
7. Cover the patient with a bath blanket. Without exposing the patient, fan-fold the top sheets to the foot of the bed. Have the patient covered only with the bath blanket.			
8. Place the disposable bed protector under the patient's hips (buttocks).			
9. Turn the patient on the left side. Bend the right knee toward the chest (left Sims' position).			
10. Place the bedpan at the foot of the bed within easy reach.			
11. Open the package. Take out the ready-to-use enema bag filled with oil. Remove the cap. Warm the oil enema, if this is the policy of the health care institution.			
12. Expose the patient's buttocks by raising the blanket in a triangle over the anal area.			
13. Raise the buttocks so you can see the anal area.			
14. Gently insert the enema tip, which is prelubricated, 2" through the anus into the rectum.			

15. Squeeze the plastic bottle gently until all the liquid goes into the patient's rectum.			
16. Remove the tube from the patient's anus. Put the empty plastic bottle back in the box. (You will discard it later.)			
17. Explain to the patient that it is necessary to retain (hold in) the oil for 20 minutes. Encourage the patient to stay in the Sims' position, if at all possible. Check on the patient every few minutes.			
18. Your instructions may require you to give a soapsuds enema after the patient has retained the oil for 20 minutes. If so, give the soapsuds enema at that time.			
19. Help the patient onto the bedpan. Raise the back of the bed, if allowed. Put the toilet tissue where the patient can reach it easily.			
20. The patient may be allowed to use a bedside commode or go to the bathroom to expel the enema. If so, assist the patient to the bathroom and stay near the bathroom to assist the patient if needed. Tell the patient not to flush the toilet. This is so the results can be observed.			
21. When the patient is in the bathroom or on the bedpan, make sure the signal cord is within reach. Check on the patient every few minutes.			
22. Discard the disposable enema equipment.			
23. Return to the patient when she is finished using the bedpan. Check the contents for color of stool, consistency, amount, unusual material, or anything abnormal. If you observe anything unusual, collect a specimen.			
24. Empty the bedpan. Clean it and put it in its proper place.			
25. Remove the disposable bed protector and discard it.			
26. Remove the bath blanket. At the same time, raise the top sheets to cover the patient.			
27. Wash the patient's hands, or have the patient wash her own hands.			
28. Make the patient comfortable.			
29. Lower the bed to a position of safety for the patient.			
30. Raise the side rails where ordered, indicated, and appropriate for patient safety.			
31. Place the call light within easy reach of the patient.			
32. Wash your hands.			

33. Report to your immediate supervisor • That you gave the patient an oil-retention enema • The time the oil-retention enema was given, the results, color of stool, consistency, flatus expelled, and any unusual material noted • How the patient tolerated the procedure			

Charting:

____

____

____

____

Date of Satisfactory Completion ____________________

Instructor's Signature ____________________

PROCEDURE 19-6: GIVING A HARRIS FLUSH (RETURN-FLOW) ENEMA

Name: ____________________ Date: ____________________

STEPS	S	U	COMMENTS
Note: Always read the package instructions for giving the enema. 1. Assemble your equipment a. Disposable enema bag, tubing, and clamp b. Lubricating jelly c. Graduated pitcher d. Bath thermometer e. Urinal (if necessary) f. Disposable plastic gloves g. Emesis basin h. Toilet tissue i. Disposable bed protector j. Paper towel k. Bath blanket l. Bedpan/bedside commode			
2. Wash your hands.			
3. Identify the patient by checking the ID bracelet.			
4. Ask visitors to step out of the room, if this is your hospital's policy.			
5. Tell the patient that you are going to give her a *Harris flush,* which is a rectal irrigation that relieves gas.			
6. Provide privacy for the patient.			
7. Cover the patient with a bath blanket. Without exposing the patient, fan-fold the top sheets to the foot of the bed. Have the patient covered only with the bath blanket.			
8. Place the disposable bed protector under the patient's hips and buttocks.			
9. Place the patient in a Sims' position (left lateral position with the right leg flexed and slightly forward, or anterior, and the left leg is extended).			
10. Put the bedpan at the foot of the bed within easy reach.			
11. Close the clamp on the enema tubing.			
12. Fill the graduated pitcher with 500 cc of water, 105°F (40.5°C). Measure the temperature of the water with the bath thermometer.			

13. Pour the water from the graduated pitcher into the enema container.			
14. Open the clamp on the enema tubing to let water run through the tubing into the bedpan. This removes any air that may be in the tubing to avoid giving the patient flatus and also warms the tube. Close the clamp.			
15. Put the lubricating jelly on a piece of toilet tissue. Lubricate the enema tip by rubbing the jelly on it with the tissue. Be sure the tip is well lubricated and the opening is not plugged.			
16. Expose the patient's buttocks by raising the blanket in a triangle over the anal area. Put gloves on now.			
17. Raise the upper buttocks so you can see the anal area.			
18. Gently insert the enema tip 2" through the anus into the rectum.			
19. Open the clamp. Hold the enema container 12" above the anus. Allow about 200 cc of water to enter the rectum. Do not clamp or remove the tubing.			
20. Lower the enema bag below the bed frame. Let the water run back into the enema bag without removing the tube from the patient's rectum.			
21. Hold the enema bag 12" above the anus. Let 200 cc of water run into the patient's rectum, then lower the bag. Allow the water to run back into the enema bag. Keep the tube in the patient's rectum.			
22. Continue letting water in and out of the rectum for 10 to 20 minutes, or as directed by the nurse.			
23. Tell the patient to take slow deep breaths. Explain that this kind of breathing helps relieve the pressure and cramps caused by the enema. It also helps the patient relax.			
24. Observe the amounts (large or small) of flatus the patient expels as the water runs out of the patient into the enema bag.			
25. Remove the tubing when the treatment is finished. Wrap the enema tip in the paper towel to avoid contamination. Place it in the disposable enema container.			
26. Help the patient onto the bedpan. Raise the back of the bed, if allowed. Put the toilet tissue where the patient can reach it easily. Give the patient the signal cord. Check on the patient every few minutes.			

27. The patient may be allowed by the nurse to go to the bathroom to expel more flatus. If so, assist the patient to the bathroom. Tell the patient to notice the amount of flatus (large or small amounts) expelled.			
28. Discard the disposable enema equipment while the patient is on the bedpan or in the bathroom.			
29. Return to the patient when she is finished using the bedpan or bathroom. Check the contents for bowel movement, color of stool, consistency, amount, unusual material, or anything abnormal. If you observe anything unusual, collect a specimen. Ask the patient if flatus was expelled.			
30. Empty the bedpan, clean it, and put it in its proper place.			
31. Remove the disposable bed protector and discard it.			
32. Remove the bath blanket. At the same time, raise the top sheets to cover the patient.			
33. Wash the patient's hands, or have the patient wash them.			
34. Make the patient comfortable.			
35. Lower the bed to a position of safety for the patient.			
36. Raise the side rails where ordered, indicated, and appropriate for patient safety.			
37. Place the call light within easy reach of the patient.			
38. Wash your hands.			
39. Report to your immediate supervisor • That you gave the patient a Harris flush • The time the Harris flush was given and how long it was continued • The results, amount of flatus expelled, and unusual material noted • Whether a specimen was obtained • How the patient tolerated the procedure • Your observations of anything unusual			

Charting:

____

____

____

____

Date of Satisfactory Completion ________________

Instructor's Signature ________________

PROCEDURE 19-7: USING DISPOSABLE RECTAL TUBES WITH CONNECTED FLATUS BAG

Name: ____________________ Date: ____________________

STEPS	S	U	COMMENTS
1. Assemble your equipment a. Disposable rectal tube with connected flatus bag (Figure 19-18) b. Small piece of adhesive tape c. Tissue d. Lubricating jelly e. Disposable gloves			
2. Wash your hands.			
3. Identify the patient by checking the ID bracelet.			
4. Ask visitors to step out of the room, if this is your hospital's policy.			
5. Tell the patient that you are going to insert a rectal tube for the purpose of relieving him of gas (flatus).			
6. Provide privacy for the patient.			
7. Turn the patient on the left side. Bend the right knee toward the chest (left Sims' position).			
8. Expose the patient's buttocks by raising the blanket in a triangle over the anal area. Put on the disposable gloves.			
9. Lubricate the tip of the rectal tube by squeezing lubricating jelly onto the tissue and rubbing the jelly on the tip. Be sure the opening at the end of the tube is not clogged. (If the rectal tube is prelubricated, this step is not necessary.)			
10. Raise the upper buttocks so you can see the anal area.			
11. Gently insert the rectal tube 2" to 4" through the anus into the rectum.			
12. Use a small piece of adhesive tape to attach the tube to the patient's buttocks in order to hold the tube in place.			
13. Let the tube remain in place for 20 minutes. Then remove and discard the equipment. (Usually this procedure is done once in a 24-hour period.)			
14. Make the patient comfortable.			
15. Lower the bed to a position of safety for the patient.			
16. Raise the side rails where ordered, indicated, and appropriate for patient safety.			

17. Place the call light within easy reach of the patient.			
18. Wash your hands.			
19. Report to your immediate supervisor • The time the rectal tube was inserted and the time it was removed • The patient's comments about the amount (small or large) of flatus expelled through the tube • How the patient tolerated the procedure • Your observations of anything unusual			

Charting:

____

____

____

____

Date of Satisfactory Completion ____________________

Instructor's Signature ____________________

PROCEDURE 19-8: CHANGING AN OSTOMY APPLIANCE

Name: ______________________ Date: ______________________

STEPS	S	U	COMMENTS
1. Assemble your equipment a. Disposable bed protector b. Bath blanket c. New pouch (may be 1 or 2 pieces) d. Toilet tissue e. Basin of warm water (115°F; 46°C) f. Non-cream-based soap or cleanser as ordered by your immediate supervisor g. Washcloth h. Disposable gloves i. Towels			
2. Identify the patient by checking the identification bracelet.			
3. Tell the patient that you will assist them in changing the ostomy appliance.			
4. Wash your hands and put on gloves.			
5. Provide privacy for the patient.			
6. Raise the bed to a comfortable working position.			
7. Place a towel over the patient's abdomen, exposing only the appliance.			
8. Place the disposable bed protector under the patient's hips to keep the bed from getting wet or dirty.			
9. Gently remove the soiled pouch. Use a push–pull method to remove barrier.			
10. Dispose of the pouch in the appropriate container. Wipe the area around the ostomy with a warm wet washcloth. This is to remove any stool from the skin.			
11. Rinse the entire area well. Be careful not to leave any soap on the skin. (Soap has a drying effect and may irritate the skin.)			
12. Dry the area gently with a bath towel.			
13. Prepare the new barrier. A colostomy stoma needs a barrier 1/8" larger than the stoma measurement. (It may need to be sized and cut out.) For urostomy and ileostomy stomas, no skin should show between the wafer and the stoma. The opening of the wafer should fit around the stoma where the skin meets the stoma. Use stoma adhesive paste if necessary. *Note:* There are 1- and 2-piece appliances. Become familiar with the supplies available to you.			

14. Apply new wafer to skin; hold in place for 30 seconds with your hand to help adhesive stick well. Apply clamp to bottom of pouch.			
15. Remove the disposable bed protector. Change any damp linen. Bag and dispose of soiled linen in the laundry hamper.			
16. Make the patient comfortable and replace the call light.			
17. Lower the bed to a position of safety.			
18. Raise the side rails when ordered or appropriate for patient safety.			
19. Remove all used equipment.			
20. Wash your hands.			
21. Report to your immediate supervisor • That you changed the ostomy wafer and pouch • The amount of drainage • The consistency of the stool • The color and appearance of the stoma and skin around it • How the patient tolerated the procedure • Your observations of anything unusual			

Charting:

____

____

____

____

Date of Satisfactory Completion ____________________

Instructor's Signature ____________________

Nutrition for the Patient

20

Key Terms Review

Match the key terms in the right column with the definitions in the left column by placing the letter of each correct answer in the space provided.

_____ **1.** Chemical substances found in foods.

_____ **2.** Person responsible for the preparation of well-balanced regular and therapeutic (special) diets to meet patients' nutritional needs.

_____ **3.** Nutrients needed for the human body to function; they must be consumed in the diet every day.

_____ **4.** Poor nutrition status.

_____ **5.** Assessment by a nurse or registered dietician as to what a patient eats and how the body uses it; determination of any special nutritional needs.

_____ **6.** Unit for measuring the energy produced when food is digested in the body.

_____ **7.** Counting or adding up a total of all calories consumed in a 24-hour period.

_____ **8.** A basic, or well-balanced, diet containing appropriate amounts of foods from each of the food groups.

_____ **9.** Any special diet.

_____ **10.** Difficulty chewing or swallowing due to damage to the nerves and muscles involved in swallowing.

Terms

A. Nutrient

B. Essential nutrient

C. Nutrition status assessment

D. Malnutrition

E. Dysphagia

F. Extra nourishment

G. Omit

H. Registered dietitian (RD)

I. Calorie

J. Calorie count

K. Regular diet

L. Therapeutic diet

M. Enterally

N. Parenteral nutrition

_____ **11.** Delivery of a nutrition formula through a tube for patients with a functional GI tract who are unable to take in adequate calories or food by mouth.

_____ **12.** Nutrition therapy delivered by an IV catheter for patients with a nonfunctioning GI tract.

_____ **13.** Snacks.

_____ **14.** Leave out.

MULTIPLE-CHOICE QUESTIONS

Circle the letter next to the word or statement that best completes the sentence or answers the question.

1. If you eat the recommended number of portions of foods from each food group on the pyramid every day, your diet will be
   a. adequate for body-builders.
   b. adequate for fast growth.
   c. adequate for good health.
   d. inadequate for patients.

2. The number and size of portions of food depend on
   a. the age of the individual.
   b. the size of the individual.
   c. the activities of the individual.
   d. all of the above.

3. Fat has _____ calories per gram of fat.
   a. 100
   b. 9
   c. 4
   d. 90

4. Alterations to the patient's diet may be necessary to
   a. increase or decrease the caloric content.
   b. change the amounts of one or more nutrients.
   c. meet cultural or religious requirements.
   d. all of the above.

5. Most patients prefer
   a. to be fed.
   b. to feed themselves.
   c. to skip meals.
   d. to eat when nauseated.

6. *Aspiration* means the patient
   a. has lost his appetite
   b. drinks thickened fluids.
   c. must be fed using a feeding tube.
   d. has fluid or food that has entered the lungs.

7. Mr. Jones is on a clear liquid diet. What should the nursing assistant remove from his tray?
   a. Cranberry juice
   b. Chicken flavored broth
   c. Lemon popsicles
   d. Plain vanilla ice cream

8. Which diet is prescribed for a patient who experiences constipation?
   a. Low residue
   b. High fiber
   c. Low calorie
   d. Bland

9. Mrs. Sellers has cancer. Her dentures are loose in her mouth from losing so much weight. What type of diet might she do best with?
   a. Mechanical soft
   b. Bland
   c. Low residue
   d. Clear liquid

10. Mr. Cox has high cholesterol and high blood pressure and has been advised to eat a _______ diet.
   a. high-protein
   b. low-fat and low-cholesterol

c. gluten-free
d. lactose-free

11. Which foods are offered on a high-protein diet?
a. A cheese omelet with bacon
b. Strawberry and rhubarb pie
c. Whole wheat bread and hot oatmeal
d. Codfish and broccoli

12. Which food should you remove before serving Mr. White his diabetic meal?
a. Lemon cake with white frosting
b. Tomato juice
c. Skinless chicken breast
d. Small apple

13. A, D, E, and K are considered
a. fat-soluble minerals.
b. fat-soluble vitamins.
c. water-soluble minerals.
d. water-soluble vitamins.

14. Calcium, phosphorous, sodium, and potassium are considered minerals and
a. help form body cells.
b. decrease energy in the body.
c. make the body processes irregular.
d. must be consumed weekly.

15. How much fluid should the average adult consume on a daily basis?
a. 6 cups a day
b. 2000–2500 mL
c. 2000 ounces
d. 8–10 ounces

16. Mr. Black returns to his room at 7 PM from some cardiac testing and missed dinner. The nursing assistant should
a. leave his tray on his overbed table for when he returns.
b. serve his tray immediately when he returns.
c. offer him a choice of either warming his tray for him or calling dietary for another meal he would enjoy.
d. remove anything that is high in fat and salt from his tray, warm the remaining food, and give it to him immediately.

17. Mrs. Cornwall is at high risk for choking. The nursing assistant should
a. feed her.
b. stay in the room and watch her eat.
c. set up her tray by opening any container she cannot open.
d. never offer her fluids.

18. Using a thickening agent in a fluid
a. changes the taste and appearance of the liquid being served.
b. maintains the criteria for keeping Kosher and gluten-free.
c. need to set for 30–60 seconds.
d. Both b and c.

19. Keeping a patient in a _______ position decreases the chance of aspiration.
a. supine
b. prone
c. Sims'
d. high Fowler's

20. When assisting a patient who has difficulty seeing, the nursing assistant should
a. feed him to make sure he does not burn himself.
b. open all containers and offer a napkin in case he drops food.
c. use the idea of a clock to orient the patient to where his food is located on his plate.
d. ask the family to help him.

21. When passing water on the unit, a nursing assistant must
a. empty the contents of the container and refill it with only ice for every patient.
b. check to see which patient is NPO.
c. take each patient container one at a time to the kitchen and refill it with clean fresh water to promote infection control measures.

d. never offer straws because they can increase the chance of choking or increase the amount of air taken in, leaving the patient feeling bloated and gassy.

22. Mrs. Miller is on bedrest. When eating, the best position for her to be in is
a. Trendelenburg.
b. semi-Fowler's.
c. to sit her up and allow her to dangle.
d. to place her in a chair at the bedside.

23. A patient has right-side weakness from a recent stroke. He is right-handed. When setting up his food tray, it is best to encourage as much independence by
a. asking dietary to puree all of his food so he does not have to chew as much or cut his food.
b. cutting all the food for him and opening all containers.
c. cutting the food into small pieces and feed him yourself.
d. asking his family to help him eat.

24. A patient will not eat the food you placed before him because of religious reasons. The nursing assistant should
a. encourage the patient to eat only the food on the tray that he is allowed to eat.
b. go shopping for him and bring back the foods he is requesting.
c. go to the nurse supervisor and explain the issue.
d. ask the family to bring in whatever foods they think might please him.

25. In an effort to promote good digestion and reduce the chance of aspiration, the nursing assistant should
a. have a patient stay seated and in an upright position for at least 30 minutes following a meal.
b. have the patient stay in the supine position for 1 hour after the meal has been eaten.
c. place the patient back to bed and in the Sims' position.
d. feed the patient small meals twice a day.

TRUE OR FALSE QUESTIONS

Determine whether each question is true or false. In the space provided, write "T" for true and "F" for false. If the statement is false, rewrite it on the line provided to make it a true statement.

_____ **1.** Calories from fat should be less than 30% of total calories.

____

_____ **2.** Water has a tremendous amount of calories.

____

_____ **3.** The nutrition status assessment may include chewing or swallowing problems.

____

_____ **4.** Providing a pleasant environment for the patient to eat may improve his appetite.

____

_____ **5.** Total parenteral nutrition (TPN) is offered when the GI tract is functioning adequately.

____

_____ **6.** When possible, children should be offered foods they like to eat.

____

_____ **7.** Beans, nuts, and peas are examples of complete essential amino acids.

____

_____ **8.** Butter is allowed to be given to a patient on a lactose-free diet.

____

_____ 9. The nursing assistant should report any complaints of nausea, constipation, and diarrhea, as this may alter the patient's nutritional intake.

____

_____ 10. Allowing a child to eat with her parents or friends who are visiting may increase the amount of food the child eats.

____

FILL-IN-THE-BLANK QUESTIONS

Provide the meaning of the following abbreviations.

1. RD _______________
2. mL _______________
3. GI _______________
4. RN _______________
5. NPO _______________

EXERCISE 20-1

Objective: To apply what you have learned about serving food to the patient.

Directions: More than one action may apply. Select the action that most closely addresses the situation. Write the letter of the correct action next to the matching situation.

Actions

A. Check the tray yourself.

B. Check the tray card against the ID band.

C. Help any patient who needs it.

D. Record this on appropriate form.

E. Correct anything that is wrong or missing.

Situations

_____ 1. Before you give a tray to a patient.

_____ 2. You find the tray for each patient.

_____ 3. A patient cannot cut his meat.

_____ 4. A patient tells you she didn't get a fork.

_____ 5. The patient ate only half his food.

_____ 6. A patient tells you she has the wrong tray.

_____ 7. The patient refuses to accept the tray and eats nothing.

_____ 8. Some food spills.

_____ 9. A patient seems too weak to pour his own coffee.

_____ **10.** A patient on a regular diet didn't get any sugar on her tray, and she would like to have some.

_____ **11.** You see a coffee pot on the patient's tray but no cup.

_____ **12.** You look to be sure everything is on the tray.

_____ **13.** A weak patient asks you to butter his bread.

_____ **14.** The patient ate all the food served to her.

_____ **15.** The patient tells you he didn't get any bread and butter, and you see none.

EXERCISE 20-2

Objective: To apply what you have learned about passing drinking water to patients.

Directions: Write "Do" or "Don't" next to each of the following statements as appropriate.

_____ **1.** Pass fresh drinking water to patients at the assigned intervals each shift or day.

_____ **2.** Give ice to a patient whose pitcher is labeled "OMIT ICE. "

_____ **3.** Check to see which patients are NPO.

_____ **4.** Check to see which patients are on restricted fluids.

_____ **5.** Check to see which patients should get water without ice.

_____ **6.** Return the same water pitcher to the patient from whom it was taken.

_____ **7.** Remember to wash your hands before passing drinking water.

_____ **8.** Wash your hands when done passing drinking water.

_____ **9.** Lower the head of bed to 10° for feeding patients.

_____ **10.** Feed patients one bite every 3 seconds.

EXERCISE 20-3

Objective: To apply what you have learned about food groups.

Directions: Beside each food, write the letter of the food group to which it belongs.

Food Groups

A. Milk, yogurt, and cheese

B. Vegetables

C. Fruits

D. Meat, poultry, fish, dried beans, eggs, and nuts

E. Breads, cereals, rice, and pasta

F. Fats, oil, and sweets

Foods

____ 1. Peas	____ 11. Nuts
____ 2. Onions	____ 12. Carrots
____ 3. Milk	____ 13. Potatoes
____ 4. Macaroni	____ 14. Cheese
____ 5. Broccoli	____ 15. Apple
____ 6. Rice	____ 16. Butter
____ 7. Bread	____ 17. Candy bar
____ 8. Dried beans	____ 18. Blueberries
____ 9. Yogurt	____ 19. Banana
____ 10. Cake	____ 20. Chicken

EXERCISE 20-4

Objective: To apply what you have learned about essential nutrients.

Directions: For each food item listed below, find the nutrient that most closely matches that food item. Select each food item only once.

Nutrients

C—carbohydrates
P—protein
F—fat
W—water
V—vitamins
M—minerals

Foods

____ 1. Margarine	____ 7. Cheese
____ 2. Beans	____ 8. Meat
____ 3. Beverages	____ 9. Calcium
____ 4. Fluoride	____ 10. Biotin
____ 5. Cereal	____ 11. Iodine
____ 6. Fruits	____ 12. Butter

EXERCISE 20-5

Objective: To apply what you have learned about the most common types of diets.

Directions: For each diet type listed, read the common purpose and then fill in the description column. You may describe the diet or give examples.

Examples of Different Types of Patient Diets		
Type of Diet	**Description**	**Common Purpose**
1. Regular		To maintain or attain optimal nutritional status in patients who do not require a special diet.
2. Clear liquid		To provide calories and fluid in a form that requires minimal digestion; commonly ordered after surgery.
3. Full liquid		For those unable to chew or swallow solid food; used as a transitional diet between clear liquids and solid foods.
4. Soft		Used for patients who are unable to chew or swallow hard or coarse foods.
5. Mechanical soft		For patients with difficulty chewing or swallowing soft food.
6. Bland		Omits food that may cause excessive gastric acid secretion (ulcers).
7. Low residue		Used for patients with acute colitis, enteritis, and diverticulitis.
8. High residue/fiber		Used for bowel regulation, high cholesterol, and high glucose; helps protect against colon cancer and diverticulosis.
9. Low calorie		For patients who need to lose weight.
10. Diabetic		For diabetic patients; matches food intake with the insulin requirements.
11. High protein		Assists in the repair of tissues wasted by disease; used for increased protein needs (wound healing).
12. Low fat, low cholesterol		For patients who have difficulty digesting fat, such as patients with pancreatitis, cholestasis, and heart and hepatic disease.
13. Lactose-free/low		Used to prevent cramping and diarrhea in patients with a lactose deficiency.
14. Low sodium (low salt)		May be needed for patients with liver, cardiac, and renal disease; used for patients with acute or chronic renal failure.
15. Gluten restricted		Used for patients with gluten-sensitive enteropathy.

THE NURSING ASSISTANT IN ACTION

1. Mrs. Vyas is from India and speaks very little English. She was visiting her daughter in America when she became ill. She was admitted to your unit 2 days ago and will not eat anything that comes from the dietary department. What should you do?

2. Mr. Walsh is receiving chemotherapy for bone cancer. He is in pain from his last treatment and from ulcers in his mouth. He has lost a significant amount of weight in the last 2 weeks and is very weak. Certain odors make him feel nauseated. His dinner tray arrives and you have been asked to assist him in setting up his tray and encouraging him to eat. What should you do?

3. Mrs. Lin was assessed by a registered dietician and placed on aspiration precautions. You are asked to feed this patient with dysphagia her noontime meal. What should you do to prevent her from choking while providing a dignified dining experience?

4. Mr. Goldstein, a Jewish man, refuses to eat anything on his tray because it is not Kosher. What should you do?

5. You are feeding Mrs. Smith, who has Alzheimer's disease. You notice she is drooling and holding food in her cheeks. You offer her some fluids, hoping she will swallow what she has in her mouth. Instead, she begins to make gurgling sounds. What should you do?

LEARNING ACTIVITIES

1. Using the Internet, locate a site such as the American Dietetic Association that explains special diets. Identify those foods and fluids a person can and cannot eat if prescribed a renal diet. Try to create a 1-day menu for breakfast, lunch, dinner, and two snacks that incorporates the foods and fluids recommended for a patient living with end stage kidney (renal) disease. What would be difficult for you if you had to follow these restrictions for the rest of your life? When taking care of a patient with kidney failure, it is important to remember to offer choices and figure out ways to make the meal appealing and tasty. What could you do in order to make the meal more palatable?
2. For 1 day, track what types of foods you eat and fluids you drink. Estimate the amount of food and fluid you ingest. Identify which foods you consume too much of and which foods you may need to add into your diet to create a more well-balanced diet. What things in your life make eating a well-balanced diet easy or difficult to do? What things might you continue to eat and drink, and what dietary changes are realistic to make?

PROCEDURE CHECKLISTS

PROCEDURE 20-1: PREPARING THE PATIENT FOR A MEAL

Name: ______________________ Date: ______________________

STEPS	S	U	COMMENTS
1. Assemble your equipment a. Bedpan or urinal b. Basin of warm water (115°F; 46. 1°C) c. Washcloth d. Towel e. Robe and slippers			
2. Identify the patient by checking the identification bracelet.			
3. Wash your hands.			
4. Tell the patient you are getting her ready for her next meal.			
5. Provide privacy for the patient.			
6. Offer the bedpan or urinal or assist the patient to the bathroom.			
7. Have the patient wash her hands or offer the patient assistance.			
8. Raise the backrest so the patient is in a sitting position, if this is allowed. If not, you might prop up her head by using several pillows.			
9. Clear the overbed table. Put it in a convenient position for the patient's meal.			
10. If the patient wants to sit in a chair to eat and this is allowed, assist her with her robe and slippers. Help the patient out of bed and to the chair.			
11. Make the patient comfortable and replace the call light.			
12. Check that the telephone is still within reach.			
13. Lower the bed to a position of safety for the patient.			
14. Raise the side rails when ordered or appropriate for patient safety.			
15. Wash your hands.			

16. Report the following to your immediate supervisor • The patient is ready for the next meal • How the patient tolerated the procedure • Your observations of anything unusual			

Charting:

____

____

____

____

Date of Satisfactory Completion ____________________

Instructor's Signature ____________________

PROCEDURE 20-2: SERVING THE FOOD

Name: ____________________ Date: ____________________

STEPS	S	U	COMMENTS
1. Wash your hands.			
2. Check the tray against the meal card before you give it to the patient to be sure the correct ordered diet and items are there. Make sure the tray looks appetizing and nothing is missing (including silverware). Make sure nothing has spilled. Correct anything that is wrong.			
3. Be sure you are giving the right tray to the right patient. Check the menu card, which will have the patient's name on it, against the patient's identification band to be sure they match.			
4. Put the tray on the overbed table. Adjust it to a height comfortable for the patient.			
5. Arrange the dishes and silverware so the patient can reach everything easily. Open containers for the patient. Be sure drinking water is handy.			
6. Help any patient who needs it. For example, if a patient seems to be weak or asks for help, you might place a clothing protector over the patient or offer to spread the napkin on his lap or tuck it under his chin. Spread butter on the bread. Cut up whatever needs cutting. Pour tea or coffee. Do not give any more help than is really needed. The more a patient can do for himself, the better.			
7. A patient may discover that he cannot eat when the food is served. Report this to your supervisor. If permitted, you may take the tray away and keep the hot food warm until the patient wants to eat.			
8. When you are sure the patient can go on with his meal by himself, leave the room.			
9. Go back for the food tray when the patient has finished eating.			
10. Note how much the patient has eaten and how much he has had to drink.			
11. Record the intake for those patients who are on calorie counts or intake and output records.			
12. Record how the patient has eaten his meal on the daily activity flow sheet. Record this information separately for breakfast, lunch, and supper: a. Did the patient eat all the food served? b. Did the patient eat about half the food served? c. Did the patient eat very little food? d. Did the patient decline to eat anything?			

13. Take the tray away and put it in its proper place.			
14. If the patient ate sitting in a chair, help him back into bed.			
15. Put personal articles back where the patient wants them.			
16. If the patient ate in bed, brush crumbs from the bed, smooth out the sheets, and straighten the bedding.			
17. Assist the patient with oral care as needed.			
18. Make the patient comfortable and replace the call light.			
19. Lower the bed to a position of safety for the patient.			
20. Raise the side rails when ordered or appropriate for patient safety.			
21. Wash your hands.			
22. Report the following to your immediate supervisor • That you have served the patient his food and fluids • The amount of food eaten (all, half, or refused to eat). Follow agency procedure for measuring and recording intake. • Your observations of anything unusual			

Charting:

____

____

____

____

Date of Satisfactory Completion ____________

Instructor's Signature ____________

PROCEDURE 20-3: FEEDING A PATIENT WITH DYSPHAGIA

Name: ______________________ Date: ______________________

STEPS	S	U	COMMENTS
1. Wash your hands.			
2. Check the tray against the meal card before you give it to the patient to be sure the correct ordered diet and all items are there. Make sure the tray looks appetizing and nothing is missing (including utensils). Make sure nothing has spilled. Correct anything that is wrong.			
3. Be sure you are giving the right tray to the right patient. Check the menu card, which will have the patient's name on it, against the patient's identification band to be sure they match.			
4. Position the patient with a 90° flexion of hips and a 45° neck flexion.			
5. Place a pillow behind the back and neck (if needed) to maintain this position. If the patient is in bed, adjust the lower section of the bed, elevating the knees to prevent the patient from slipping down.			
6. Foods should be served right away so the cold foods remain cold and the hot foods remain hot. Add a thickening product if instructed to do so.			
7. Sit while feeding the resident with dysphagia to avoid giving the feeling you are rushing him.			
8. Allow the resident to feed himself any food items she can. When feeding the resident requiring assistance, present food from the midline and below. Allow for choices, and ask the resident what food item they prefer you to offer.			
9. If available, use a cut-out cup to make it easier to feed liquids.			
10. Remind the resident to keep his head down, suck in a small amount of liquid, swallow, then rest.			
11. Place solid food on the tongue with a spoon.			
12. Wait and be sure the mouth is empty before offering more food. Provide liquids every few bites, or more often if desired.			
13. Offer very cold foods or Italian ices between every five or six bites. Doing so can make it easier for some patients to eat.			
14. Avoid offering dry foods, for example, bread, waffles, and pancakes. Extra honey, syrup, butter, or applesauce can help make these foods easier to swallow for patients who desire them.			

15. Encourage the patient to swallow twice after each bite.			
16. Be patient, and offer verbal cues as needed.			
17. Check that the mouth is empty after the feeding and have the patient remain sitting up for 30 minutes. Assist the resident or patient with oral care as needed.			
18. Make the resident or patient comfortable and replace the call light.			
19. Lower the bed to a position of safety for the patient.			
20. Raise the side rails when ordered or appropriate for patient safety.			
21. Wash your hands.			
22. Report the following to your immediate supervisor • That you fed the resident or patient his food • The amount of food eaten (all, half, or refused to eat) • Your observations of anything unusual or difficulty encountered.			

Charting:

____

____

____

____

Date of Satisfactory Completion ____________________

Instructor's Signature ____________________

PROCEDURE 20-4: FEEDING A PHYSICALLY CHALLENGED PATIENT OR THE PATIENT WHO IS UNABLE TO FEED HIMSELF

Name: ______________________ Date: ______________________

STEPS	S	U	COMMENTS
1. Assemble your equipment on the overbed table a. Patient's tray			
2. Check the name on the card on the tray against the patient's identification bracelet.			
3. Tell the patient you are going to feed him or assist with the meal.			
4. Wash your hands.			
5. If allowed, the patient should be in high-Fowler's position.			
6. If you plan to be seated while you feed the patient, bring a chair to a convenient position beside the bed.			
7. Check the tray to make sure everything is there. If anything is missing, have it brought in or get it yourself.			
8. Tuck a napkin under the patient's chin.			
9. Season the food the way the patient likes it. However, do this only if his request agrees with the prescribed diet.			
10. For most patients unable to feed themselves, you will use a spoon. Fill the spoon only half full. Give the food to the patient from the tip of the spoon, not the side. Put the food in one side of the patient's mouth so he can chew it more easily. If a patient is paralyzed on one side of his body, make sure you feed him on the side of his mouth that is not paralyzed.			
11. If the patient cannot see the tray, name each mouthful of food as you offer it. Offer the different foods in a logical order, for example, soup or juice before the main course. Alternate between liquids and solid foods throughout the meal. Feed the patient as you yourself would want to eat. Or follow the patient's suggestions about how he wants to alternate between various kinds of foods and a beverage.			
12. If the patient is unable to see and would like to feed himself, you can describe the position of the food on the tray. For example, cold liquids are in the left corner, hot liquids in the right corner. Describe the food on the plate in terms of a clock face. For example, "Baked potato at 2 o'clock, peas at 4 o'clock, carrots at 5 o'clock, roast beef at 8 o'clock, and bread at 11 o'clock."			

13. Try to maintain the patient's independence as much as possible.			
14. Warn the patient if you are offering something hot. Never offer extremely hot liquids; allow them to cool. Use a straw for giving liquids. Use a new straw for each beverage.			
15. Feed the patient slowly. Remember that he may chew and swallow very slowly. Allow plenty of time between mouthfuls.			
16. Encourage the patient to finish the meal, but do not use force.			
17. When the patient has finished eating, help him to wipe his mouth with the napkin, or do this for the patient.			
18. Note how much the patient has eaten and how much he has had to drink.			
19. Record fluid intake on the intake and output (I&O) sheet or as directed by your supervisor, when the patient is on intake and output.			
20. Record how the patient has eaten his meal on the daily activity sheet or as directed by your supervisor. Record this information separately for breakfast, lunch, and supper. a. Did the patient eat all the food served? b. Did the patient eat about one-half the food served? c. Did the patient eat very little food? d. Did the patient refuse to eat anything?			
21. As soon as you are sure the patient is finished with the tray, take it away. Put it in its proper place.			
22. Adjust the backrest of the bed to make the patient comfortable, if this is allowed.			
23. Brush crumbs from the bed, smooth the sheets, and straighten the bedding.			
24. Assist the patient with oral care, or provide oral care as needed.			
25. Make the patient comfortable and replace the call light.			
26. Lower the bed to a position of safety for the patient.			
27. Raise the side rails when ordered or appropriate for patient safety.			

28. Wash your hands.			
29. Report the following to your immediate supervisor • That you fed the patient • Your observations of anything unusual			

Charting:

____

____

____

____

Date of Satisfactory Completion ____________________

Instructor's Signature ____________________

PROCEDURE 20-5: SERVING BETWEEN-MEAL NOURISHMENT

Name: ______________________ Date: ______________________

STEPS	S	U	COMMENTS
1. Wash your hands.			
2. Assemble your equipment on a tray or a cart a. Nourishment b. Cup, dish, and a spoon or straw c. Napkin			
3. Identify the patient by checking the identification bracelet.			
4. If the patient has a choice of items, ask what the patient prefers.			
5. Prepare the nourishment.			
6. Take the nourishment to the patient on a tray or cart.			
7. Encourage the patient to take the nourishment, assisting as needed. Offer a straw, if this is more convenient.			
8. After the patient has finished, collect the tray.			
9. Discard the disposable equipment.			
10. Record the intake for those patients who are on intake and output (I&O) records or calorie counts.			
11. Make the patient comfortable and replace the call light.			
12. Lower the bed to a position of safety for the patient.			
13. Raise the side rails when ordered or appropriate for patient safety.			
14. Wash your hands.			
15. Report the following to your immediate supervisor • That you served the between-meal nourishment • Your observations of anything unusual			

Charting:

____

____

____

____

Date of Satisfactory Completion ______________________

Instructor's Signature ______________________

PROCEDURE 20-6: PASSING DRINKING WATER

Name: ______________________ Date: ______________________

STEPS	S	U	COMMENTS
1. Assemble your equipment a. Moving table (cart) with small ice chest and cover or disposable water pitcher liners b. Ice cubes c. Scoop d. Paper or disposable cups e. Disposable water pitchers f. Straws g. Paper towels			
2. Wash your hands.			
3. Fill the disposable water pitcher liners or ice chest with ice cubes and cover it.			
4. Put all the equipment on the cart.			
5. Before you pass drinking water, be sure you know a. Which patients are NPO (nothing by mouth) b. Which patients are on restricted fluids and get only a measured amount of water c. Which patients get only tapwater (**omit** ice) d. Which patients may have icewater e. Which patients may not have a straw f. Which patients require a thickening product added to their water			
6. Roll the moving table into the hall outside the patient's room.			
7. Go into the room and pick up one patient's water pitcher/container. Record the patient's intake. Empty it in the sink in the room.			
8. Remove and discard the disposable liner.			
9. Walk to the water table in the hall. Insert a new water pitcher liner into the pitcher/container. Fill it half full with tapwater.			
10. Fill the pitcher to the brim with ice cubes, *being sure the scoop does not touch the water pitcher.*			
11. Replace the water pitcher on the same patient's table from which it was taken. If the pitcher is labeled with the patient's name, check it against the identification bracelet.			

12. Throw away used paper cups.			
13. Wipe the table with a clean paper towel. Discard the towel.			
14. Place several clean paper cups next to the water pitcher.			
15. Place several straws next to the water pitcher.			
16. Be sure the patient can reach the water pitcher easily.			
17. Offer to pour a fresh glass of water for the patient.			
18. Wash your hands.			
19. Report the following to your immediate supervisor • That you passed fresh drinking water to the patient • Your observations of anything unusual			

Charting:

____

____

____

____

Date of Satisfactory Completion ____________________

Instructor's Signature ____________________

The Urinary System and Related Care

21

Key Terms Review

Match the key terms in the right column with the definitions in the left column by placing the letter of each correct answer in the space provided.

_____ **1.** The group of body components including the kidneys, ureters, bladder, and urethra that removes wastes from the blood and produces and eliminates urine.

_____ **2.** A body opening or passage, such as the opening of the ear or the urethral canal.

_____ **3.** To urinate.

_____ **4.** Small tube that serves to empty urine from the bladder to the external environment.

_____ **5.** Waves of involuntary contractions.

_____ **6.** To discharge urine from the body; other terms for this function are *void, micturate,* and *pass water.*

_____ **7.** The fluid secreted by the kidneys, stored in the bladder, and excreted through the urethra.

_____ **8.** To urinate or pass water.

_____ **9.** A stretching out of the bladder when urine produced is not excreted.

_____ **10.** Painful voiding.

_____ **11.** Inability to urinate; no urine output.

_____ **12.** Fluid that is lost from the body without being noticed, such as in perspiration or air breathed out.

Terms

A. Catheter
B. Indwelling urinary catheter
C. Calibrated
D. Cubic centimeter (cc)
E. Convert
F. Graduate
G. Perspiration
H. Fluids
I. Restrict fluids
J. Parenteral intake
K. Nothing by mouth (NPO)
L. Fluid intake
M. Fluid output
N. Force fluids
O. Fluid balance
P. Fluid imbalance
Q. Eliminate
R. Void
S. Micturate
T. Urinate

_____13. Stability of all body functions at normal levels.

_____14. To pass off as vapor, as water evaporating into the air.

_____15. To take or soak in, up, or through.

_____16. Flowing out of material (secretion or excretion) from any part of the body, such as pus, feces, urine, or drainage from a wound.

_____17. To rid the body of waste products; to excrete, expel, remove, put out.

_____18. Unable to control urine or feces.

_____19. A watery environment around each cell that acts as a place of exchange for gases, food, and waste products between the cells and the blood.

_____20. Abnormal swelling of a part of the body caused by fluid collecting in that area; usually the swelling is in the ankles, legs, hands, or abdomen.

_____21. To keep or hold in.

_____22. Remaining or left over.

_____23. A decrease in the amount of water in the tissues occurring when fluid output exceeds input or intake.

_____24. Inflammation of the urinary bladder.

_____25. Acute or chronic inflammation of the kidneys.

_____26. A process used to remove waste products from the blood.

_____27. Use of an artificial kidney machine that filters a person's blood to remove waste products; lifesaving treatment required when a person has defective kidneys or chronic renal failure.

_____28. Fluids limited to certain amounts.

_____29. Cannot eat or drink anything at all.

_____30. Fluids taken in intravenously.

_____31. Liquid substances.

_____32. The same amount of fluid that is taken in by the body is given out by the body.

_____33. Occurs when too much fluid is kept in the body or when too much fluid is lost.

_____34. The fluid taken into the body, from whatever source, including IV fluids.

_____35. The fluid passed or excreted out of the body; for example urine, vomit, diarrhea.

_____36. Encouraging extra fluids to be taken in by a patient according to the doctor's orders.

_____37. Sweat.

U. Evaporate
V. Absorb
W. Incontinent
X. Discharge
Y. Retain
Z. Residual
AA. Urinary system (excretory system)
BB. Urethra
CC. Meatus
DD. Peristaltic waves
EE. Urine
FF. Bladder distention
GG. Homeostasis
HH. Dysuria
II. Anuria
JJ. Insensible fluid loss
KK. Edema
LL. Tissue fluid
MM. Dehydration
NN. Cystitis
OO. Nephritis
PP. Dialysis
QQ. Hemodialysis

_____38. A device for draining urine out of the body.

_____39. A bladder drainage tube that is allowed to remain in place within the bladder

_____40. To change from one form to another.

_____41. Having a volume equal to a cube whose edges are 1 centimeter long; 1 cc = 1 mL.

_____42. Marked with lines and numbers for measuring.

_____43. A measuring cup marked along its side to show various amounts so that the material placed in the cup can be measured accurately; the marks are called *calibrations*.

MULTIPLE-CHOICE QUESTIONS

Circle the letter next to the word or statement that best completes the sentence or answers the question.

1. Homeostasis is the body's attempt to
- a. keep its internal environment stable or in balance.
- b. increase its fluid intake.
- c. gain weight through fluid intake.
- d. stand very still.

2. Diagnostic studies of the urinary system are
- a. body fat analysis and QID urinalysis.
- b. difficult to interpret.
- c. key to predicting growth rates in children.
- d. able to indicate kidney function.

3. Some body fluid is lost through
- a. perspiration.
- b. delegation.
- c. undulation.
- d. constipation.

4. Cubic centimeters is a unit of measurement that can be used to measure fluids. Often _____ is the acceptable alternative to use.
- a. cb. ctr.
- b. mL.
- c. cubo cento.
- d. cbcmtr.

5. The best time to record the patient's fluid intake is
- a. when you have time.
- b. when your immediate supervisor tells you to record ASAP.
- c. 20 minutes before the end of your shift.
- d. as soon as the patient consumes the fluids.

6. When measuring and recording intake and output, __________ __________and __________ __________ are very important.
- a. good vision; good will
- b. exact observations; working fast
- c. disposable gloves; inline skates
- d. exact observations; accurate recordings

7. Fluids taken _______ are recorded by the nurse.
- a. intravenously
- b. secretly
- c. copiously
- d. daily

8. The indwelling catheter bag must always be kept
- a. above the head.
- b. above the waist.
- c. below the knee.
- d. below hip level.

9. The urinary system is responsible for
- a. placing waste back into the blood.
- b. making urine and plasma.

c. getting rid of unwanted materials though diarrhea.
d. reabsorbing essential materials and getting rid of waste through the production of urine.

10. The _______ is a storage container for urine and contains stretch receptors that send messages to the brain, allowing micturition to occur.
a. bladder
b. ureter
c. urethra
d. meatus

11. The _______ are tubes that allow urine to pass from the kidney to the bladder using peristaltic action.
a. ureters
b. urethras
c. meatus
d. valves

12. Because the _______ is in close proximity to the anus, bladder infections are more likely to occur in females.
a. ureters
b. urethral opening
c. bladder
d. kidneys

13. If cystitis is not treated correctly, __________ may occur.
a. nephritis or kidney damage
b. bladder tonicity
c. enlarged prostate
d. cancer

14. Men who are 50 years and older may have an enlarged prostate gland, which causes changes in the urinary system. They may experience ________________ because of this.
a. concentrated urine
b. decreased bladder tone
c. a feeling of pressure and urinary frequency
d. the ability to void normally with good force and flow

15. When observing urine, it is important for the nursing assistant to report any unusual finding such as
a. clear, straw-colored urine.
b. a slight ammonia smell.
c. urine that turns cloudy when left to stand for a few minutes.
d. blood or white fragments floating in the urine.

16. Normal fluid intake and output for most adults is approximately _____ of fluid per day.
a. 100–200 mL
b. 2000 mL
c. 1/5 of the approximate body weight
d. approximately 3 quarts, or 3300 mL

17. Which condition in infants and the elderly is dangerous and should be reported immediately?
a. Constipation
b. Not voiding in 4 hours
c. Diarrhea
d. Diaphoresis

18. Retaining fluid in the lower extremities is called _______ and can indicate a fluid imbalance.
a. diaphoresis
b. dehydration
c. edema
d. perspiration

19. Vomiting, bleeding, excess sweating, and diarrhea can lead to
a. fluid loss and dehydration.
b. fluid maintenance and good hydration.
c. wound drainage and perspiration.
d. all of the above.

20. If a patient is on I&O and has an incontinent episode in bed, the nursing assistant should
a. estimate how much urine was lost in milliliters and document this on the flow sheet.
b. strip the linens off the bed and then weigh them using a patient scale and

then document the weight of the urine lost.

c. tell the supervisor the patient is incontinent and needs an indwelling catheter placed for accurate I&O measurement.

d. document what time an incontinent episode occurred and note urine could not be measured so the physician can see that the patient is capable of voiding.

21. When a doctor writes an order that a patient must be NPO because surgery is scheduled for the next day, the nursing assistant should

a. remove the water pitcher from the room and explain to the patient he should not drink anything after midnight.

b. allow the patient to brush his teeth frequently.

c. post a sign outside the patient's door alerting staff not to refill the patient's water pitcher.

d. all of the above.

22. A nursing assistant could persuade a patient to drink fluids by offering

a. broth.

b. ice cream.

c. custard.

d. all of the above.

23. Indwelling catheters should

a. be hung on the bedframe or a non-moveable part of the bed lower than the patient's waist.

b. placed higher than the patient's bladder to insure gravity helps urine drain correctly.

c. pinned to the bed sheets so tearing of the meatus does not occur.

d. never be cleaned as this can lead to a urinary tract infection.

24. When caring for an indwelling catheter, the nursing assistant should

a. empty the drainage bag only at the end of her shift.

b. kink the tubing so no back flow of urine occurs in the kidneys.

c. loosely tape or strap the tubing to the patient's inner thigh to avoid tearing of the meatus.

d. allow the tubing to touch the floor to ensure proper drainage of urine from the bladder.

25. Should the drainage port touch the floor when emptying a catheter, the nursing assistant should

a. report this to the supervisor immediately.

b. wipe the port off with an alcohol swab immediately.

c. cut the tubing at the place it touched the floor.

d. remove the catheter and insert a new one immediately.

TRUE OR FALSE QUESTIONS

Determine whether each question is true or false. In the space provided, write "T" for true and "F" for false. If the statement is false, rewrite it on the line provided to make it a true statement.

_____ **1.** When measuring the capacity of serving containers, be sure to hold them at waist level while observing the amount of fluid carefully.

____

_____ **2.** *NPO* means "Note Patient Order."

____

_____ 3. When a woman is pregnant, she may experience pressure on her bladder and urinary frequency.

____

_____ 4. A nursing assistant should report if a patient has not voided in an 8-hour period.

____

_____ 5. *Nocturia* means the patient has blood in the urine.

____

_____ 6. Another word for *vomitus* is *emesis*.

____

_____ 7. Gelatin is considered a solid and should not be counted on the I&O sheet.

____

_____ 8. Offering frequent mouth care is acceptable practice when a patient has been ordered to restrict fluids.

____

_____ 9. A nursing assistant should report any patient complaint of burning, tenderness, pain, or change in the appearance of the urine when an indwelling catheter is in place.

____

_____ 10. When discontinuing an indwelling catheter, it is acceptable for any nursing assistant to cut the tubing below the valve and pull the tubing out of the bladder.

____

FILL-IN-THE-BLANK QUESTIONS

Provide the meaning of the following abbreviations.

1. NPO ______________________________
2. mL ______________________________
3. I&O ______________________________
4. L ______________________________
5. FF ______________________________

EXERCISE 21-1

Objective: To recognize and be able to correctly spell the parts of the urinary system.

Directions: Label the diagram in Figure 21-1 with the correct words from the following word list.

Word List

Ureters	Nephron	Left kidney
Urethra	Bowman's capsule	Right kidney
Bladder	Glomerulus	Tubule

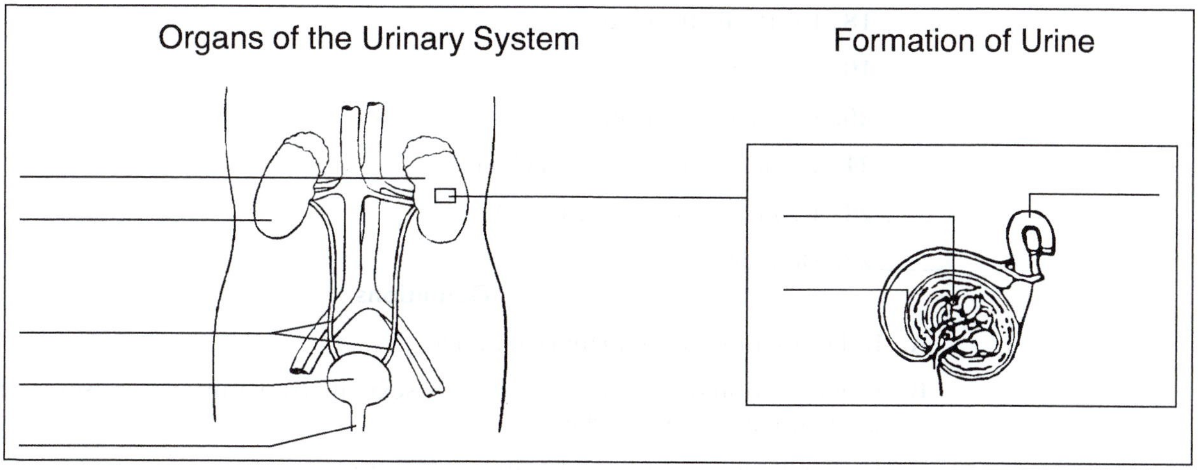

FIGURE 21-1

EXERCISE 21-2

Objective: To define correctly words that refer to diseases and disorders of the urinary system.

Directions: Label each disease or disorder with the letter of its correct definition.

Disease or Disorder

_____ **1.** Acute renal failure

_____ **2.** Anuria

_____ **3.** Cancer of the urinary bladder

_____ **4.** Chronic renal failure

_____ **5.** Cystitis

_____ **6.** Dysuria

_____ **7.** Hematuria

_____ **8.** Hydronephrosis

_____ **9.** Injury to the bladder

_____ **10.** Nocturia

_____ **11.** Oliguria

_____ **12.** Polyuria

_____ **13.** Pyelonephritis

_____ **14.** Pyuria

_____ **15.** Renal colic

_____ **16.** Tuberculosis of the kidney

_____ **17.** Tumors of the kidney

_____**18.** Urethral stricture

_____**19.** Urethritis

_____**20.** Urinary retention

_____**21.** Urinary tract infection (UTI)

_____**22.** Urolithiasis (renal calculi)

_____**23.** Dehydration

Definitions

A. Inflammation of the urinary bladder

B. Inflammation of the urethra often by sexually transmitted diseases such as chlamydia or gonorrhea.

C. Unusually large volume of urine in 24 hours

D. Painful voiding

E. Frequency of urination at night

F. Loss of kidney function

G. Presence of pathogenic microorganisms in the urinary tract

H. Sharp, severe pain in lower back over kidney, accompany forcible dilation of a ureter because of a stone or urinary calculus

I. Presence of stones in the urinary (excretory) system

J. Distention of the pelvis or one or both kidneys (urine being made but cannot be excreted because of urinary backup)

K. Inability to urinate

L. Very small amount of urine in 24 hours

M. Caused by *Mycobacterium tuberculosis* in the kidney

N. Pus in the urine infection

O. Infection of the kidney (acute or chronic)

P. Malignant tumor

Q. No urine

R. Narrowing of the urethra caused by infection or instrumentation; results in frequent voiding, dysuria, and hematuria (blood in the urine)

S. Blood in the urine

T. Progressive deterioration of kidney function

U. Considered malignant until proved otherwise

V. The result of trauma

W. Insufficient water in the tissues because of inadequate fluid intake or excessive fluid output

EXERCISE 21-3

Objective: To demonstrate the correct placement of intake and output information on the Intake and Output sheet.

Directions: Record the information in each statement in the correct place on the Intake and Output sheet in Figure 21-2. Total the amount for your shift. Refer to Figure 21-3 for the capacities of the serving containers.

PRACTICE STATEMENT: Mrs. Stavros, a patient, is dehydrated. You are her nursing assistant from the 7 AM to 3 PM shift. The doctor has ordered that she be put on a liquid diet, force fluids, and that her fluid intake and output be measured for the next 24 hours. The nurse communicates to you in the morning report meeting that Mrs. Stavros is on Intake and Output (I&O). The patient has not been taking fluids well. The nurse would like you to encourage her to increase her fluid intake. If her fluid intake does not improve in the next 24 hours, the doctor stated that she will order that an IV be started. She would prefer that the patient try to take her fluids orally, if possible. Mrs. Stavros has an indwelling catheter.

INTAKE				OUTPUT			
				URINE		GASTRIC	
ITEM	BY MOUTH	TUBE	PARENTERAL	VOIDED	CATHETER	EMESIS	SUCTION
TOTAL							

FIGURE 21-2

Statements

1. Your patient drank one 6-oz cup of juice, drank one-half of a 12-oz bowl of broth, and ate one 6-oz gelatin cup for breakfast.
2. Between breakfast and lunch, with your encouragement, she drank one 12-oz can of ginger ale.
3. Your patient drank one 8-oz cup of milk, drank one-half of a 12-oz bowl of broth, and ate one 6-oz gelatin cup for lunch.
4. Between lunch and the time your shift was over, you convinced her to drink one 8-oz cup of water.
5. When you measured the amount of urine in the catheter bag, you determined that it filled the graduate container to the one-quart level.

FIGURE 21-3

Examples of Capacities of Serving Containers	
4-oz juice cup	120 mL
6-oz cup	180 mL
8-oz cup	240 mL
12-oz cup	360 mL
1-cup milk carton	240 mL
4-oz ice cream cup	120 mL
6-oz Jell-O cup	180 mL
6-oz coffee cup	180 mL
1-qt water pitcher	1000 mL

EXERCISE 21-4

Directions: Circle the correct answer after reading the following word problem. Use scrap paper to do the math if needed.

1. Mrs. Jones is on I&O. At 9 AM, she drank a 4-oz container of orange juice, a 6-oz cup of coffee, and 80 mL of water with her medication. How much fluid did she drink during the morning meal?
   a. 380 mL
   b. 90 oz
   c. 380 oz
   d. 250 mL
2. At 11:30 AM, Mrs. Jones uses the bathroom after she eats breakfast. She uses the specipan as you directed and voids 9 ounces of clear, light straw-colored urine. On the I&O sheet, you document the volume of urine she voided as
   a. 9 oz.
   b. 270 mL.
   c. 39 mL.
   d. 3 mL.
3. For lunch, Mrs. Jones drinks one-half of an 8-ounce soda and one-third of a 6-ounce bowl of broth. She asks for a 6-ounce cup of coffee and drinks only half of it. How much fluid did she drink?
   a. 20 oz
   b. 18 oz
   c. 9 mL
   d. 270 mL
4. Using the results from questions 1–3, how much fluid did Mrs. Jones drink in an 8-hour shift?
   a. 650 mL
   b. 21 mL
   c. 920 mL
   d. 30 oz

5. At 2:45 PM, you tally Mrs. Jones' I&O and note that in your 8-hour shift her intake was _____ and her output was ______.
   a. 650 mL; 270 mL
   b. 270 mL; 650 mL
   c. 540 mL; 380 mL
   d. 540 mL; 270 mL

THE NURSING ASSISTANT IN ACTION

1. Your shift is starting. As you check on your patients, you notice the nursing assistant from the night shift forgot to empty and record the output on all the indwelling catheter drainage bags for your patients. What should you do?

   ____
   ____
   ____
   ____

2. You just started your 12-hour shift at 7 PM. In report, the nurse tells you that the doctor just wrote an NPO order for the patient in room 101 because this patient will go into surgery at 8 AM tomorrow. What should you do?

   ____
   ____
   ____
   ____

3. You empty urine into a graduate from an indwelling catheter. You go to set a barrier down on a flat surface and knock the graduate filled with urine onto the floor before getting a chance to read the volume of urine. The patient is on I&O. What should you do?

   ____
   ____
   ____
   ____

4. A patient who is on I&O uses the bathroom to void. You enter the bathroom to record the output and clean the specipan when you realize there is toilet paper in the specipan. What should you do?

   ____
   ____
   ____
   ____

5. You are asked by your supervisor to change an indwelling catheter bag to a leg bag. What should you do?

____

____

____

____

LEARNING ACTIVITIES

1. It is very important that you observe the exact amounts of fluids taken in by the patient and that you record them accurately. You must measure the amount of liquid contained in each serving container, bowl, glass, or cup used by the patient. If your institution does not have a list of the amounts contained in each container, bowl, glass, or cup, make such a list yourself. See Table 21–3 in the textbook to help you create a "cheat sheet" which you can then laminate or glue to a 3" × 5" index card and keep in the pocket of your uniform.
2. Take a sealable plastic bag and fill it halfway with water. Using paper tape, secure it to the outside of your upper leg. Wear it for a 24-hour period and even when you sleep. Identify what felt strange about this exercise, what types of clothes you wore that helped conceal the bag, and what difficulties you encountered. Using this information, apply it the next time you have a patient who has a urinary drainage bag to help the patient adjust and cope with this new appliance.

PROCEDURE CHECKLISTS

PROCEDURE 21-1: MEASURING THE CAPACITY OF SERVING CONTAINERS

Name: ______________________ Date: ______________________

STEPS	S	U	COMMENTS
1. Assemble your equipment in the utility room a. Complete set of dishes, bowls, cups, and glasses used by the patients b. Graduate (measuring cup) c. Water d. Pen and paper			
2. Fill the first container with water.			
3. Pour this water into the graduate.			
4. Place the graduate on a flat surface for accuracy in measurement.			
5. At eye level, carefully look at the level of the water and determine the amount in mL.			
6. Write this information on the paper. For example, one carton of milk = 240 mL.			
7. Repeat these steps for each dish, glass, bowl, or cup used by the patient.			
8. You will have a complete list to use when measuring intake.			

Charting:

____

____

____

____

Date of Satisfactory Completion ______________________

Instructor's Signature ______________________

PROCEDURE 21-2: MEASURING FLUID INTAKE BY DETERMINING THE AMOUNTS CONSUMED

Name: ____________________ Date: ____________________

STEPS	S	U	COMMENTS
1. Assemble your equipment on the bedside table a. Graduate b. Pen and paper c. Leftover liquids in their serving containers			
2. Pour the leftover liquid into the graduate.			
3. Look at the level and determine the amount in mL.			
4. From your list (see Procedure 21-1), determine the amount in the full serving container.			
5. Subtract the leftover amount from the full-container amount. This figure is the amount the patient actually drank.			
6. Immediately record this amount on the intake side of the intake and output sheet.			

Charting:

____

____

____

____

Date of Satisfactory Completion ____________________

Instructor's Signature ____________________

PROCEDURE 21-3: MEASURING URINARY OUTPUT

Name: ____________________ Date: ____________________

STEPS	S	U	COMMENTS
1. Assemble your equipment in the patient's bathroom a. Bedpan, cover, urinal, or specipan b. Graduate (measuring container or calibrated container) c. Intake and output sheet d. Pencil or pen e. Disposable gloves			
2. Wash your hands and put on gloves.			
3. Pour the urine from the bedpan or urinal into a graduate.			
4. Place a barrier or paper towel first and then the graduate on a flat surface for accuracy in measurement.			
5. At eye level, carefully look at the level of urine in the graduate to see the number reached by the level of the urine.			
6. Record this amount in mL, as well as the time, on the output side of the intake and output sheet.			
7. Discard paper towel. Wash, rinse, and return the graduate to its proper place.			
8. Wash, rinse, and return the urinal or bedpan to its proper place.			
9. Dispose of gloves and wash your hands.			
10. Report to your immediate supervisor • That you measured the output for the patient. • Your observations of anything unusual.			

Charting:

____

____

____

____

Date of Satisfactory Completion ____________________

Instructor's Signature ____________________

PROCEDURE 21-4: EMPTYING, MEASURING, AND RECORDING URINARY OUTPUT FROM AN INDWELLING CATHETER DRAINAGE BAG

Name: ______________________ Date: ______________________

STEPS	S	U	COMMENTS
1. Assemble your equipment a. Calibrated graduate b. Alcohol swab c. Disposable gloves			
2. Wash your hands and put on gloves.			
3. Check for and unbend any kinks in tubing. Be sure the urine bag is hanging lower than the bladder. (The bag should be hanging with the hook connected to the bedframe or a non-moveable section of the bed.)			
4. Open the drain at the bottom of the plastic urine drainage bag and let the urine run into the graduate; after the bag has emptied, close the drain, wipe with alcohol swab, and replace in the holder on the bag.			
5. Measure the amount of urinary output.			
6. Record the amount immediately on the output side of the intake and output sheet.			
7. Wash and rinse the graduate and put it in its proper place.			
8. Dispose of gloves and wash your hands.			
9. Document or report to your immediate supervisor • That you emptied the urine drainage bag and measured the amount of output. • That you recorded the amount on the output side of the intake and output sheet. • Your observations of anything unusual.			

Charting:

____

____

____

____

Date of Satisfactory Completion ______________________

Instructor's Signature ______________________

PROCEDURE 21-5: CHANGING A LEG BAG TO A DRAINAGE BAG

Name: ____________________ Date: ____________________

STEPS	S	U	COMMENTS
1. Assemble your equipment a. Drainage bag and tubing b. Alcohol swab c. Disposable gloves d. Sterile cap and plug e. Waterproof pad f. Catheter clamp g. Bedpan h. Bath blanket i. Paper towels j. Waterproof pad or barrier			
2. Identify the patient by checking the identification bracelet.			
3. Arrange waterproof barrier, paper towels, and equipment on the overbed table.			
4. Tell the patient you are going to change his leg bag to a drainage bag.			
5. Provide privacy for the patient.			
6. Have the patient sit on the side of the bed.			
7. Wash your hands and put on gloves.			
8. Expose the catheter and leg bag. Clamp the catheter to prevent urine from draining from the catheter into the drainage tubing.			
9. Allow any urine below the clamp placed on the tubing to empty into the collection bag.			
10. Assist the patient to lie down. Raise the side rails on the opposite side of the bed before adjusting the height of the bed to a comfortable working position.			
11. Cover the patient with the bath blanket, leaving the catheter and leg bag exposed.			
12. Place the waterproof pad or barrier under the patient's leg.			
13. Open the alcohol or antiseptic wipes and place them on the paper towel.			
14. Open the package with the sterile plug and cap. Place the opened package on the paper towel. Do not allow anything to touch the cap or plug.			

15. Open the package with the drainage bag and tubing. Attach the drainage bag to the bedframe.			
16. Disconnect the catheter from the drainage tubing; do not allow anything to touch the end.			
17. Hold on to the plug end and insert the sterile plug into the retention catheter end. Should you touch anything with the end of the catheter, wipe the end with the antiseptic before inserting the sterile plug.			
18. Place the sterile cap on the end of the leg drainage bag tubing. (Should you touch anything with the tubing end, wipe the end with the antiseptic before putting on the sterile cap.)			
19. Remove the sterile cap from the end of the new drainage bag tubing.			
20. Remove the sterile plug from the catheter and insert the of the drainage tubing into the catheter.			
21. Remove the clamp from the catheter.			
22. Loop the drainage tubing on the bed and secure the tubing to the bottom bed linens.			
23. Remove the leg bag and place it in the bedpan.			
24. Remove and discard the waterproof pad and any disposable items.			
25. Cover the patient, remove the bath blanket, and make the patient comfortable. Readjust bed height and lower side rails as needed.			
26. Take the bedpan to the bathroom.			
27. Open the drain at the bottom of the plastic urine leg drainage bag and allow the urine to run into the graduate container. After the bag has emptied, close the drain.			
28. Measure the amount of urine in the graduate container and record the amount of urinary output.			
29. Discard leg bag and tubing following the agency's policy.			
30. Wash and rinse the graduate and put it in its proper place.			
31. Dispose of gloves and wash your hands.			
32. Record the amount immediately on the output align side of the intake and output sheet.			

33. Document or report to your immediate supervisor • That you changed the leg bag to a drainage bag, emptied the urine drainage bag, and measured the amount of output. • That you recorded the amount on the output side of the intake and output sheet. • Your observations of anything unusual.			

Charting:

____

____

____

____

Date of Satisfactory Completion ____________________

Instructor's Signature ____________________

PROCEDURE 21-6: PROVIDING MALE AND FEMALE INDWELLING CATHETER CARE

Name: ____________________ Date: ____________________

STEPS	S	U	COMMENTS
1. Assemble your equipment a. Disposable catheter care kit (or use washcloths and soap or cleaning solution as directed) b. Disposable gloves c. Disposable bed protector			
2. Identify the patient by checking the identification bracelet.			
3. Wash your hands.			
4. Tell the patient you are going to clean the area around his catheter tube. Make sure the patient's genital area has already been washed or that perineal care has been done.			
5. Provide privacy for the patient.			
6. Raise the bed to a comfortable working position. Raise the side rail on opposite side of the bed.			
7. Make sure there is plenty of light.			
8. Cover the patient with a bath blanket. Without exposing him, fan-fold the top sheets to the foot of the bed. Have the patient covered with only the blanket.			
9. Open the catheter kit. Put on the disposable gloves. Place the disposable bed protector under the patient's buttocks.			
10. Observe for crusting, lesions, discharge, or anything else abnormal.			
11. Take the applicators from the kit. The applicators are covered with antiseptic solution. Female patient: With your gloved thumb and forefinger (index finger), gently separate the labia on female patients. Male patient: If the male patient has not been circumcised and has a foreskin, gently pull it back to apply antiseptic solution to the entire area. Apply antiseptic solution on the entire area where the catheter enters the patient's body. Work from the cleanest area to the dirtiest. Use a circular motion when washing the meatus and glans. Gently replace the male's foreskin if you have pulled it back.			

12. Hold the catheter near the meatus. Using one stroke, clean the catheter from the meatus down the catheter about 4". If the catheter is not clean, repeat as needed. (You may be instructed to use a clean soapy washcloth to perform catheter care. If so, rinse the catheter with a clean wet washcloth from the meatus down the catheter about 4".) Avoid pulling or tugging on the catheter.			
13. Pat the perineal area dry from front to back.			
14. Check the strap or tape to be sure the tubing is taped correctly in place.			
15. Remove the disposable bed protector.			
16. Cover the patient with the top sheets. Remove the bath blanket.			
17. Make the patient comfortable and replace the call light.			
18. Lower the bed to a position of safety for the patient.			
19. Lower or raise the side rails as ordered or appropriate for patient safety.			
20. Discard disposable equipment.			
21. Remove gloves and wash your hands.			
22. Report to your immediate supervisor • That catheter care was given. • The time it was given. • How the patient tolerated the procedure. • Your observations of anything unusual.			

Charting:

____

____

____

____

Date of Satisfactory Completion ______________

Instructor's Signature ______________

PROCEDURE 21-7: APPLYING A CONDOM CATHETER ON A MALE PATIENT

Name: ____________________ Date: ____________________

STEPS	S	U	COMMENTS
1. Assemble your supplies a. Condom catheter kit b. Drainage bag or leg bag and cap c. Basin of warm water d. Soap, washcloth, and towel e. Gloves f. Bed protector g. Paper towels			
2. Identify the patient by checking the identification bracelet.			
3. Explain the procedure to the patient.			
4. Ask about any allergies, including latex.			
5. Provide privacy for the patient.			
6. Wash your hands.			
7. Cover the patient with a bath blanket. Fan-fold top bed linens to the patient's lower legs.			
8. Ask the patient to raise his buttocks to enable you to slide the bed protector under him. (Turn the patient on his side to place the bed protector under his buttocks if he is unable to lift himself.)			
9. Assemble the equipment, making sure the drainage bag or leg bag is ready with the drain closed and cap in place.			
10. Arrange the bath blanket to expose the genital area.			
11. Put on gloves.			
12. Remove condom catheter if patient has one in place by removing elastic tape and rolling the condom sheath off the penis. Disconnect the drainage tubing from the condom and cap the drainage tube. Discard the tape and condom.			
13. Provide male perineal care. Check the penis for signs of skin breakdown, redness, or irritation.			
14. Prepare the new condom by removing the protective backing and exposing the adhesive strip. Remove the fenestrated drape from the kit, and using your nondominant hand, place the penis through the hole in the drape. Keep your dominant hand sterile.			

15. (Optional; depends on agency and manufacturer product.) Secure the condom with the elastic tape applied in a spiral. Do not apply the tape completely around the penis, as it can prevent circulation.			
16. Connect the condom with the drainage bag or attach the leg bag.			
17. Remove bed protector and bath blanket. Position the patient for comfort and replace the linens.			
18. Measure and record the amount of urine in the bag.			
19. Firmly hold the penis as you roll the condom over the penis. Be sure to leave a 1" space at the end of the condom catheter.			
20. Clean the basin and return items to their proper place. Remove and discard gloves and all disposable items used.			
21. Wash hands.			
22. Document and report the results to your supervisor.			

Charting:

____

____

____

____

Date of Satisfactory Completion ____________________

Instructor's Signature ____________________

PROCEDURE 21-8: REMOVING OR DISCONTINUING AN INDWELLING CATHETER

Name: ______________________ Date: ______________________

STEPS	S	U	COMMENTS
1. Assemble your supplies a. 10 cc syringe b. Gloves c. Basin of warm water d. Soap, washcloth, and towel e. Bed protector			
2. Identify the patient by checking the identification bracelet.			
3. Explain the procedure to the patient.			
4. Provide privacy for the patient.			
5. Wash your hands.			
6. Cover the patient with a bath blanket. Fan-fold the top bed linens to the patient's lower legs.			
7. a. Ask the female patient to raise her buttocks to enable you to slide the bed protector or towel under her. (Turn the patient on her side to place the bed protector under her buttocks if she is unable to lift herself.) b. Drape the towel or bath blanket over the male patient's thighs and under the scrotum.			
8. Assemble the equipment.			
9. Arrange the bath blanket to expose the genital area.			
10. Put on gloves.			
11. Remove any tape securing the catheter tube to the patient.			
12. Attach the syringe to the balloon port on the catheter.			
13. Tell the patient that you are ready. Slowly withdraw all the contents of the inflated balloon (usually about 10 cc of sterile saline). This allows the balloon to deflate and the catheter can easily be removed from the urethra. Call your supervisor if you experience difficulty removing the water.			
14. Ask the patient to take a deep breath as you gently but firmly pull the catheter out. Do not use force to remove the catheter. If you encounter resistance, stop and check with your supervisor.			
15. Clean up any urine that may have dripped.			

16. Provide perineal care. Check the penis or female's urethra for signs of skin breakdown, redness, or irritation.			
17. Remove the bed protector and bath blanket. Position the patient for comfort and replace the linens.			
18. Measure and record the amount of urine in the bag.			
19. Clean the basin and return items to their proper place. Remove and discard gloves, the catheter, drainage bag and all disposable items used.			
20. Wash your hands.			
21. Document and report the results to your supervisor.			

Charting:

____

____

____

____

Date of Satisfactory Completion________________

Instructor's Signature________________________

Specimen Collection

22

Key Terms Review

Match the key terms in the right column with the definitions in the left column by placing the letter of each correct answer in the space provided.

_____ **1.** A sample of material taken from the patient's body; examples are urine, stool, and sputum.

_____ **2.** Free of disease-causing microorganisms.

_____ **3.** Special practices and procedures for preventing the conditions that allow disease-producing bacteria to live, multiply, and spread.

_____ **4.** Solid waste material discharged from the body through the rectum and anus. Other names include *stool, excrement, bowel movement,* and *fecal matter.*

_____ **5.** To cough up and spit out matter from the lungs, trachea, or bronchial tubes.

_____ **6.** Means the urine for this specimen is not contaminated by anything outside the patient's body.

_____ **7.** Catching the urine specimen between the time the patient begins to void and the time he stops.

_____ **8.** Urine collected from a patient over a 24-hour period that is studied to determine kidney function.

_____ **9.** A substance found in urine when your body converts fats into energy; can indicate diabetes or diet problems.

_____ **10.** Waste material coughed up from the lungs or trachea.

Terms

A. Asepsis

B. Medical asepsis

C. Specimen

D. Ketone

E. Sputum

F. Expectorate

G. Clean catch

H. 24-hour urine

I. Midstream

J. Feces or stool

MULTIPLE-CHOICE QUESTIONS

Circle the letter next to the word or statement that best completes the sentence or answers the question.

1. Most of the body's waste materials are discharged in the
   a. blood and sputum.
   b. sweat and mucus.
   c. urine and feces.
   d. stool and emesis.

2. Specimens are to be collected
   a. within 2 hours of the ordered collection time.
   b. when the nursing assistant or nurse has time.
   c. at the time that is indicated by the medical order.
   d. whenever.

3. The specimen collection procedure must be followed exactly
   a. or the specimen may not be useful.
   b. for the right patient.
   c. or the patient may be misdiagnosed.
   d. all of the above.

4. The specimen must be ____________ immediately to avoid mistakes.
   a. tested
   b. labeled
   c. stored
   d. shaken

5. If the specimen has the wrong name on it,
   a. the right treatment may be ordered.
   b. the correct medication may be ordered.
   c. the wrong problem may be identified.
   d. the patient will receive effective treatment.

6. It is important to wash your hands before and after collecting a specimen to avoid
   a. contamination of the specimen with your bacteria.
   b. spreading disease to the patient.
   c. contaminating yourself with disease-producing bacteria.
   d. all of the above.

7. The urine specimen that is the most common is the
   a. routine urine specimen.
   b. stool specimen.
   c. common specimen.
   d. 24-hour specimen.

8. A clean-catch specimen must be free from
   a. contamination.
   b. harm.
   c. cost.
   d. high temperatures.

9. Before a 24-hour urine specimen is started, the patient must
   a. shower for 24 minutes.
   b. be NPO for 24 hours.
   c. empty her bladder.
   d. measure her weight.

10. *Sputum* is a substance collected from the patient's
   a. axilla.
   b. navel.
   c. sputola structures.
   d. lungs.

11. The most common reason to test stool is to look for the presence of
   a. blood or parasites.
   b. stones or calculi.
   c. *E. coli* bacteria.
   d. bile.

12. It is important to explain to the patient
   a. the reason for the test.
   b. the results of the test.
   c. what you are going to do before you do it.
   d. all the steps to be followed in collecting specimens.

13. When obtaining a specimen from an older person who has memory loss, the nursing assistant should
   a. explain all the steps all at once.

b. place many signs all over the room to remind the person that a specimen must be obtained.
c. offer simple steps and stay with the patient while the specimen is obtained.
d. keep the curtain open to maintain privacy.

14. During the collection of a routine urine specimen, the nursing assistant must
a. fill the collection container at least half full.
b. squeeze urine from any toilet paper left in the bedpan to ensure correct measurement.
c. place the label on the container while the urine is being collected.
d. wash the patient's genitals for him prior to collecting the specimen.

15. When obtaining a _______ urine specimen, it is important that the patient begins to void, stops voiding, collects the urine, and then completely finishes voiding.
a. clean-catch
b. midstream
c. 24-hour
d. Both a and b

16. A 24-hour urine specimen has been ordered for a female patient. As a nursing assistant, you explain the reason for the test, place a specipan in the toilet, and then
a. place signs over the bed and in the bathroom to help remind the patient and staff that 24-hour urine is in progress.
b. have the patient void regardless of whether she has to do so, collect this specimen, and begin the test immediately.
c. have the patient clean her genitals, start voiding, stop voiding, collect the urine in the container, and finish voiding.
d. measure each time the patient voids and record the amount on the intake and output flow sheet and discard the urine.

17. When a 24-hour urine specimen is in progress, ice may be placed in a second container to
a. help dilute the urine in the container used to collect the urine.
b. increase the amount of bacteria that will grow during that time.
c. keep the specimen cool during the time it takes to collect all of the urine and ensure better test results.
d. rule out diabetes and renal failure.

18. When checking urine for kidney stones (calculi), the nursing assistant must
a. place all urine collected in a container and send it to the lab immediately.
b. strain the urine using gauze, place any particles found in a bag and send the specimen to the lab.
c. have the patient void directly into the graduate with the strainer in place so no stone gets missed.
d. look closely at the urine for anything unusual floating in the waste.

19. When working with reagent test strips, the nursing assistant should
a. store the strips at room temperature.
b. keep the strips out of direct sunlight.
c. discard any container that is expired.
d. all of the above.

20. Reagent test strips are used for many reasons. The most common reason a nursing assistant uses a reagent test strip is to test for
a. glucose in urine.
b. ketones in urine.
c. pH in urine.
d. all of the above.

21. A sputum sample was ordered for a patient. The nursing assistant enters a room to find what looks like spit in the sputum container. The nursing assistant should
a. bring the specimen to the nurse supervisor and ask what to do next.
b. send the specimen with the accurate information written on the label to the lab immediately.
c. note the color, amount, odor, and consistency of the specimen and send it to the lab at once.
d. bring another container to the patient, have him cough deeply upon the third exhale, and try to obtain another specimen.

22. A stool sample can be obtained
a. to diagnose the presence of glucose.
b. to rule out the existence of parasites in feces.
c. using a gloved finger.
d. from 1–2 teaspoons of fecal matter.

23. If a warm stool sample is ordered, the nursing assistant must
a. ask the patient to defecate immediately.
b. take the sample to the lab as soon as the sample is obtained.
c. place the stool sample on ice to ensure bacteria does not grow.
d. wrap the specimen in toilet paper to keep it warm while it is being transported to the lab.

24. If the solution used on the Hemoccult slide turns blue, the nursing assistant should
a. report a guiac positive result to the nurse.
b. hand the Hemoccult slide to the nurse and have her retest the stool.
c. assume there is no blood in the stool.
d. wait 1 minute and then report a guiac negative result to the nurse.

25. Allowing a nursing assistant to perform a Hemoccult test
a. is allowed in all types of facilities.
b. is allowed in some states.
c. is never allowed and should be performed at all times by a nurse.
d. can only be done under the direct supervision of a doctor.

TRUE OR FALSE QUESTIONS

Determine whether each question is true or false. In the space provided, write "T" for true and "F" for false. If the statement is false, rewrite it on the line provided to make it a true statement.

_____ **1.** If a person is sick, there are noticeable changes in the body wastes when they are tested.

____

_____ **2.** It is very important to identify the patient by name, ID number, and room number before obtaining the specimen.

____

_____ **3.** A clean-catch specimen procedure requires careful washing of the abdominal area.

____

_____ **4.** It is important to wear personal protective equipment while collecting patient specimens.

____

_____ **5.** The best time to obtain a sputum specimen is in the early morning after the patient has been sleeping all night.

____

_____ **6.** Some stool specimens must be kept cold until tested.

____

_____ **7.** It may be necessary to remain with a small child to talk them through the process as a specimen is being collected.

____

_____ **8.** A nursing assistant should wait approximately 30 minutes for accurate Hemoccult results.

____

_____ **9.** Approximately 1–2 tablespoons of feces is needed when obtaining a stool specimen.

____

_____ **10.** A specimen must be ordered by a doctor before collection can occur.

____

FILL-IN-THE-BLANK QUESTIONS

Provide the meaning of the following abbreviations.

1. ID ______________________________
2. pH ______________________________
3. BM ______________________________
4. neg ______________________________

EXERCISE 22-1

Objective: To apply what you have learned about specimen collection.

Directions: Read the following carefully before writing the correct answer on the blank line.

1. What process is done to urine samples to detect solids in the urine?

   ____

2. What word describes a clean-catch urine specimen?

   ____

3. Feces are placed on this what item when collected?

   ____

4. What can be found when the urine is strained?

   ____

5. When collecting a specimen, what item must be filled out with the proper information and sent to the laboratory with the specimen?

   ____

EXERCISE 22-2

Directions: Practice filling out the example of a specimen label (Figure 22-1) using your own personal information.

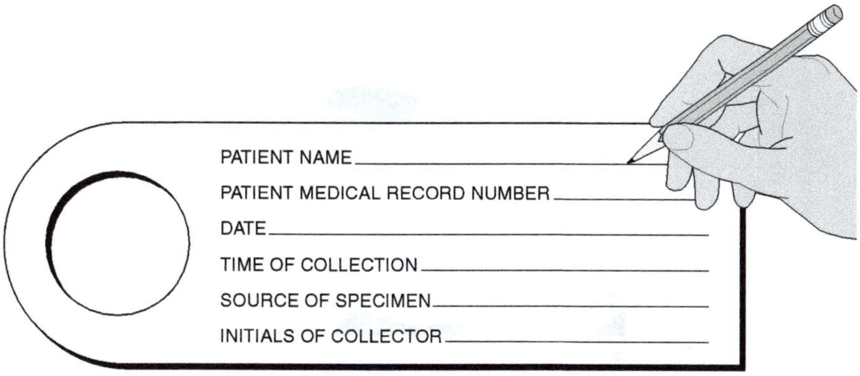

FIGURE 22-1

EXERCISE 22-3

Directions: Using the following word list, label each specimen container or piece of equipment.

Word List

A. Strainer used for straining calculi from urine
B. Reagent test strip and color chart comparison
C. Equipment for collecting stool specimen
D. Infant urine collection bag
E. Container used for adult urine specimen

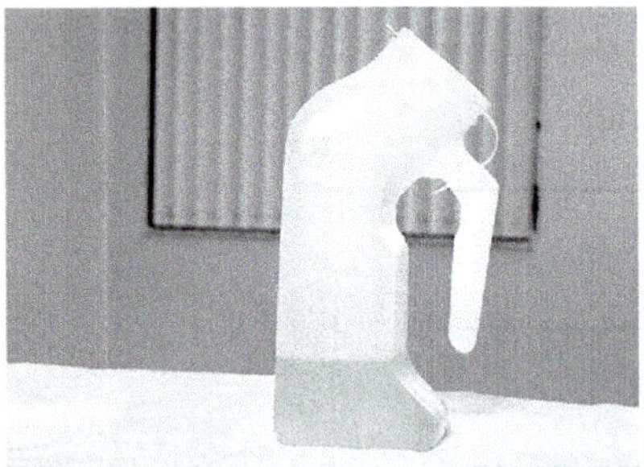

1. ____________________

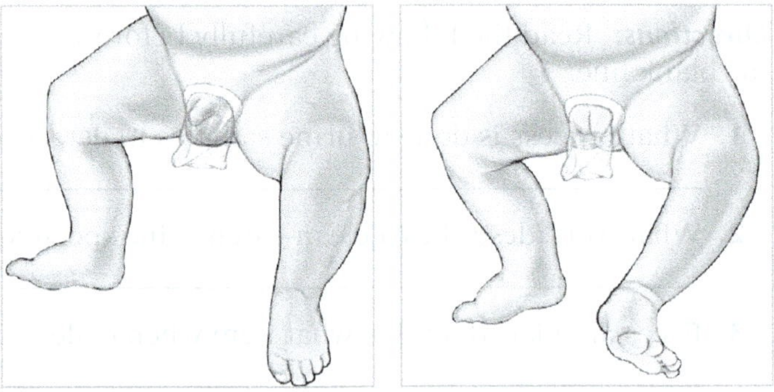

2. ____________________

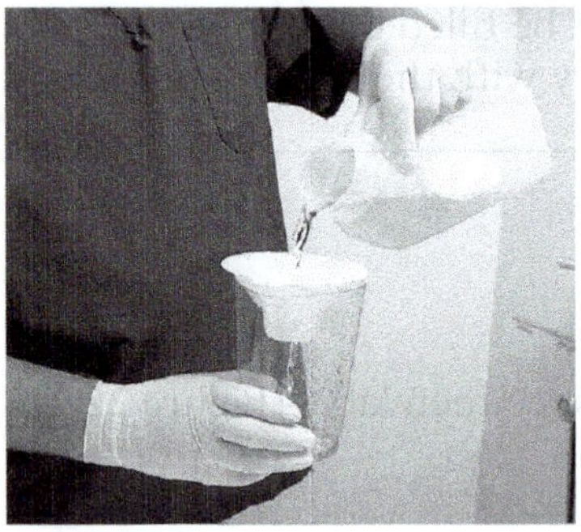

3. ____________________

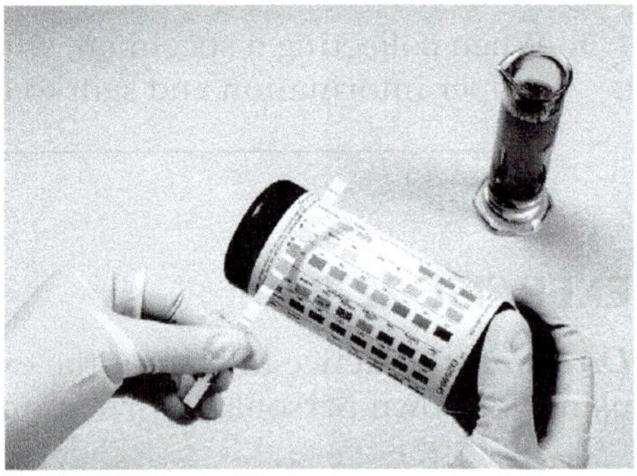

4. ____________________

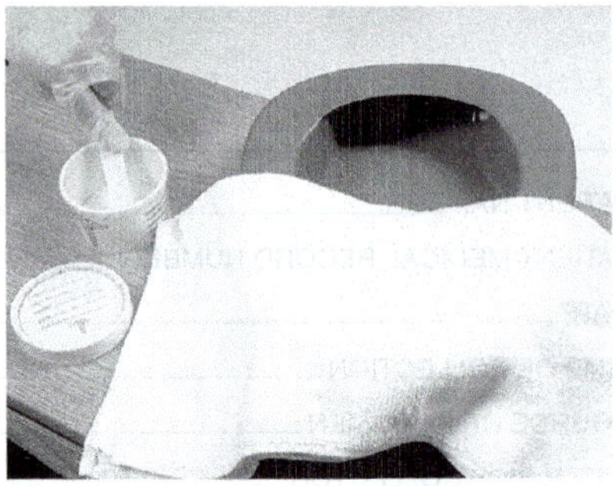

5. ____________________

EXERCISE 22-4

Directions: Select from the following list of procedures the letter of the procedure that best answers each question. Write the correct letter(s) on the blank line next to the question. Letters may be used more than once, and each procedure may have more than one answer.

A. Collecting a 24-hour urine sample

B. Collecting a stool sample

C. Collecting urine using an infant urine collection bag

D. Collecting a midstream urine sample

E. Collecting a sputum sample

_____ **1.** During which procedure(s) must the specimen label be filled out accurately?

_____ **2.** In which procedure(s) must the nursing assistant observe the amount, color, and odor of the specimen?

_____ **3.** Which procedure(s) should a bedpan be used to collect the specimen before transferring it into the proper specimen container?

_____ **4.** Which procedure(s) might a doctor ask that the specimen be sent to the lab as soon as it is obtained?

_____ **5.** Which procedure(s) is important to collect again if the nursing assistant suspects the specimen has been obtained inaccurately?

THE NURSING ASSISTANT IN ACTION

1. Your nursing supervisor asks you to obtain a routine urine specimen from a patient. You enter the patient's bathroom and find that there is toilet paper and feces in the specipan. You have all your supplies ready. What should you do?

____

____

____

____

2. You are assigned to obtain a routine urine specimen from a child who is 6 months old. What would you do?

____

____

____

____

3. A midstream urine specimen must be obtained on a male patient who has severe rheumatoid arthritis that has left his fingers deformed. He has difficulty using his hands and cannot hold a urinal. He is on bedrest and cannot walk to the bathroom. You find out he is uncircumcised. What should you do?

____

____

____

____

4. A 24-hour urine specimen was started on a patient at 7 AM yesterday and will end and be sent to the lab at 7 AM today. You are working the night shift and find this patient in the bathroom at 4 AM. She forgot that this test was being done and emptied her specipan into the toilet. What should you do?

____

____

____

____

5. A patient just defecated in the specipan and it is your responsibility to obtain a Hemoccult test. What should you do?

____

____

____

____

LEARNING ACTIVITIES

1. Sometimes a Hemoccult test can show false results because the patient ate or drank something that reacted with the solution. Using the Internet, research which foods and fluids can change a Hemoccult test result to a false positive. Share these results with classmates. Make a small "cheat sheet" that you can keep in your pocket and use the next time you are asked to perform a Hemoccult on a patient. Remember to ask your patient about diet and fluid intake should you get a positive result.
2. Gather all the equipment necessary to collect a mid-stream urine sample. If you do not have a pre-packaged container, use a small disposable paper drinking cup. Cleanse your perineal area the same way you would if you were explaining the procedure to a patient. Try to obtain your own midstream urine sample in this container. Go through the process and practice the steps of collecting, observing, and recording the results. Note what was awkward for you to do and anything you felt was uncomfortable about the procedure. Use this experience the next time you work with a patient and have to explain and collect a midstream urine sample to help reduce embarrassment and the chance of contamination of the sample.

PROCEDURE CHECKLISTS

PROCEDURE 22-1: COLLECTING A ROUTINE URINE SPECIMEN

Name: ____________________ Date: ____________________

STEPS	S	U	COMMENTS
1. Assemble your equipment a. Bedpan and cover, or urinal, or specipan b. Graduate used for measuring output c. Urine specimen container and lid d. Label, if your institution's procedure is not to write on the lid e. Laboratory requisition or request slip, which should be filled out by the patient's primary nurse f. Gloves			
2. Identify the patient by checking the ID bracelet.			
3. Inform the patient that you are going to obtain a urine specimen.			
4. Wash your hands.			
5. Prepare the label by copying all necessary information from the patient's ID bracelet or using the addressograph. Record the date and time.			
6. Provide privacy and comfort for the patient.			
7. Explain the procedure to the patient. If the patient is able, have him collect the specimen himself.			
8. Put on gloves prior to handling the bedpan or urinal.			
9. Have the patient urinate into a clean bedpan, urinal, or specipan, or directly into a specimen cup.			
10. Ask the patient not to put toilet tissue into the specimen collection container.			
11. Take the bedpan or urinal to the patient's bathroom or dirty utility room.			
12. Pour the urine into a clean graduated container that is used for that patient only.			
13. If the patient is on output measurement, note the amount of urine and record it on the intake and output sheet.			
14. Pour urine from the graduated container into a specimen container, filling it at least half full, if possible.			
15. Put a lid on the specimen container. Place the correct label on the container for the correct patient.			

16. Pour the remaining urine into the toilet.			
17. Clean and rinse the graduated container. Put it in its proper place in the patient's bathroom.			
18. Clean the bedpan or urinal and put it in its proper place.			
19. Dispose of gloves and wash your hands.			
20. Make the patient comfortable and replace the call light.			
21. Lower the bed to a position of safety.			
22. Raise the side rails when ordered or indicated.			
23. Send or take the labeled container to the laboratory with a requisition or request slip.			
24. Report to your immediate supervisor • That a routine urine specimen was obtained • That the specimen was sent to the laboratory • The date and time of collection • Any abnormal or unusual observations			

Charting:

____

____

____

____

Date of Satisfactory Completion ____________________

Instructor's Signature ____________________

PROCEDURE 22-2: COLLECTING A ROUTINE URINE SPECIMEN FROM AN INFANT

Name: ______________________ Date: ______________________

STEPS	S	U	COMMENTS
1. Assemble equipment a. Urine specimen bottle or container b. Plastic disposable urine collector c. Label for specimen container d. Laboratory request slip, which should be filled out by the patient's primary nurse			
2. Wash your hands.			
3. Identify the patient by checking the ID bracelet.			
4. Ask all visitors, except the parents, to step out of the room.			
5. Inform the parents or guardian that you are going to collect a urine specimen.			
6. Provide privacy and comfort for the patient.			
7. Put on gloves.			
8. Take off the child's diaper.			
9. Make sure the child's skin is clean and dry in the genital area. This is where you are going to apply the urine collector, which is a small plastic bag.			
10. Remove the outside piece that surrounds the opening of the plastic urine collector. This leaves a sticky area, which is placed over the entire genital area on the child.			
11. Put the diaper back on as usual.			
12. Dispose of gloves and wash your hands.			
13. Return and check every half hour to see if the infant has voided. Put on gloves, open the diaper, and look at the urine collector to see if there is urine in it.			
14. When the infant has voided, carefully remove the plastic urine collector. Wash off any sticky residue, rinse, and pat dry.			
15. Replace the child's diaper.			
16. Put the specimen in the specimen container and cover it immediately.			
17. Label the container properly, using the ID bracelet or addressograph.			
18. Dispose of gloves and wash your hands.			

19. The labeled specimen container must be sent or taken to the laboratory with the requisition or request slip.			
20. Make the baby comfortable.			
21. Lower the crib to a position of safety.			
22. Raise the side rails to assure patient safety.			
23. Report to your supervisor • That a routine urine specimen was obtained • That the specimen was sent to the lab • The date and time of collection • Any abnormal or unusual observations			

Charting:

____

____

____

____

Date of Satisfactory Completion ____________________

Instructor's Signature ____________________

PROCEDURE 22-3: COLLECTING A MIDSTREAM, CLEAN-CATCH URINE SPECIMEN

Name: ____________________ Date: ____________________

STEPS	S	U	COMMENTS
1. Assemble equipment a. Obtain a midstream, clean-catch collection kit from your supervisor b. Label and container c. Gloves d. Laboratory request slip e. Patient's bedpan or urinal, if the patient is unable to go to the bathroom			
2. Identify the patient by checking the ID bracelet.			
3. Inform the patient that you need a midstream, clean-catch urine specimen.			
4. Wash your hands.			
5. Provide privacy and comfort for the patient.			
6. Explain the procedure, and if the patient is able, allow him to collect his own specimen.			
7. If the patient is not able to collect the specimen himself, help him with the procedure.			
8. Open the kit.			
9. Explain to the patient that she is able to start to urinate into the bedpan, urinal, or toilet. After the flow of urine has started, she is to stop urinating. The specimen container is then placed under the patient and she is to begin urinating again, directly into the specimen container. After obtaining the specimen, remove the container before the flow of urine stops. This procedure catches the urine that is passed in the middle of the void. If the patient cannot stop urinating once having started, move the container into the stream of urine to collect the middle of the stream specimen into the container.			
10. For male patients a. Put on gloves. b. If the patient is not circumcised, pull back the foreskin on the penis to clean it, and hold it back during urination. c. Use a circular motion to clean the head of the penis. Discard each towelette after use.			
11. Remove the towelettes and the urine specimen container from the kit.			

12. For female patients a. Put on gloves. b. Use all three towelettes to clean the genital area. c. Separate the folds of the labia and wipe with one towelette from the front to the back on one side. Discard the towelettes. d. Wipe the other side with a second towelette, again, from front to back. Discard the towelettes. e. Wipe down the middle from front to back, using the third towelette. Discard the towelettes.			
13. Cover the urine container immediately with the lid. Be careful not to allow anything to touch the inside of the container.			
14. Label the container right away. Record the date and time of collection.			
15. Clean the bedpan or urinal and store in its proper place.			
16. Discard all used disposable equipment.			
17. Dispose of gloves and wash your hands.			
18. Make the patient comfortable and replace the call light.			
19. Lower the bed to a position of safety.			
20. Raise the side rails if ordered or indicated.			
21. Send the labeled specimen container to the laboratory with a requisition or lab request slip.			
22. Report to your supervisor • That a midstream, clean-catch urine specimen was obtained • That it was sent to the laboratory • The date and time of collection • Any abnormal or unusual observations			

Charting:

____

____

____

____

Date of Satisfactory Completion ____________________

Instructor's Signature ____________________

PROCEDURE 22-4: COLLECTING A 24-HOUR URINE SPECIMEN

Name: ____________________ Date: ____________________

STEPS	S	U	COMMENTS
1. Assemble your equipment a Large container, usually a 1-gallon plastic disposable bottle b. Funnel, if the neck of the bottle is small c. Grated container used to measure output d. Patient's bedpan, urinal, or specipan e. Label for the container f. Laboratory request slip, which should be filled out by the patient's primary nurse g. Sign to be placed over the patient's bed or in the patient's room to indicate that a 24-hour urine specimen is being collected h. Disposable gloves			
2. Identify the patient by checking the ID bracelet.			
3. Inform the patient that a 24-hour urine specimen is needed.			
4. Explain the procedure. Tell the patient that you will place the large container in the bathroom.			
5. Wash your hands.			
6. Fill in the label for the large container. Copy all needed information from the patient's ID bracelet. Record the date and time of the first collection. Attach the label to the urine specimen container.			
7. Post the sign over or on the patient's bed and in the patient's bathroom. This is so all personnel are aware that a 24-hour urine specimen is being collected.			
8. Provide privacy and comfort each time the patient voids, if she uses a urinal or bedpan.			
9. If the patient is on intake and output measurement, measure all urine each time the patient voids. Write the amount on the intake and output sheet.			
10. When the collection starts, have the patient void. Discard this first amount of urine to ensure that the bladder is completely empty. The first voiding should not be included in the specimen.			
11. You may be instructed to refrigerate the urine or place it on ice. If so, fill a large bucket with ice. Keep the large urine container in the ice in the patient's bathroom. All nursing assistants for the next 24 hours are responsible for keeping the bucket filled with ice.			

12. For the next 24 hours, save all urine voided by the patient. Pour urine from each voiding into the large container.			
13. At the end of the 24-hour period, have the patient void at the same time the test was started the previous day. Add this to the collection of urine in the large container. This will be the last time you will collect the urine for this test.			
14. The large labeled container with the 24-hour collection of urine is taken to the laboratory with a requisition or laboratory request slip.			
15. Clean the equipment and put it in its proper place. Discard disposable equipment.			
16. Remove the 24-hour specimen sign from the patient's bed.			
17. Make the patient comfortable and replace the call light.			
18. Lower the bed to a position of safety.			
19. Raise the side rails when ordered or indicated.			
20. Wash your hands.			
21. Report to your supervisor • That a 24-hour urine specimen was obtained • That the specimen was sent to the laboratory • The date and time of collection • Any abnormal or unusual observations			

Charting:

____

____

____

____

Date of Satisfactory Completion ____________________

Instructor's Signature ____________________

PROCEDURE 22-5: STRAINING THE URINE

Name: ______________________ Date: ______________________

STEPS	S	U	COMMENTS
1. Assemble equipment a. Disposable paper strainer or gauze squares b. Specimen container with cover or small plastic bag to be used as a specimen container c. Label for specimen container d. Patient's bedpan, urinal, or specipan e. Laboratory request slip, filled out by the patient's primary nurse f. Sign to be placed in the patient's room indicating that all urine must be strained g. Disposable gloves			
2. Identify the patient by checking the ID bracelet.			
3. Inform the patient that each time she urinates, it must be into a urinal, bedpan, or specipan, because all urine must be strained. Caution the patient not to put any tissue into the container.			
4. Provide privacy whenever the patient voids.			
5. Wash your hands and put on gloves.			
6. When the patient voids, take the bedpan or urinal to the patient's bathroom. Pour the urine through the strainer into the measuring container.			
7. If any particles show up on the strainer, place the particles in a plastic bag or specimen container.			
8. Label the specimen container immediately. Copy information from the patient's ID bracelet. Record the date and time of collection.			
9. Measure the amount of the voiding and record it on the intake and output sheet, if the patient is on intake and output.			
10. Discard the urine.			
11. Clean and rinse the bedpan and graduated container and put them in the proper places.			
12. Dispose of gloves and wash your hands.			
13. Make the patient comfortable and replace the call light.			
14. Lower the bed to a position of safety.			

15. Raise the side rails when ordered or indicated.			
16. Report to your supervisor • That urine was strained and particles were obtained • That a specimen was collected • Date and time of collection • Any abnormal or unusual observations			

Charting:

____

____

____

____

Date of Satisfactory Completion ______________

Instructor's Signature ______________

PROCEDURE 22-6: TESTING URINE WITH REAGENT STRIPS

Name: ____________________ Date: ____________________

STEPS	S	U	COMMENTS
1. Assemble equipment a. Urine collection container b. Urine reagent strips c. Disposable gloves			
2. Identify the patient by checking the ID bracelet.			
3. Inform the patient that a urine specimen is needed.			
4. Wash your hands and put on gloves.			
5. Remove a urine reagent strip from the bottle and replace the cap tightly.			
6. Completely immerse the reagent strip in the fresh urine sample.			
7. Remove the reagent strip from the urine after immersing. While removing, gently tap excess urine from the strip by touching the side of the reagent strip against the urine container. You may blot the lengthwise edge of the reagent strip on absorbent paper to remove excess urine.			
8. Obtain results by comparing the colors on the reagent strip with the color chart on the bottle of the testing strips.			
9. Record the results of the reading.			
10. Discard the reagent strip in the appropriate receptacle.			
11. Dispose of your gloves and wash your hands.			
12. Report to your supervisor • That the patient's urine was tested using a urine reagent strip • Date and time of test was performed • The results of the urine reagent strip testing • Any abnormal or unusual observations			

Charting:

____

____

____

____

Date of Satisfactory Completion ____________________

Instructor's Signature ____________________

PROCEDURE 22-7: COLLECTING A SPUTUM SPECIMEN

Name: ______________________ Date: ______________________

STEPS	S	U	COMMENTS
1. Assemble equipment a. Sputum container with cover and tissues b. Label for container c. Laboratory request slip, filled out by the patient's primary nurse d. Disposable gloves			
2. Identify the patient by checking the ID bracelet.			
3. Inform the patient that a sputum specimen is needed.			
4. Wash your hands and put on gloves.			
5. Have the patient rinse out her mouth if she has eaten recently.			
6. Give the patient a sputum container.			
7. Ask her to take three consecutive deep breaths and on the third exhalation, to cough deep from within the lungs to bring up sputum.			
8. The patient may have to cough several times to bring up enough sputum for the specimen.			
9. Cover the container immediately, being careful not to touch the inside of the container or the cover.			
10. Label the container right away, using information from the patient's ID bracelet.			
11. The labeled specimen container must be sent or taken to the laboratory with a requisition or request slip.			
12. Make the patient comfortable and replace the call light.			
13. Lower the bed to apposition of safety.			
14. Raise the side rails when ordered or appropriate for patient safety.			
15. Dispose of gloves and wash your hands.			

16. Report to your supervisor • That a sputum specimen was obtained • The color, amount, odor, and consistency of the specimen • That the specimen was sent to the laboratory • The date and time of collection • How the patient tolerated the procedure • Any abnormal or unusual observations			

Charting:

____

____

____

____

Date of Satisfactory Completion ____________________

Instructor's Signature ____________________

PROCEDURE 22-8: COLLECTING A STOOL SPECIMEN

Name: ______________ Date: ______________

STEPS	S	U	COMMENTS
1. Assemble equipment a. Patient's bedpan b. Stool specimen container c. Wooden tongue depressor d. Label for container e. Laboratory request slip, usually filled out by the patient's primary nurse f. Plastic bag for specimen, if ordered g. Disposable gloves			
2. Identify the patient by checking the ID bracelet.			
3. Wash your hands.			
4. Inform the patient that a stool specimen is needed. Explain that the patient should notify you when he feels he must move his bowels so you can collect the specimen.			
5. Provide privacy and comfort for the patient.			
6. Have the patient move his bowels into the bedpan or into a specipan placed in the back half of the toilet.			
7. Ask the patient NOT to urinate or place toilet tissue in the bedpan.			
8. Prepare the label immediately, using information from the patient's ID bracelet.			
9. Put on gloves.			
10. After the patient has had a bowel movement, cover the container and take it to the bathroom or soiled utility room.			
11. Using the wooden tongue depressor, take about 1–2 tablespoons of feces from different areas in the stool and place them in the specimen container. Label the container.			
12. Cover the container immediately, being careful not to touch the inside of the container or lid.			
13. Wrap the tongue depressor in a paper towel and discard it.			
14. Empty the remaining feces into the toilet.			
15. Clean the bedpan and return it to its proper place.			
16. Dispose of the gloves and wash your hands.			

17. If the nurse has told you this is a warm specimen, it must be taken to the laboratory while it is still warm from the patient's body. Place the container in a plastic bag and take it immediately to the laboratory.			
18. Make the patient comfortable and replace the call light.			
19. Lower the bed to a position of safety.			
20. Raise the side rails when ordered or indicated.			
21. Wash your hands.			
22. Report to your supervisor • That a stool specimen was obtained • That the specimen was sent to the laboratory • The date and time of collection • Any abnormal or unusual observations			

Charting:

____

____

____

____

Date of Satisfactory Completion ______________

Instructor's Signature ______________

PROCEDURE 22-9: PREPARING A HEMOCCULT SLIDE

Name: ____________________ Date: ____________________

STEPS	S	U	COMMENTS
1. Assemble equipment a. Patient's bedpan b. Hemoccult slide c. Wooden tongue depressor d. Label e. Specimen bag f. Disposable gloves			
2. Identify the patient by checking the ID bracelet.			
3. Wash your hands and put on your gloves.			
4. Inform the patient that you are going to prepare a Hemoccult slide for stool testing.			
5. Ask the patient to move her bowels into a bedpan or specipan, whenever possible.			
6. Label the outside of the Hemoccult slide with the patient's name and the date the specimen is collected.			
7. Collect a small amount of stool on a tongue depressor.			
8. Open side 1.			
9. Apply a small amount in Box A on Hemoccult slide.			
10. From a different area of stool, collect a small amount of stool on the tongue depressor.			
11. Apply a small amount in Box B on Hemoccult slide.			
12. Close cover of slide card and secure it.			
13. Check information with the patient's identification bracelet.			
14. Dispose of gloves and wash your hands.			
15. Place the Hemoccult slide in a specimen bag and send it to the laboratory (or give to a nurse to check, if this is policy).			

16. Report to your supervisor • That the Hemoccult specimen was collected • The time and date it was collected • Any abnormal or unusual observations.			

Charting:

____

____

____

____

Date of Satisfactory Completion ____________________

Instructor's Signature ____________________

PROCEDURE 22-10: TESTING A STOOL SPECIMEN FOR BLOOD

Name: ____________________ Date: ____________________

STEPS	S	U	COMMENTS
1. Assemble the equipment a. Bedpan or commode b. Disposable gloves c. Specimen cup d. Hemoccult stool slide e. Wooden applicator f. Developing solution			
2. Identify the patient by checking the ID bracelet.			
3. Wash your hands and put on your gloves.			
4. Inform the patient that you are going to prepare a Hemoccult slide and test it for the presence of blood.			
5. Obtain uncontaminated stool specimen.			
6. Label the outside of the Hemoccult slide with the patient's name, the date, and time that the specimen is collected.			
7. Collect a small amount of stool on a tongue depressor.			
8. Open side 1 of the Hemoccult slide.			
9. Apply a small amount in Box A on Hemoccult slide.			
10. From a different area of stool, collect a small amount of stool on the tongue depressor.			
11. Apply a small amount in Box B on Hemoccult slide.			
12. Close the cover of the Hemoccult slide. Turn the Hemoccult slide over, to the reverse side.			
13. Open the cardboard flap and apply two drops of Hemoccult developing solution on each box of guiac paper.			
14. Wait 30–60 seconds to read the results, noting any color changes. Bluish discoloration indicates the presence of occult blood in the stool and is recorded as *guiac positive*. No change in color of the guiac paper indicates an absence of occult blood in the stool and is recorded as *guiac negative*.			
15. Discard test slide in proper receptacle.			
16. Remove and dispose of contaminated gloves.			
17. Wash hands.			

18. Report to your supervisor • The date and time Hemoccult testing was done • The Hemoccult test results • Any abnormal or unusual observations.			

Charting:

____

____

____

____

Date of Satisfactory Completion ____________________

Instructor's Signature ____________________

23

The Endocrine System and Related Care of Diabetics

Key Terms Review

Match the key terms in the right column with the definitions in the left column by placing the letter of each correct answer in the space provided.

_____ **1.** An organ that is able to make and discharge a chemical that will be used elsewhere in the body.

_____ **2.** Ductless glands that make hormones and secrete them directly into the bloodstream.

_____ **3.** Glands that make hormones and secrete them either directly or through a duct to the system that is affected by that hormone.

_____ **4.** Produce and release into the body; glands secrete hormones.

_____ **5.** The process through which food elements are converted into energy for use in the human body.

_____ **6.** Basic food element used by the body; includes sugars and starches.

_____ **7.** A sugar formed during metabolism of carbohydrates; also called *blood sugar*.

_____ **8.** Protein substance secreted by endocrine glands directly into the blood to stimulate increased activity.

_____ **9.** Hormone that regulates the sugar content of the blood.

_____ **10.** Disorder of carbohydrate metabolism; this happens when the body cannot change sugar into energy because of a lack of production of or ability to use insulin.

Terms

A. Diabetes mellitus
B. Hyperglycemia
C. Hypoglycemia
D. Insulin shock
E. Diabetic coma
F. Insulin
G. Hormone
H. Gland
I. Exocrine glands
J. Endocrine glands
K. Carbohydrate
L. Glucose
M. Metabolism
N. Secrete

_____ 11. An abnormally deep stupor that can occur in a diabetic patient from lack of insulin.

_____ 12. Abnormally high blood sugar.

_____ 13. Abnormally low blood sugar.

_____ 14. Serious complication related to diabetes, when too much insulin is present in the blood. May occur when the diabetic person has received too much insulin, misses a meal, or has too much physical activity.

MULTIPLE-CHOICE QUESTIONS

Circle the letter next to the word or statement that best completes the sentence or answers the question.

1. The "master gland" of the body is the __________ gland.
   a. adrenal
   b. thyroid
   c. captain
   d. pituitary
2. The gland that is thought to be the link between our thinking, our emotions, and our body functions is the
   a. thinking link gland.
   b. hypothalamus gland.
   c. hippopotamus gland.
   d. emoto gland.
3. Insulin is produced in the
   a. hypoinsulin gland.
   b. sugar gland.
   c. parathyroid.
   d. pancreas.
4. In an emergency, the adrenal glands produce __________, which gives the body large amounts of energy.
   a. sugar
   b. insulin
   c. adrenalin
   d. progesterone
5. Two female hormones are __________ and __________
   a. insulin; protectin.
   b. estrogen; testosterone.
   c. testosterone; insulin.
   d. estrogen; progesterone.
6. The __________ produces a hormone that regulates growth.
   a. pancreas
   b. thyroid
   c. heart
   d. stomach
7. Insulin-dependent diabetes mellitus is
   a. also known as type I diabetes.
   b. also known as juvenile-onset diabetes.
   c. rapidly increasing in occurrence in the United States.
   d. all of the above.
8. Male hormones are produced in the
   a. ovaries.
   b. testes.
   c. pancreas.
   d. liver.
9. A common sign and symptom of diabetes is
   a. excessive thirst.
   b. fast-healing wounds.
   c. weight gain.
   d. chest pain.
10. __________ is a male hormone.
    a. Estrogen
    b. Progesterone

c. Testosterone
d. Insulin

11. Cushing's syndrome occurs when the adrenal glands are
a. not active.
b. too active.
c. reactive.
d. absent.

12. The most common disorder caused by endocrine problems is
a. diabetes.
b. obesity.
c. pulmonary edema.
d. Cushing's syndrome.

13. Gangrene can occur when a body part does not get enough
a. insulin.
b. circulating blood.
c. gangrenite.
d. pituitrin.

14. A sign and symptom of diabetes can be
a. polydipsia.
b. hypocalcemia.
c. apnea.
d. polyinsulin.

15. Symptoms of insulin shock are
a. faintness and dizziness.
b. excessive sweating and fast breathing.
c. irritability and nervousness.
d. all of the above.

16. Signs of diabetic coma are
a. increased urination and dry mouth.
b. loss of appetite and fruity breath.
c. confusion and difficult time paying attention.
d. all of the above.

17. ____________ care is very important for diabetic health.
a. Foot
b. Hair
c. Car
d. Home

18. Good awareness of blood sugar levels is dependent on use of
a. foot meters.
b. insulin meters.
c. carbohydrate meters.
d. blood glucose meters.

19. For diabetics, shoes and stockings should fit correctly and not be
a. too tight.
b. white.
c. washed.
d. cotton.

20. When using a blood glucose meter for several patients, the nursing assistant should
a. use a pipet to prevent contamination of the patient.
b. wash his or her hands between patients.
c. be sure to record the blood level after each test.
d. all of the above.

21. Whenever testing the urine for glucose, use a sample that is
a. fresh.
b. from the Foley bag.
c. from the last test.
d. from the toilet.

22. When performing foot care on a patient living with diabetes, it is important for the nursing assistant to
a. remember to keep the toe nails clipped as short as possible.
b. soak the feet in very hot water and remove any dead skin with a file.
c. avoid placing lotion between toes to prevent bacteria from growing.
d. provide deep massage to promote circulation.

23. A patient is experiencing insulin shock. The nursing assistant should provide basic emergency care by
a. sitting the patient up and calling 911.
b. feeding the patient something like honey and crackers if a blood glucose reading cannot be obtained.

c. offering the patient diet soda immediately.
d. not feeding the patient anything as he may choke.

24. A blood glucose reading greater than 250 mg/dL indicates
a. hyperglycemia and should be reported to the nurse.
b. hypoglycemia and 15–20 grams of sugar should be offered.
c. the person should not eat anything when the next meal is offered.
d. the diabetic is doing fine and should continue his exercise and diet routine.

25. A blood sugar reading less than 70 mg/dL is considered an emergency and the nursing assistant should
a. hold all foods because the body has too much insulin and the patient can experience diabetic ketoacidosis.
b. immediately give the patient 4 teaspoons of sugar and get the nurse.
c. check the patient in 15 minutes because the machine may not have been calibrated correctly.
d. give an insulin shot to help stabilize the patient.

TRUE OR FALSE QUESTIONS

Determine whether each question is true or false. In the space provided, write "T" for true and "F" for false. If the statement is false, rewrite it on the line provided to make it a true statement.

_____ **1.** The thymus gland gets larger with age.

____

_____ **2.** It is important that the patient learn to use a blood glucose meter and to administer his own insulin.

____

_____ **3.** The nursing assistant must always wear disposable gloves when testing the patient's blood.

____

_____ **4.** Regardless of age, a patient living with diabetes needs good information and emotional support when learning how to care for himself.

____

_____ **5.** The pituitary gland controls the hypothalamus.

____

_____ **6.** Both the thyroid and the parathyroid glands help regulate calcium and potassium in the blood.

____

_____ **7.** Estrogen and testosterone are the two major sex hormones that help to maintain pregnancy.

____

_____ **8.** The adrenal glands are categorized as both endocrine and exocrine glands.

____

_____ **9.** African Americans, Latinos, and American Indians are at higher risk for diabetes than other cultures.

____

_____ **10.** Polyphagia is not a sign or symptom of insulin shock.

____

FILL-IN-THE-BLANK QUESTIONS

Provide the meaning of the following abbreviations.

1. CDC ______
2. IDDM ______
3. NIDDM ______
4. FBS ______
5. GTT ______
6. PPBS ______
7. mg/dL ______
8. DKA ______
9. PC ______

EXERCISE 23-1

Objective: To recognize and correctly spell words related to the endocrine system and related care.

Directions: Label the diagram in Figure 23-1 with the correct words from the following word list.

Word List

Pineal	Pituitary	Parathyroid
Thymus	Thyroid	Testes (in men)
Pancreas	Adrenals	Ovaries (in women)

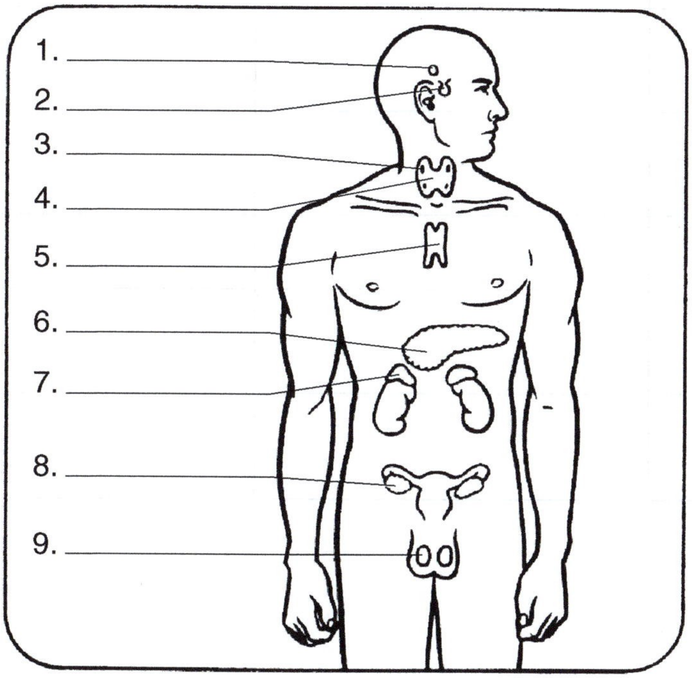

FIGURE 23-1

EXERCISE 23-2

Objective: To apply what you have learned about the endocrine system and related care of the diabetic patient.

Directions: Read the following riddles carefully before writing the correct answer on the blank line.

1. What are three classic symptoms of diabetes? (*Hint:* The beginnings of all three words are the same and sound like a girl's name.)

   ____

2. What sounds like something you would write with, but it contains a point much sharper than a pen? (*Hint:* It contains a lancet.)

   ____

EXERCISE 23-3

Directions: Using what you learned from the textbook reading, complete the following table. Write the answer(s) in the blank provided.

	Insulin Shock	**Diabetic Coma**
What would a blood sugar reading be to indicate an emergency?		
What behavioral changes might occur?		
What skin changes would you observe?		
What might the patient complain about related to gastrointestinal issues?		
What changes might occur in the respiratory system?		
What changes might occur with the patient's vision and urine status?		
What changes in the nervous system might be observed or might the patient complain about?		
What can you do if a diabetic patient were to experience this?		

THE NURSING ASSISTANT IN ACTION

1. A 7-year-old child has been admitted to your unit. The doctor told the parents and the child earlier this morning that the test results prove the child has diabetes. Later in the day, while you are taking care of the child, she grabs your hand and asks, "What is diabetes? Will my friends want to play with me still since they can get diabetes from me?" What should you do?

____

____

____

2. A 15-year-old girl living with type I diabetes is assigned to your care. You enter the room about an hour after she ate her lunch to find she is eating pizza, potato chips, and drinking soda with her friends who came to visit. What should you do?

____

____

____

3. Mrs. Jones, a type I diabetic, arrives back to her room around 9 AM from physical therapy. She missed breakfast this morning. She begins to scream and yell at you for not helping her fast enough. Usually, Mrs. Jones is rather quiet and very polite. You notice her skin is pale, she is sweating, breathing fast, and her hands are shaking. What should you do?

____

____

____

4. Mr. Black, a diabetic, complains this morning he feels very weak and he barely touched his breakfast. You set his personal hygiene equipment up on his overbed table and realize he is not following your directions very well, so you help him with his morning care rituals. While providing oral care, you realize his mouth is very dry and his breath smells like sweet chewing gum. What should you do?

____

____

____

5. Mrs. Schultz was diagnosed with diabetes. Today, she will be discharged to her home and will care for herself. You notice while you are packing her belongings that she is wearing knee-high hose, very pointy high heels, and is sitting cross-legged in her chair. What kind of advice should you give to Mrs. Schultz to help her maintain good skin integrity and care for her feet once she is discharged?

____

____

____

LEARNING ACTIVITIES

1. Find an old pair of gloves, sunglasses, and tape. Place a handful of uncooked macaroni in the gloves and using tape place small pieces randomly on the sunglasses. Now try to dress, eat, and read the newspaper. What did you experience? What was difficult for you to do? Sometimes persons living with neuropathy experience pain, tingling, and the decreased ability to perform certain activities of daily living. The next time you care for someone living with diabetes who has neuropathy or significant changes in vision, use what you learned to help them stay independent and while providing emotional support to them.
2. Some diabetics must perform finger sticks on themselves more than once a day. If available, use a blood glucose monitoring device and stick your own finger. Try sticking the tip, the side, and then the finger pad. Which place was the least painful? What area did the blood come out the fastest? What did you find difficult about the experience? Use this information when performing finger sticks on your patients and when teaching them how to care for themselves.

PROCEDURE CHECKLIST

PROCEDURE 23-1: MEASURING BLOOD GLUCOSE USING THE ACCU-CHECK® AVIVA GLUCOMETER

Name: ________________ Date: ________________

STEPS	S	U	COMMENTS
1. Wash your hands.			
2. Inform the patient that you are going to test his blood sugar level.			
3. Make the patient comfortable, and wash his hands with soap and water.			
4. Assemble equipment a. ACCU-CHEK® Aviva glucometer (Figure 23-2) b. ACCU-CHEK® Aviva test strips c. ACCU-CHEK® Multiclix lancing device d. Disposable pipet e. Disposable gloves f. Bandage			
5. Check the expiration date on the test strips. Discard them if they have expired.			
6. Remove a test strip from the container. Close the container.			
7. Insert the test strip into the opening of the meter. This turns on and activates the meter. Test strip and blood drop symbols appear on the display.			
8. Observe the number displayed by the meter and compare to the code on the test strip canister to be certain they are the same. Follow manufacturer's instructions to calibrate the meter with the test strips every time you change to another canister of test strips.			
9. Put on disposable gloves.			
10. Place the clear plastic ACCU-CHEK® Multiclix cap on the lancing device and press until it clicks.			
11. Firmly press the clear cap of the lancing device against the side of a fingertip of the patient.			
12. Press the button on the lancing device to prick the fingertip.			
13. Squeeze the finger to obtain a large drop of blood.			

14. Using a disposable pipet, slowly draw up the drop of blood and apply the blood sample to front edge of the yellow window on the test strip. This method prevents contamination of the patient and is preferred in a hospital or nursing home setting where several different patients use the same meter. In a home setting, it is acceptable to apply the blood sample directly to the strip.			
15. A flashing hourglass indicates that enough blood has been applied to the test strip. Wait a short time for the results to appear on the blood glucose meter.			
16. Apply a bandage to the patient's finger, if needed.			
17. Remove the test strip from the meter.			
18. Discard the test strip and lancet in the proper receptacles.			
19. Remove gloves and wash your hands.			
20. Record the results. Notify your supervisor of the results or follow your institution's policy for reporting blood glucose results.			
21. Show the patient how she can use the memory function of the meter to review past test results. If desired, and given the appropriate software and cable, the patient can download the test results to a personal computer (PC). This data can be used to identify trends in glucose levels and to prepare reports to share with healthcare professionals.			

Charting:

____

____

____

____

Date of Satisfactory Completion ____________________

Instructor's Signature ____________________

24

The Reproductive System and Related Care

Key Terms Review

Match the key terms in the right column with the definitions in the left column by placing the letter of each correct answer in the space provided.

_____ **1.** The group of body organs that makes possible the creation of a new human life.

_____ **2.** The area of the body between the thighs; includes the area of the anus and the external genital organs.

_____ **3.** A female hormone that causes a buildup of the lining of the uterus to prepare it for possible pregnancy. It is also responsible for the development of secondary sexual characteristics.

_____ **4.** Patient being treated for diseases or conditions of the female reproductive organs, including the breasts.

_____ **5.** Diseases acquired as a result of oral, anal, or vaginal sexual encounters or intercourse with an infected person.

_____ **6.** Infection and inflammation of the female reproductive organs. This disease can spread to all structures in the pelvic cavity causing scarring of the tubes that carry eggs from the ovary to the uterus which can lead to infertility, ectopic pregnancy, and pelvic pain.

_____ **7.** Human immunodeficiency virus; the microorganism that causes AIDS.

_____ **8.** Viral infection characterized by decreased immunity to opportunistic infections.

Terms

A. Sexually transmitted diseases (STDs)

B. HIV

C. AIDS

D. Pelvic inflammatory disease (PID)

E. Gynecological (GYN) patient

F. Estrogen

G. Menstruation

H. Menopause

I. Sperm

J. Testosterone

K. Vagina

L. Ovulation

M. Ova/ovum

N. Fertile

O. Fertilization

P. Transurethral resection of the prostate (TURP)

_____ 9. Periodic (monthly) loss of some blood and a small part of the lining of the uterus when a woman is not pregnant.

_____ 10. Time during which menstruation stops, resulting in decreased hormone production and an end of fertility.

_____ 11. Able to become pregnant; capable of reproduction.

_____ 12. Joining of a sperm and ovum to form a new cell.

_____ 13. The female reproductive cell(s) produced in the ovaries that is capable of uniting with a sperm cell and developing into a new organism.

_____ 14. Process whereby an ovum is released from one ovary into the opening of the fallopian tube and moves to the uterus.

_____ 15. The male reproductive cell produced in the testes, which is released from the male during intercourse.

_____ 16. The primary male sex hormone; manufactured in the testes.

_____ 17. Non-cancerous enlargement of the prostate gland; commonly seen in males over age 50.

_____ 18. A urological surgical procedure removal of the prostate gland by inserting a surgical instrument through the urethra and removing prostate tissue.

_____ 19. Organ in the female reproductive system that receives the penis and semen and serves as the birth canal.

_____ 20. The canal leading from the cervix to the outside of the female body; serves as the organ for intercourse and as the birth canal.

_____ 21. Discharge of blood, clots, and fluids that occur several days following a vaginal delivery.

Q. Benign prostatic hypertrophy (BPH)

R. Lochia

S. Vaginal canal

T. Perineal area

U. Reproductive system

MULTIPLE CHOICE QUESTIONS

Circle the letter next to the word or statement that best completes the sentence or answers the question.

1. There are several female organs of reproduction, but the primary reproductive organs are the
  a. uterus and the vagina.
  b. two ovaries.
  c. fallopian tubes.
  d. testes and the penis.

2. The primary reproductive organs of the male are the
  a. two testes.
  b. penis and the prostate gland.
  c. sperm cells.
  d. urethra and the penis.

3. The process whereby an ovum is released from an ovary into the fallopian tubes and travels to the uterus is called
   a. conception.
   b. climax.
   c. menstruation.
   d. ovulation.

4. There is only one duct in the penis that is used for the flow of urine and the flow of
   a. blood.
   b. milk.
   c. testosterone.
   d. semen.

5. *Sexuality* refers to the group of characteristics that identify the differences between
   a. sex and reproduction.
   b. good and bad.
   c. right and wrong.
   d. male and female.

6. Sexually transmitted diseases (STDs) can be 100% prevented
   a. by luck and timing.
   b. through abstinence.
   c. by the use of male condoms.
   d. by the use of female condoms.

7. Three examples of STDs are
   a. chlamydia, pneumonia, and gonorrhea.
   b. chlamydia, gonorrhea, and amenorrhea.
   c. HSV, HPV, and HIV.
   d. syphilis, BPH, and SBE.

8. Genital herpes simplex (HSV) can be contracted
   a. only if sores are visible.
   b. only if sores are open and draining.
   c. from anyone having HSV.
   d. only during menstruation.

9. Examples of female reproductive disorders are
   a. cystocele and rectocele.
   b. tumors of the breast and hydrocele.
   c. prostatitis and BPH.
   d. varicocele and varicose veins.

10. Examples of male reproductive disorders are
   a. prostatitis and benign prostatic hyperplasia (BPH).
   b. tumors of the breast and cancer of the uterus.
   c. vaginitis and pelvic inflammatory disease (PID).
   d. menorrhagia and backaches.

11. Another word for *vaginal irrigation* is
   a. constipation.
   b. enema.
   c. douche.
   d. perineal care.

12. Postpartum perineal care is important to prevent
   a. infection.
   b. herpes.
   c. HIV.
   d. chlamydia.

13. Early ambulation is important to prevent circulation problems after childbirth, but before the patient gets up, the nursing assistant must check with her immediate supervisor to see if the patient
   a. has hard sole shoes to wear.
   b. has numbness in her legs from the anesthesia.
   c. has orders to walk more than a mile a day.
   d. can request that her husband walk for her.

14. Some female patients develop a severe _______ if they ambulate when they have doctor's orders to lie flat or at a reduced angle for several hours after receiving spinal anesthesia.
   a. rash
   b. headache
   c. clot
   d. pressure ulcer

15. The way a patient expects to be treated by a health care worker is influenced by
   a. the time of day.
   b. the nurse.

c. pain.
d. the cultural characteristics of that patient.

16. The last stage of labor and delivery is when the ______ is expelled.
a. fetus
b. infant
c. newborn
d. placenta

17. When a female ages, a decrease in estrogen can lead to many changes in her body. Which is a normal part of aging because of hormone levels decreasing?
a. Breast cancer
b. Decrease of vaginal secretions
c. Excessive ovulation
d. Decreased episodes of vaginitis

18. Stress incontinence can be decreased when a woman
a. performs exercises to strengthen pelvic floor muscles.
b. drinks lots of water.
c. stops having sexual intercourse.
d. enters menopause.

19. Which signs and symptoms can be reported by a patient when BPH occurs?
a. Urinary dribbling and decreased force of urine
b. Nocturia and urinary retention
c. Having a feeling to want to void and experiencing urinary urgency
d. All of the above

20. What is an acceptable treatment for BPH?
a. Taking drugs that help shrink the growth of the prostate
b. Having laser treatment that helps destroy excessive tissue in the prostate
c. Having a prostatectomy
d. All of the above

21. A pelvic examination is performed
a. to assess the female reproductive system and collect specimens.
b. to assess the male reproductive organs and offer breast examination.
c. by a nursing assistant and a nurse.
d. before the patient has emptied her bladder.

22. When caring for a women after she has delivered a baby, the nursing assistant may be asked by the supervisor to
a. count the number of pads the patient uses
b. observe the amount of blood on each pad
c. describe the color and amount of blood on the pad
d. all of the above.

23. Lochia rubra
a. is red in color and lasts 2–4 days after giving birth.
b. is pink in color and occurs within the first 2 days after giving birth.
c. is white in color and can last 2–6 weeks after delivery.
d. should appear thick and without clots.

24. When performing postpartum perineal care, the water should
a. be cool to the touch.
b. be at least 100°F.
c. chilled with ice to reduce swelling.
d. be mixed with rubbing alcohol to kill bacteria.

25. After a cesarean section is performed, the nursing assistant should
a. get the patient up immediately to prevent clots forming in the legs.
b. encourage the patient to cough and breathe deeply.
c. rub the abdominal incision to promote wound healing.
d. offer the baby to the mom so they can sleep together and bond.

TRUE OR FALSE QUESTIONS

Determine whether each question is true or false. In the space provided, write "T" for true and "F" for false. If the statement is false, rewrite it on the line provided to make it a true statement.

_____ **1.** Males may be unaware they have human papillomavirus and can spread it to their partners.

____

_____ **2.** During intercourse, the sperm travel up the vas deferens to a point where they enter the urethra.

____

_____ **3.** Menstruation diminishes around age 45–55, leading to menopause.

____

_____ **4.** Females may have no symptoms of gonorrhea and still spread the diseases to sexual partners.

____

_____ **5.** Sexuality is a normal part of growth and development and ends when women enter menopause.

____

_____ **6.** A person can carry the HIV virus for many years before developing AIDS.

____

_____ **7.** Some forms of human papillomavirus (HPV) infection (genital warts) can be cancerous.

____

_____ **8.** Men being treated for impotence as a result of erectile dysfunction should see a dermatologist before taking topical or internal remedies.

____

_____ **9.** An *episiotomy* is a small cut in the vagina made during childbirth to make the opening larger and to prevent tearing.

____

_____ **10.** Postpartum perineal care is performed each time after the patient urinates or defecates.

____

FILL-IN-THE-BLANK QUESTIONS

Provide the meaning of the following abbreviations.

1. AIDS _______________________________
2. HIV _______________________________
3. BPH _______________________________
4. GYN _______________________________
5. PID _______________________________
6. STDs _______________________________
7. TURP _______________________________
8. CDC _______________________________
9. HSV _______________________________
10. HPV _______________________________
11. C-section _______________________________

EXERCISE 24-1

Objective: To recognize and be able to correctly spell the parts of the female reproductive system.

Directions: In Figure 24-1, label the parts of the female reproductive organs and specialized cells with the words from the following word list.

Word List

Labia majora	Urethral meatus	Uterus
Ovary tube	Ovary	Cervix
Uterine neck	Fallopian tube	Vaginal orifice
Clitoris	Hymen	Labia minora
Ovum escaping	Vagina or birth canal	

FIGURE 24-1

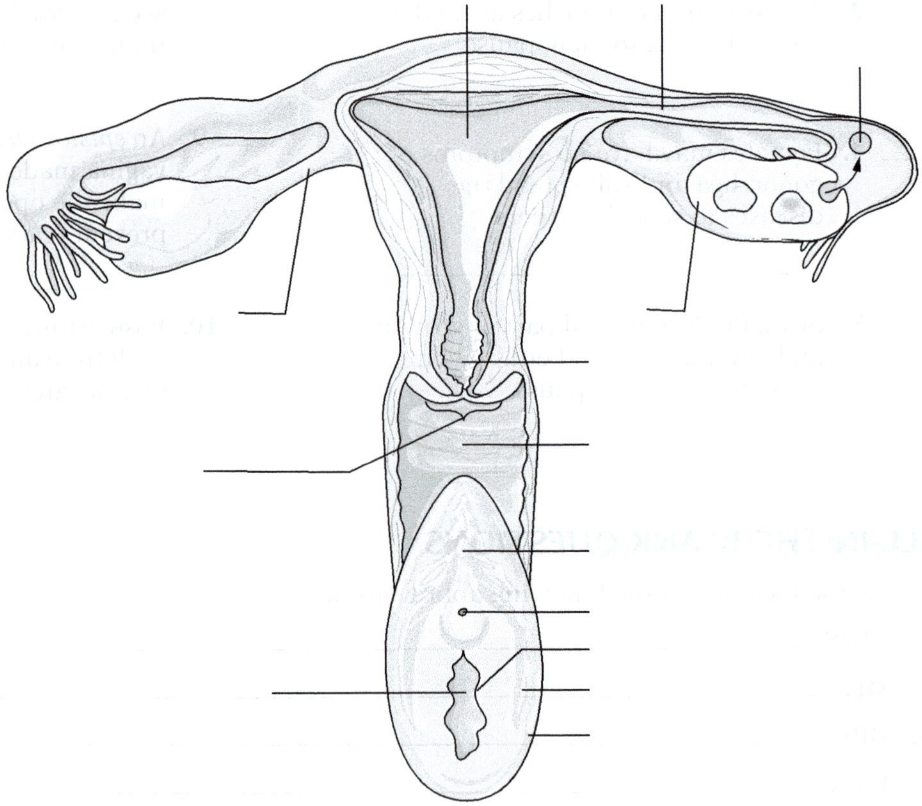

EXERCISE 24-2

Objective: To recognize and be able to correctly spell the parts of the male reproductive organs.

Directions: In Figure 24-2, label the parts of the male reproductive organs and specialized cells with the words from the following word list.

Word List

Bladder	Testicle (testis)	Glans penis
Vas deferens	Prostate	Epididymis
Ejaculatory duct	Seminal vesicle	Rectum
Urethral meatus	Prepuce	Scrotum
Bulbo-urethral gland or Cowper's gland		

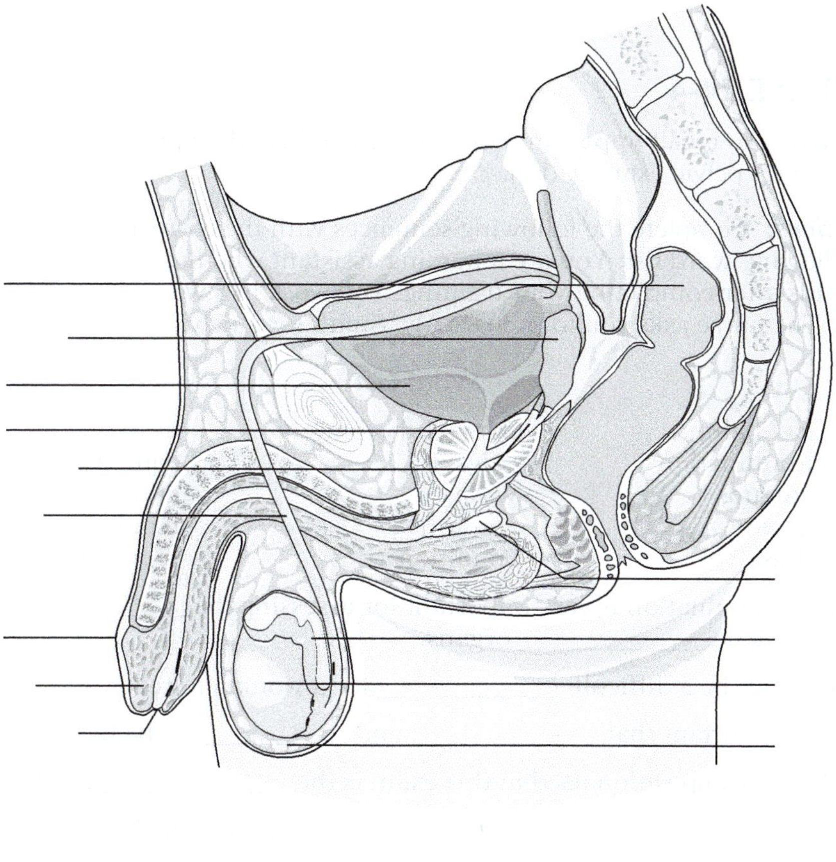

FIGURE 24-2

EXERCISE 24-3

Objective: To associate sexually transmitted diseases (STDs) with their responsible organisms.

Directions: Draw a line to connect the disease with the correct organism.

Disease	Organism
Pelvic inflammatory disease	HPV virus
Gonorrhea	Herpes simplex virus
AIDS	Chlamydia
Syphilis	Gonococcus
Genital warts	HIV virus
Genital herpes simplex	*Treponema pallidum*

EXERCISE 24-4

Objective: To recall important points to remember when preparing a female patient for a pelvic examination.

Directions: Complete the following sentences with the correct words from the following word list. You are a nursing assistant who has been working for 6 months after completing your training. You work in a women's health clinic. The nurse asks you to prepare Ms. Smith for a pelvic exam.

Word List

call light	dorsal lithotomy	drape
examination	privacy	equipment
stirrups	wash	gloves
gown	comfort	hands
dress	condition	reproductive

1. This examination is very important for assessing the ______________ of the female ______________ organs.
2. This can be a difficult ______________ for a woman to receive.
3. It is important that ______________ and ______________ be maintained.
4. The typical position used in this exam is the ______________ position.
5. ______________ may be used to position the legs and the feet.
6. An additional ______________ may be used to cover the feet.
7. If the nursing assistant leaves the patient alone in the room, she should make sure to leave the ______________ within the patient's reach.
8. ______________ your ______________ before and after handling equipment or specimens and use disposable ______________.

9. Care for the ____________ according to the clinic's policy.

10. After the examination, assist the patient to ____________ or put on a ____________. If she is able to dress herself, leave the room so that the patient can dress herself in private.

THE NURSING ASSISTANT IN ACTION

1. You are helping Mr. Smith shower when he reaches out and fondles you and tells you, "You make me feel so good." What should you do?

____

____

____

2. A woman who had a baby 6 weeks ago is admitted to your unit. She confides in you and tells you she does not want to get out of bed in the morning and cannot find the energy to care for her baby. Sometimes she has a fear she will hurt her child. What should you do?

____

____

____

3. An 18-year-old woman is getting ready to be discharged from your unit with her new infant who was born 2 days ago. As you are helping her pack her belongings she tells you she thinks she is bleeding too much. She has never had a period that is so red and with so many clots. What should you do?

____

____

____

4. Mr. Cecil expresses concern about his ability to perform sexually and the possibility of being impotent now that he has had a prostatectomy. What should you do?

____

____

____

5. A new mother asks that her baby be left with her all night long. She wants to cuddle with the baby and have the newborn sleep with her. What should you do?

____

____

____

LEARNING ACTIVITIES

1. Find a Well Woman Clinic or an obstetric/gynecological (OB/GYN) office in the area you live and ask for a tour or to shadow a health care provider for part of the day. Report back to your class about what you observed, the type of population seen in this facility and the services offered.
2. Explore the Internet to find a video of a **TURP** or prostatectomy being performed. Or, find information about equipment used to help correct erectile dysfunction.

PROCEDURE CHECKLISTS

PROCEDURE 24-1: PREPARING A PATIENT FOR A PELVIC EXAM

Name: ____________________ Date: ____________________

STEPS	S	U	COMMENTS
1. Assemble the equipment a. Disposable gloves b. Microscope slides c. Cotton applicators d. Cotton balls e. Pap smear fixative f. Vaginal speculum g. Uterine dressing forceps h. Lubricant i. Wooden tongue blade			
2. Wash your hands and put on disposable gloves.			
3. Provide privacy for the patient.			
4. Tell the patient you are going to prepare her for a pelvic exam.			
5. Have the patient empty her bladder in the bathroom or assist with a bedpan.			
6. Help the patient undress while providing coverage with a blanket.			
7. Position the patient on her back with her knees separated and legs flexed. Stirrups may be used to position the legs and feet. An additional drape may be used to cover the legs.			
8. If you leave the room before the exam, place the call light within easy reach of the patient. However, you may be asked to remain during the exam.			
9. After the exam, assist the patient to dress or put on a gown.			
10. Make sure the patient is comfortable.			
11. Care for the equipment according to the institution's policy.			
12. Remove your gloves and wash your hands.			

13. Report to the supervisor • That the exam was performed. • What time the exam was performed.			

Charting:

____

____

____

____

Date of Satisfactory Completion ____________________

Instructor's Signature ____________________

PROCEDURE 24-2: POSTPARTUM PERINEAL CARE

Name: ______________________ Date: ______________________

STEPS	S	U	COMMENTS
1. Assemble your equipment a. Disposable bed protector b. Bedpan and cover c. Squirt bottle (peri bottle) d. Toilet paper e. Disposable gloves			
2. Wash your hands.			
3. Identify the patient by checking the identification bracelet.			
4. Ask visitors to leave the room, if this is your hospital's policy.			
5. Tell the patient you are going to clean the genital area.			
6. Provide privacy for the patient.			
7. Be sure there is plenty of light. Raise the bed to a comfortable working position.			
8. Cover the patient with a bath blanket. Without exposing her, fan-fold the top sheets to the foot of the bed. Have the patient covered only with the blanket. Put on gloves.			
9. Fill the squirt bottle with warm water at 100°F (37.7°C) or use the solution provided in your institution.			
10. Place the disposable bed protector under the patient's hips (buttocks).			
11. Help the patient to get on the bedpan.			
12. Put on disposable gloves.			
13. Spray the perineum with solution, working from anterior to posterior.			
14. Dry the patient gently with the toilet paper. Remove and discard the disposable gloves.			
15. Remove the bedpan and disposable bed protector. Place them on a chair.			
16. Cover the patient with the top sheets. Remove the bath blanket.			
17. Make the patient comfortable.			
18. Lower the bed to a position of safety for the patient.			

19. Raise the side rails where ordered, indicated, and appropriate for patient safety.			
20. Place the call light within easy reach of the patient.			
21. Discard disposable equipment.			
22. Empty, rinse, and put the equipment back where it belongs.			
23. Remove your gloves and wash your hands.			
24. Report to your immediate supervisor • That postpartum perineal care was given • Your observations of anything unusual • How the patient tolerated the procedure			

Charting:

____

____

____

____

Date of Satisfactory Completion ____________________

Instructor's Signature ____________________

The Nervous System and Related Care

25

Key Terms Review

Match the key terms in the right column with the definitions in the left column by placing the letter of each correct answer in the space provided.

_____ **1.** The part of the peripheral nervous system that carries messages and functions without conscious thought.

_____ **2.** The portion of the nervous system that is outside of the brain and spinal cord. These nerves control the automatic functions, such as the heart and kidneys. They also control the sensory organs, hearing, smell, touch, vision, and taste.

_____ **3.** Blood clot or mass of other undissolved matter that travels through the circulatory system from its place of formation to another site and lodges in a small blood vessel, causing an obstruction.

_____ **4.** Excessive bleeding.

_____ **5.** A blood clot that remains at its site of formation.

_____ **6.** To break open.

_____ **7.** Pertaining to blood vessels.

_____ **8.** Fatty deposits attached to vessel walls within blood vessels.

_____ **9.** Stroke; blockage or bleeding of blood vessels in the brain, interrupting the blood supply to that part of the brain and damaging the surrounding area of the brain.

_____ **10.** A temporary or permanent negative change in a patient's usual neurologic function.

Terms

A. Osteoporosis
B. Normal pressure hydrocephalus
C. Autonomic nervous system
D. Peripheral nervous system
E. Convulsive
F. Seizure
G. Complex partial seizure
H. Simple partial seizure
I. Spasm
J. Contracture
K. Canthus
L. Environment
M. Respond
N. Involuntary
O. Stimuli
P. Voluntary
Q. Nervous system
R. Thrombus
S. Embolus

_____11. The partial or total loss of producing language or understanding speech.

_____12. Paralysis of one-half of the body.

_____13. Involving *convulsions,* which are rhythmic and involuntary muscle contractions.

_____14. Seizure with motor and possible sensory symptoms (such as muscle twitching and smelling a foul odor) and a change in the level of consciousness.

_____15. An episode, either partial or generalized, that may include altered consciousness, motor activity, or sensory phenomena or convulsions.

_____16. A seizure when the patient is aware of his surroundings but experiences either motor (muscle twitching or movement) or sensory changes (see or hear things not present).

_____17. An involuntary sudden movement or convulsive muscular contraction.

_____18. The inner aspect of the eye closest to the nose.

_____19. The fluid that circulates around and within the brain and spinal cord.

_____20. The material between the vertebral bodies that cushions the spinal column.

_____21. The covering of the brain and spinal cord; there are three layers: the dura mater, the arachnoid, and the pia mater.

_____22. Protective covering around most nerves.

_____23. The bones around the spinal cord.

_____24. Final vertebra in the spinal column; referred to as the tailbone.

_____25. Drawing together, bunching up, or shortening of muscle tissue because of spasm or paralysis, either permanently or temporarily.

_____26. All the surrounding conditions and influences affecting the life and development of an organism.

_____27. Half of a sphere; in the nervous system, one-half of the brain.

_____28. Area of the brain responsible for control of the pituitary gland.

_____29. An electrical or chemical charge transmitted through certain tissues, especially nerve fibers and muscles.

_____30. A type of nerve cell in the nervous system.

_____31. To react; begin, end, or change activity in reaction to stimulation.

T. Hemorrhage

U. Rupture

V. Vertebral bodies

W. Myelin sheath

X. Coccyx

Y. Meninges

Z. Cerebral spinal fluid

AA. Cerebrovascular accident (CVA)

BB. Vascular

CC. Plaque

DD. Deficit

EE. Hemiplegia

FF. Aphasia

GG. Intervertebral discs

HH. Hemisphere

II. Hypothalamus

JJ. Neuron

KK. Impulse

_____**32.** Changes in the external or internal environment strong enough to set up a nervous impulse or other responses in an organism.

_____**33.** Under control of the will; with conscious decision.

_____**34.** Without conscious will, control, or decision.

_____**35.** The group of body organs consisting of the brain, spinal cord, and nerves that controls and regulates the activities of the body and the functions of the other body systems.

_____**36.** A disorder caused by enlargement of the *ventricles,* fluid-filled spaces in the brain.

_____**37.** Condition in which bones become brittle or thin and break easily.

MULTIPLE-CHOICE QUESTIONS

Circle the letter next to the word or statement that best completes the sentence or answers the question.

1. CVAs may be caused by
   a. plaque build up occluding the blood vessel.
   b. rupture of a hemorrhaging blood vessel.
   c. a thrombus or an embolus.
   d. all of the above.

2. For the patient who has a(n) __________, cleaning it is part of daily personal hygiene.
   a. artificial eye
   b. pacemaker
   c. wheelchair
   d. shunt

3. Hemiplegia may result in which of the following?
   a. Loss of sensation
   b. Loss of movement
   c. Loss of pain
   d. All of the above

4. __________________ is a weakness or paralysis of one side of the face.
   a. Bell's palsy
   b. Bob's palsy
   c. Paul's belsy
   d. Belle's palsy

5. ____________________ may be related to cerebral trauma.
   a. Osteoporosis
   b. Alopecia
   c. Dermatitis
   d. Epilepsy

6. A disease that is a type of dementia is
   a. glaucoma.
   b. vertigo.
   c. Alzheimer's.
   d. a detached retina.

7. Blisters along the path of certain nerves is known as
   a. shingles (Herpes zoster).
   b. quadriplegia.
   c. cataracts.
   d. Meniere's disease.

8. A transient ischmetic attack (TIA) is
   a. a permanent condition.
   b. a sign of cancer.
   c. a mini stroke.
   d. an endocrine condition.

9. To provide safe care for a patient having a seizure,
a. put the patient in bed.
b. move furniture or equipment the patient may bump.
c. put a tongue depressor in the patient's mouth.
d. put the patient's head between his knees.

10. The brain and spinal cord
a. nerves cannot regenerate once they are damaged.
b. have a protective sheath called *myelin* surrounding them.
c. are controlled by the hypothalamus.
d. receive motor sensations and are continually contracting.

11. The ______ controls ________________.
a. midbrain; incontinence.
b. cerebellum; balance and coordination.
c. cerebrum; involuntary movement, like muscle jerking.
d. pituitary gland; the hypothalamus.

12. A(n) __________ is a doctor who specializes in the diagnosis and treatment of problems in the nervous system.
a. neurologist
b. anesthesiologist
c. podiatrist
d. urologist

13. When cleaning an artificial eye, the nursing assistant should
a. transport the eye in a cup filled to the top with cold water to ensure the eye does not dry out.
b. sit the patient up in bed to make it easier for the eye to be removed.
c. cleanse the canthus starting from the nose and working out and changing the cotton ball with each swipe.
d. keep the water running in the sink and keep the drain open.

14. When caring for patient's eyeglasses, the nursing assistant should
a. hold the glasses by the lenses, making sure not to drop them.
b. use alcohol to cleanse the lenses.
c. cleanse the lenses using a soft cloth and solution if it is provided.
d. dry the lenses using her uniform.

15. If a nursing assistant hears a high-pitched squealing noise coming from a patient's hearing aid, she should
a. turn the volume off to make the sound stop.
b. turn the volume slightly lower and ask the patient if he can still hear.
c. remove the hearing aid and place it in the bedside table, because the sound can damage the patient's ability to hear.
d. clean the hearing aid with water because it is clogged with ear wax.

16. An easy way to tell if the batteries on a patient's hearing aid are working correctly is to
a. hold the hearing aid in a slightly closed hand and listen for a whistling sound.
b. submerge the hearing aid in a container filled with liquid cleanser.
c. have the nursing assistant place the hearing aid in her own ear to see if the hearing aid is working.
d. turn the volume to the highest level, place the hearing aid in the patient's ear, and wait to hear a high-pitched squeal.

17. During the aging process, an older person may
a. have more than 50% decrease in the size and weight of their brain.
b. experience difficulty walking and have incontinent episodes.
c. have the same response time as when he was in his early adulthood.
d. feel hotter because of changes in his body fat.

18. Which change may occur when a person ages?
a. Dysphagia
b. Saliva production increases
c. The amount of taste buds stay the same
d. None of the above

19. If a patient is quadriplegic, he
   a. cannot move his arm and legs.
   b. can move only his arms but not his legs.
   c. can move only one side of his body.
   d. will not need any help with his activities of daily living.

20. Which diseases or disorders are associated with a change in vision?
   a. Meniere's disease and otitis media
   b. Retinal detachment and glaucoma
   c. Shingles and Parkinson's disease
   d. Multiple sclerosis and cataracts

21. Spinal cord problems can result from
   a. the way heat, cold, and pain are perceived.
   b. wearing pantyhose too tightly.
   c. having a diagnosis of Parkinson's or Alzheimer's
   d. lifting heavy objects incorrectly and dislocating a vertebral disc.

22. During a generalized tonic-clonic seizure, the patient may
   a. have stiffness in the limbs.
   b. lose control of urine or stool.
   c. be very tired afterward and want to sleep.
   d. all of the above.

23. Which two things can cause a CVA?
   a. Increase in oxygen and blood to the brain
   b. Myocardial infarction and benign positional vertigo
   c. Occlusion of an artery supplying blood to the brain and a hemorrhage of a vessel in the brain
   d. Parkinson's and Alzheimer's diseases

24. Mr. Walls is a hemiplegic. He has become withdrawn and tells the nursing assistant, "I cannot do anything for myself anymore. I am half the man I used to be." An appropriate response is:
   a. "You are right. You have had many setbacks since you had your stroke."
   b. "Don't worry about it. You have a loving wife who will take care of your every need."
   c. "Groveling will get you nowhere with me. Now come on, let's get to it!"
   d. "It must be difficult to go through what you have gone through. Would you like to talk about it?"

25. During a TIA, a patient may experience
   a. a change in vision.
   b. weakness in the arms and legs.
   c. short-lived aphasic episodes.
   d. all of the above.

TRUE OR FALSE QUESTIONS

Determine whether each question is true or false. In the space provided, write "T" for true and "F" for false. If the statement is false, rewrite it on the line provided to make it a true statement.

_____ **1.** A hearing aid will restore full, normal hearing ability.

____

_____ **2.** The weight and size of the brain decrease as a person ages.

____

_____ **3.** Parkinson's disease is a progressive disorder, leading to loss of control of movement.

____

_____ **4.** *Hypoxia* means there is an increase of oxygen to the brain.

____

_____ **5.** The purpose of the myelin sheath is to protect and insulate nerve cells and to help an injured nerve regenerate.

____

_____ **6.** The spinal cord is one of the five components that make up the brain.

____

_____ **7.** There are 40 pairs of cranial and spinal nerves in the nervous system.

____

_____ **8.** The spinal cord can be found in all four sections of the spine.

____

_____ **9.** A young boy is being chased by a dog. During this "fight or flight" experience, the boy's pupils contract, he has a decreased heart rate, and his breathing changes.

____

_____ **10.** During a simple seizure, a patient may tell you later that she experienced an unusual humming sound and saw gold and green lights dancing before her.

____

FILL-IN-THE-BLANK QUESTIONS

Provide the meaning of the following abbreviations.

1. CNS ______________________________
2. PNS ______________________________
3. CVA ______________________________
4. TIA ______________________________
5. Sections of the vertebrae: C, T, L, and S ______________________________
6. F ______________________________
7. C ______________________________
8. MRI ______________________________
9. GTC ______________________________

EXERCISE 25-1

Objective: To apply what you have learned about the nervous system and related care.

Directions: Read the following riddles carefully before writing the correct answer on the blank line.

1. I often form on the inside of vessel walls. Who am I? (*Hint:* My name sounds like an engraved award.)

   ____

2. When I occur, I can cause the patient to become unconscious. Who am I? (*Hint:* Under different circumstances, I would take your possessions away.)

   ____

EXERCISE 25-2

Objective: To recognize the structures and functions of the nervous system.

Directions: Label the drawings in Figure 25-1 using the words from the following word list. (Some answers may be used more than once.)

Word List

Cerebrum	Cerebellum	Brain	Spinal nerves
Axon	Muscle tissue	Nucleus	Dendrite
Motor neuron	Pons	Neuron	Spinal cord
Medulla	Myelin sheath	Motor message from the brain	
	sensory message to the brain		

FIGURE 25-1

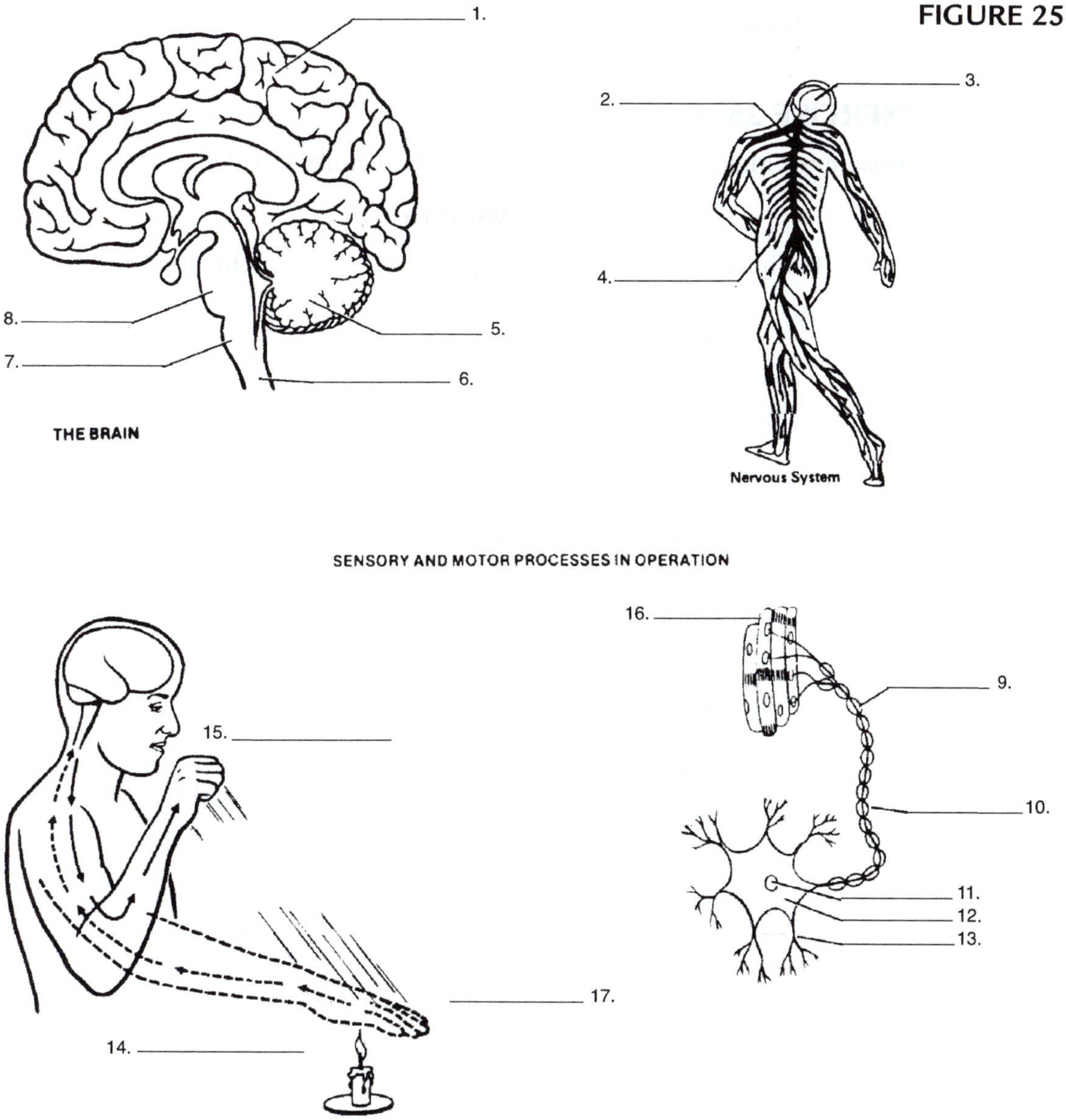

EXERCISE 25-3

Directions: Select from the list of procedures the letter of the procedure that best answers each question. Write the correct letter(s) on the blank line next to the question.

a. Artificial eye care

b. Hearing aid care

c. Eyeglass care

_____**1.** Which procedure(s) could involve the use of a special solution?

_____**2.** Which procedure(s) would the nursing assistant observe for damage to the patient's equipment?

_____**3.** Which procedure(s) involve helping the patient clean a part of his body?

EXERCISE 25-4

Directions: Match the correct answer to the picture provided.

Word List

Hemiplegia Paraplegia Quadriplegia

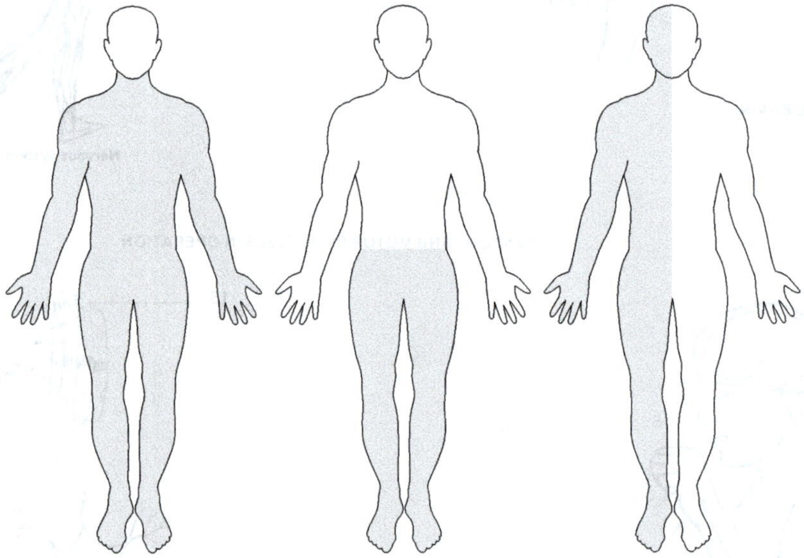

_______________ _______________ _______________

THE NURSING ASSISTANT IN ACTION

1. Mr. Selleck is walking in the hallway. You stop to converse with him and ask, "Did you take your meds today?" He answers, "No, I did not bump my head today." What should you do?

____

____

____

2. Mrs. Jansen is sitting in the back of the living room in the nursing home while a guest speaker is lecturing. Her hearing aid begins to make a high-pitched squealing noise. She is unaware of the sound. However, the other residents wave to you to come over. They whisper to you that Mrs. Jansen's hearing aid is making noises. What should you do?

____

____

____

3. You are working with a group of teens when you suddenly notice one young man is staring and not responding to a question his friend asks him. His arms and legs begin to shake. The friend tells you that his friend is epileptic. What should you do?

____

____

____

4. You call for help when a patient of yours begins having myoclonic seizures. Your colleague helps you get the patient to the floor and places a pillow under her head. The other nursing assistant insists on taking a tongue blade and forcing into the patient's mouth so the patient does not bite her tongue off. What measures should you take when a patient has a seizure? Also, how should you deal with this colleague's persistence to use a tongue blade?

____

____

____

5. Mrs. Warrington recently had a stroke and is frustrated because no one seems to be able to understand what she says. She presents with garbled language and frequently has problems finding the words she wants to use. However, you notice there is a stack of mystery novels next to her bed. She is an avid reader. What methods could you use to improve communication between Mrs. Warrington and the staff?

____

____

____

LEARNING ACTIVITIES

1. Using a piece of paper, randomly write down 10 sentences you think you use frequently each day. For the next 12 hours, you may only use these 10 sentences throughout the day. At the end of this experience, journal about your experiences and the reaction you received from family, friends, colleagues, and strangers. What other methods of communication did you have to rely on to get others to understand what you wanted or needed? What did you feel during this experience? Using what you learned about yourself and the frustration and difficulties associated with your communication deficit, jot some notes to yourself about how you can help your patients who live with aphasia. Share these ideas with classmates.
2. Using a scarf or belt, secure your dominant hand to your waist. Move through your day living with hemiplegia and only using your nondominant hand. At the end of this experience, journal about your experiences and the tasks you could and could not do correctly. How did you feel during this experience? Using what you learned about yourself and the frustration and difficulties associated with your ability to move about freely, jot some notes to yourself about how you can help your patients who live with paralysis. Share these ideas with classmates.

PROCEDURE CHECKLISTS

PROCEDURE 25-1: CARING FOR AN ARTIFICIAL EYE

Name: ______________________ Date: ______________________

STEPS	S	U	COMMENTS
1. Assemble your equipment on the bedside table a. An eyecup half-filled with lukewarm water at 98° to 100°F (36.6° to 37.7°C) and labeled with the patient's name and room number (or, if no eyecup is available, use a clean denture cup) b. Gauze, 4" × 4" (3–4 pieces), for the bottom of the cup (or per your institution's policy) c. Small basin with lukewarm water d. Four cotton balls e. Special cleansing solution, if ordered by the doctor			
2. Wash your hands.			
3. Ask visitors to step out of the room, if this is your hospital's policy.			
4. Identify the patient by checking the identification bracelet.			
5. Tell the patient you are going to take care of his eye.			
6. Pull the curtain around the bed for privacy.			
7. Help the patient lie down on the bed. This is to prevent accidental dropping of the artificial eye.			
8. Put on gloves.			
9. Have the patient close his eyes. Clean any external secretions from the patient's upper eyelid. Use cotton balls and warm water from the basin. Clean from the canthus (the inner aspect of the eye closest to the nose) to the outside of the eye area. This means you move from the nose to the outside of the eye. If you need to wipe more than once, use a clean (new) cotton ball each time. Use gentle strokes.			
10. Remove the artificial eye. To do this, carefully depress the lower eyelid with your thumb. Lift the upper lid gently with your forefinger. The eye should slide out and down, into your hand. Have the patient do this, if he is able.			

11. Place a 4" × 4" gauze in the cup and place the eye on the gauze. Let it soak in the water.			
12. Wash off external matter and encrustations from the outside of the eye socket with cotton balls and warm water. Using gentle strokes, clean from the inner canthus to the outside of the eye.			
13. Take the eyecup to the patient's bathroom. Close the drain in the sink. Fill the sink one-half full with water to prevent breakage if the eye is dropped.			
14. Take the eye in your gloved hand and wash with running lukewarm water 98°–100°F (36.6°–37.7°C). Use plain water unless the doctor orders a special solution. Place the eye in the gauze from the eyecup and rub gently between your thumb and forefinger. *Do not use alcohol, ether, or acetone. These may dissolve the plastic of the artificial eye or dull the luster.*			
15. Rinse the eye under running lukewarm water at 98°–100°F (36.6°–37.7°C), then dry it using the second 4" × 4" gauze. Discard the water from the eyecup. Place the slightly moistened eye on dry gauze in the eyecup. (A slightly moistened eye is easier to insert.) Return to the patient's bedside.			
16. If the patient cannot wear the eye immediately, store it by adding water to the eyecup and placing it in the bedside table drawer. Label the cup with the patient's name and room number.			
17. Before inserting the artificial eye, remove your gloves and wash your hands thoroughly a second time. Put on clean gloves. If the patient is to insert the eye, have him wash his hands.			
18. Insert the eye in the patient's eye socket. Have the notched edge toward the nose. Raise the upper lid with your forefinger. With your other hand, insert the eye. Place the eye under the upper lid. Then depress the lower lid. The eye should settle in place.			
19. Make the patient comfortable.			
20. Lower the bed to a position of safety for the patient.			
21. Pull the curtains back to the open position.			
22. Raise the side rails where ordered, indicated, and appropriate for patient safety.			

23. Place the call light within easy reach of the patient.			
24. Remove your gloves and wash your hands.			
25. Report at once to your immediate supervisor • That you completed care of the artificial eye. • The time the procedure was done. • How the patient tolerated the procedure. • Your observations of anything unusual.			

Charting:

____

____

____

____

Date of Satisfactory Completion ____________

Instructor's Signature ____________

PROCEDURE 25-2: CARING FOR EYEGLASSES

Name: ____________________ Date: ____________________

STEPS	S	U	COMMENTS
1. Knock or ask permission to enter the patient's room.			
2. Assemble your equipment on the bedside table or in the bathroom a. A soft cloth b. Cleaning solution if needed			
3. Wash your hands.			
4. Identify yourself.			
5. Identify the patient.			
6. Explain what you are going to do. Remove the patient's eyeglasses from the case or take them off the patient's face with the patient's permission and assistance. Handle the glasses by the frame only.			
7. Inspect the eyeglasses. Do this by holding them up to the light and looking for scratches, smears, or soiling. Look for any loose screws in the hinges of the frame.			
8. Clean the eyeglasses by polishing them with a soft cloth. If more cleaning solution is needed, run them under warm water or use the cleaning solution provided by your institution. Dry the eyeglasses with a soft cloth.			
9. Return the eyeglasses to the case or to the patient. Assist the patient with putting them on as needed.			
10. Remember to always keep eyeglasses in the case when the patient is not wearing them to avoid breaking or scratching them.			
11. Wash your hands.			
12. Report at once to your immediate supervisor • That you completed care of the eyeglasses. • The time the procedure was done. • How the patient tolerated the procedure. • Your observations of anything unusual, such as scratches on the eyeglasses or loose hinge screws.			

Charting:

____

____

____

____

Date of Satisfactory Completion ____________________

Instructor's Signature ____________________

Emergency Care

26

Key Terms Review

Match the key terms in the right column with the definitions in the left column by placing the letter of each correct answer in the space provided.

_____ **1.** Event that calls for immediate action.

_____ **2.** Terrorist attacks using chemical or biological materials.

_____ **3.** Circulatory system, which includes heart, arteries, veins, and capillaries.

_____ **4.** The first action taken to help a person who is in crisis.

_____ **5.** The extreme or unexpected loss of blood; heavy bleeding.

_____ **6.** Tissue damage caused by excessive heat, regardless of the source.

_____ **7.** When the airway is closed or blocked and a person cannot breathe or speak.

_____ **8.** Procedure used on a choking patient that lifts the diaphragm and forces air from the lungs to expel the object blocking the airway.

_____ **9.** An emergency procedure used to reestablish effective circulation and respiration in order to prevent irreversible brain damage.

_____ **10.** The unexpected stopping of the heartbeat and circulation.

Terms

A. First aid

B. Burn

C. Choking

D. Abdominal thrust

E. Hemorrhage

F. Cardiovascular system

G. Fainting

H. Shock

I. Poison control center

J. Poison

K. Seizure

L. Cardiac arrest

M. Cardiopulmonary resuscitation (CPR)

N. Bag–valve mask

O. Emergency

P. Bioterrorism

Q. Cerebrovascular accident (CVA) or stroke

R. Myocardial infarction

_____**11.** A hand-held device used to provide ventilations to a patient who is not breathing or who is breathing inadequately; ambu bag.

_____**12.** A sudden, brief loss of consciousness; "passing out."

_____**13.** The failure of the cardiovascular system to provide sufficient blood circulation to every part of the body.

_____**14.** Any substance ingested, inhaled, injected, or absorbed into the body that interferes with normal physiological function.

_____**15.** A free telephone service where poison experts are available to assist people with questions about poisoning emergencies 24 hours a day, 7 days a week, 365 days a year by dialing 1-800-222-1222.

_____**16.** An episode (either partial or generalized) that may include altered consciousness, motor activity, or sensory phenomena, as well as convulsions.

_____**17.** Interruption or damage to the blood supply to the brain.

_____**18.** Interruption or damage to the blood supply to the heart muscle.

MULTIPLE-CHOICE QUESTIONS

Circle the letter next to the word or statement that best completes the sentence or answers the question.

1. Which of the following must you determine before you take any action in an emergency?
   a. What is the problem or emergency?
   b. Is there anyone available to help you?
   c. What must be done immediately to maintain life for the person in crisis?
   d. All of the above.

2. The emergency plan for home-care patients should contain the telephone numbers for which of the following?
   a. Fire rescue squad
   b. Physician
   c. Poison control center
   d. All of the above

3. Guidelines for assisting a victim in an emergency do include
   a. bleeding control.
   b. preventing further injury or harm.
   c. preventing shock.
   d. all of the above.

4. In an emergency, you may be called on to perform _______ until medical help arrives.
   a. OBRA
   b. RACE
   c. PASS
   d. CPR

5. ________ are used to dislodge an object and open the airway of a choking victim.
   a. Push hard and fast compressions
   b. Look, listen, and feel techniques
   c. Abdominal thrusts
   d. Last chance techniques

6. Placing your hands in the wrong position while doing chest compressions
   a. can improve the circulation.
   b. strengthens your hands.

c. is not a major problem.
d. can cause broken ribs and other problems for the victim.

7. A _________ is an episode, either partial or generalized, that may include alteration of consciousness, body movements, and convulsions.
a. seizure
b. stroke
c. shock
d. hemorrhage

8. A(n) _______ is a site where a main artery lies near the surface of the body, directly over a bone.
a. vein
b. airway
c. artery
d. pressure point

9. __________ can be a sign of internal bleeding.
a. Dilated pupils
b. Extreme hunger
c. Slow pulse
d. Headache

10. A burn from steam, chemicals, excessive heat, or sun can cause
a. choking.
b. hemorrhagic shock.
c. tissue damage.
d. anaphylactic shock.

11. Complications of a burn may include
a. infection, shock, and growth.
b. pain, infection, and death.
c. promotion, infection, and death.
d. tanning, sleepiness, and death.

12. Pale, moist, and cold skin may be a sign of
a. death.
b. birth.
c. post-shower syndrome.
d. internal bleeding.

13. When speaking with a 911 operator, the caller should
a. give the address where the emergency occurred.
b. state the phone number where the crisis is occurring.
c. tell the operator how many people are injured.
d. all of the above.

14. Loss of __________ and body _________ is a complication of burns.
a. mobility; image
b. heat; temperature
c. heat; fluids
d. heat; flexibility

15. A __________ is any substance that is toxic to the body.
a. vitamin
b. mineral
c. radical
d. poison

16. The wrong medication or an incorrect dose of a prescribed medication may occur for which reason?
a. Adults ignoring warning labels.
b. Teens experimenting with others' prescription drugs.
c. No child-proof locks exist on cabinets containing medications.
d. All of the above.

17. When assisting the patient who has been poisoned, the nursing assistant should
a. check the mouth for burns.
b. look for a container from which the poison may have come.
c. note the odors on the person's breath.
d. all of the above.

18. The interruption of the blood supply to the heart muscle is called a
a. muscle cramp.
b. heart attack.
c. pneumothorax.
d. cerebrovascular accident.

19. When a person is having a seizure, you should protect him from injury and maintain a(n) _______ airway.
a. closed
b. patent/open

c. fluid
d. obstructed

20. What is a sign or symptom of shock?
a. Pulse is slow and steady.
b. Pulse is rapid and weak.
c. Respirations are regular and deep.
d. Pupils are constricted.

21. When a patient experiences chest pain from a possible myocardial infarction he might complain of
a. pain in the jaw.
b. a heavy feeling in his chest.
c. tightness in his chest.
d. all of the above.

22. Hands-Only™ CPR for an untrained person was introduced so lay persons
a. can do mouth to mouth without fear of getting an infection.
b. can report an accident and then leave the scene immediately.
c. would be more likely to perform CPR.
d. would perform the steps and sequence of CPR without making a mistake.

23. Adult CPR should be performed
a. only by a healthcare professional.
b. on a smooth and soft surface so injury does not occur.
c. with both hands interlaced and placed on the victim's abdomen.
d. with shoulders over the victim's sternum and with straight arms.

24. How deep should compressions be when performing adult CPR?
a. 1½"
b. 100 per minute
c. 2"
d. 30:2

25. When helping an infant who is choking, you should
a. place the infant's head higher than his feet.
b. give 5 back blows and then 5 chest thrusts until the object is expelled.
c. place your finger in the infant's mouth and try to get the infant to vomit the object out.
d. give mouth to mouth immediately and then call 911.

TRUE OR FALSE QUESTIONS

Determine whether each question is true or false. In the space provided, write "T" for true and "F" for false. If the statement is false, rewrite it on the line provided to make it a true statement.

_____ **1.** Deliver approximately 50 compressions in a minute while giving CPR to an adult.

____

_____ **2.** Open the airway of the patient using the head-tilt/chin-lift technique.

____

_____ **3.** After calling for medical assistance, a victim who has been poisoned can be left alone.

____

_____ **4.** The American Heart Association and the Red Cross are agencies that can recertify a healthcare professional in CPR and First Aid.

____

_____ **5.** If the person who has been poisoned is unconscious, give fluids by mouth to minimize the effect.

____

_____ **6.** The Good Samaritan Law protects a person from being sued in court for stopping to help a person in crisis.

____

_____ 7. If you suspect that a person has had a stroke, call Poison Control.

____

_____ 8. When caring for a patient who was just burned, you should remove their clothing immediately and then dress the wound with sterile dressing.

____

_____ 9. The medical term for fainting is *syncope*.

____

_____ 10. Status epilepticus can last for hours.

____

FILL-IN-THE-BLANK QUESTIONS

Provide the meaning of the following abbreviations.

1. CPR __________________________________
2. PPE __________________________________
3. DNR __________________________________
4. MI __________________________________
5. CAD __________________________________
6. AHA __________________________________
7. ECC __________________________________
8. "CAB" sequence of CPR __________________________________
9. EMS __________________________________
10. AED __________________________________
11. cm __________________________________

EXERCISE 26-1

Objective: To recognize and correctly spell words related to emergency care.

Directions: Fill in the missing letters to correctly spell the following medical terms. The total number of letters is listed next to each word.

1. ______MER__CY (9)
2. H_________RRH__GE (10)
3. S_________CK (5)
4. F_________T A__(8)
5. _____TRO__E (6)
6. C_____RDIO_LMONY (15)
7. CA__I_____AR___S_____(13)
8. RES__ITA__ON (13)
9. _____RD___V_____S___LAR (14)

10. P_____SO___(6)

11. S_____Z____E (7)

12. ______N____HYL__T_____C(12)

13. B____T____RR_____ISM(12)

14. ______EI____IC_____(8)

EXERCISE 26-2

Directions: When performing CPR using an AED, certain steps must occur in the correct sequence. Place the following choices in the correct order by placing the numbers 1–7 in the spaces provided.

_____A. Shock the patient if the AED advises to do so.

_____B. Check for unresponsiveness.

_____C. Do not touch the patient.

_____D. Position the AED next to the patient and closest to the nursing assistant so reaching over the patient does not occur.

_____E. The machine states, "Analyzing heart rhythm. Do not touch the patient."

_____F. Turn the machine on.

_____G. Place pads to chest.

EXERCISE 26-3

Objective: To recognize the symptoms of shock.

Directions: Draw a line to connect the correct type of shock that matches the cause.

Type of Shock	Shock Causes
1. Hemorrhagic	Fear
2. Respiratory	Changes in body chemistry
3. Psychogenic	Insufficient oxygen in the blood
4. Septic	Spinal cord damage
5. Cardiogenic	Insect stings
6. Neurogenic	Infection
7. Anaphylactic	Heart not functioning well
8. Metabolic	Extreme blood loss

EXERCISE 26-4

Directions: Select from the following list the letter of the poison that best answers each question. Write the correct letter(s) on the blank line next to the question. There may be more than one letter used for each question.

Poisons

A. Petroleum products

B. Iodine

C. Metals (copper, lead, mercury, zinc)

D. Food poisoning

E. Arsenic (rat poison)

F. Acetaminophen

G. Bleach

_____**1.** Which poison(s) produce a garlic smell on the breath?

_____**2.** Which poison(s) may produce vomiting?

_____**3.** For which type of poisoning could Poison Control be contacted?

_____**4.** For which type of poisoning can a "soapy" appearance in the mouth occur?

_____**5.** Which type of poisoning can present with gastrointestinal changes?

THE NURSING ASSISTANT IN ACTION

1. You are the first to arrive at the scene of an automobile accident. There are two people who present with injuries. Both have gotten out of the car and are sitting on the curb. You notice one has lost an arm and blood is spurting onto the pavement. The other is holding his head, blood has trickled down his cheek and he is moaning loudly. What should you do?

____

____

____

____

2. You are picnicking in a local park and the child with you gets stung by a bee on the finger. Her finger, lips, and eyelids begin to swell. You have a cell phone with you and other people are picnicking at a table near yours. What should you do?

____

____

____

____

3. Uncle Ernie has removed himself from the Thanksgiving dinner feast and goes to lie down on the couch. As you pass the living room, you notice he is sweating profusely, has opened his shirt, and his skin is very pale. You ask him if he is feeling all right. He tells you, "Your mama sure knows how to cook. I just ate too much and have a little indigestion. Just let me rest a while and I will be able to finish off that pumpkin pie in a minute." What should you do?

4. You are babysitting for your neighbor's 11-month-old baby. The child is with you in the kitchen and sitting in a highchair, eating a piece of baloney. You notice that she stops eating, is turning blue, and is making a high-pitched squealing sound. What should you do?

5. You have been invited to chaperone a school trip your child's class is taking. During the ride, an 11-year-old on the school bus has a seizure. What should you do?

LEARNING ACTIVITIES

1. Enroll in a course for CPR and First Aid if your course or place of employment does not offer this and receive certification.
2. Using your textbook, copy the table of Common Poisons (Table 26-1) located on page 631 and post it in your kitchen inside a cabinet door. If you do not have access to a photocopy machine, then use the Internet and print a list for yourself.
3. Create a list of emergency numbers and post it in a visible spot, like your refrigerator, in case an emergency should occur. Include your address and land-line phone number where your reside, the Poison Control number, your physician's number, the local police and fire department numbers, and a nearby neighbor's number. Include the names of each family member along with their birthdates, weight, height, and any medical problems or medication they are taking. Tell people in your family or any babysitter/caregiver you use, where this list is located. In case an emergency does occur, everyone is ready to provide the 911 operator with this information so proper care can be administered.

PROCEDURE CHECKLISTS

PROCEDURE 26-1: ADULT CPR WITH ONE RESCUER

Name: ______________________ Date: ______________________

STEPS	S	U	COMMENTS
1. Determine responsiveness of the person by tapping the shoulder and shouting, "Are you all right?"			
2. If the person is unresponsive, not breathing or not breathing normally (e.g., gasping), activate the EMS (emergency medical system) by calling 911, or if in an institution with an emergency response system, call that facility's emergency response number.			
3. Position the person on his back. Logroll the person to avoid twisting the spine. Place the person on a firm surface, if possible, with his arms alongside his body.			
4. Kneel beside the person's chest if the person is on the ground, or stand beside the bed if the person is in bed. If a backboard is available, place it under the person, being careful not to delay the initiation of CPR.			
5. The health care provider only should take no more than 10 seconds to check for a carotid pulse to see if the heart is beating. If no heartbeat is detected, proceed to chest compressions.			
6. Begin chest compressions immediately by placing the heel of one hand on the center (middle) of the person's chest (the lower half of the sternum) and the heel of the other hand on top of the first so that the hands are overlapped and parallel.			
7. Depress the chest at least 2" (5 cm) with each chest compression and with chest compression recoil/relaxation times approximately equal. Allow the chest to completely recoil after each compression. Perform 30 chest compressions at a rate of at least 100 compressions per minute. a. Count out loud: "1 and 2 and 3 and 4 . . .," continuing to 30.			
8. Open the airway using the head-tilt/chin-lift method or the jaw-thrust method if a cervical spine injury is suspected.			

9. If the person is not breathing, give two rescue breaths. Each rescue breath should be delivered over 1 second, with sufficient tidal volume to produce visible chest rise, being careful not to overinflate the lungs. Allow the chest to deflate before delivering the second breath. If the chest does not rise with the first rescue breath, reposition the head by performing the head-tilt/chin-lift maneuver again and then give a second rescue breath. If available, use your bag–valve-mask device, pocket face-breathing mask, or barrier device on the patient's mouth.			
10. Repeat chest compressions and ventilations using a compression-to-ventilation ratio of 30 chest compressions to 2 ventilations. a. Count out loud: "1 and 2 and 3 and 4 . . .," continuing to 30. b. Open the airway and give two breaths. c. Repeat the cycle of 30 compressions followed by 2 breaths.			
11. Continue CPR until help arrives to relieve you, the patient resumes breathing and has a heart rate, or the person begins to move.			
12. Wash your hands.			
13. Document and report the results to the EMS and your supervisor.			

Charting:

____

____

____

____

Date of Satisfactory Completion ____________________

Instructor's Signature ____________________

PROCEDURE 26-2: ADULT CPR WITH TWO RESCUERS

Name: ______________________ Date: ______________________

STEPS	S	U	COMMENTS
1. First determine unresponsiveness by gently tapping the person on the shoulder. Shout, "Are you all right?" If there is no response, the person is considered unresponsive.			
2. The first rescuer should instruct the second rescuer to activate the EMS system by calling 911, or if in an institution with an emergency response system, call that facility's emergency response number.			
3. The first rescuer should also check for no breathing or no normal breathing (e.g., gasping) while checking for responsiveness; if the health care provider finds that the victim is unresponsive with no breathing or no normal breathing (e.g., gasping), the health care provider should consider the person in cardiac arrest.			
4. Position the person on his back. Logroll the person to avoid twisting the spine. Place the person on a firm surface, if possible, with his arms alongside his body.			
5. Kneel beside the person's chest if the person is on the ground, or stand beside the bed if the person is in bed. If a backboard is available, place it under the person, being careful not to delay the initiation of CPR.			
6. The health care provider only should take no more than 10 seconds to check for a carotid pulse to see if the heart is beating. If no heartbeat is detected, proceed to chest compressions.			
7. The first rescuer should begin chest compressions immediately by placing the heel of one hand on the center (middle) of the person's chest (the lower half of the sternum) and the heel of other hand on top of the first so that the hands are overlapped and parallel.			
8. Depress the chest at least 2" (5 cm) with each chest compression and with chest compression recoil/relaxation times approximately equal. Allow the chest to completely recoil after each compression. The first rescuer should perform 30 chest compressions at a rate of at least 100 compressions per minute. a. Count out loud: "1 and 2 and 3 and 4 . . ." continuing to 30.			
9. The second rescuer should open the airway using a head-tilt/chin-lift method, or the jaw-thrust method if a cervical spine injury is suspected.			

10. If the person is not breathing, the second rescuer should give two rescue breaths. Each rescue breath should be delivered over 1 second, with sufficient tidal volume to produce visible chest rise, being careful not to overinflate the lungs. Allow the chest to deflate before delivering the second breath. If the chest does not rise with the first rescue breath, reposition the head by performing the head-tilt/chin-lift again, and then give a second rescue breath. Use your bag-valve-mask device, pocket face-breathing mask, or barrier device on the patient's mouth, if available.			
11. Repeat chest compressions and ventilations. With two rescuers, the first rescuer delivers chest compressions and the second rescuer delivers breaths at a ratio of 30 chest compressions to 2 breaths. a. Count out loud: "1 and 2 and 3 and 4 . . ." continuing to 30. b. Open the airway and give 2 breaths. c. Repeat the cycle of 30 compressions followed by 2 breaths.			
12. After approximately 2 minutes (5 cycles) of chest compressions and ventilations, the rescuers should switch positions to help prevent rescuer fatigue and a decrease in the quality of compressions.			
13. Continue CPR until help arrives to relieve you, the patient resumes breathing and has a heart rate, or the patient begins to move.			
14. Wash your hands.			
15. Document and report the results to the EMS crew and your supervisor.			

Charting:

____

____

____

____

Date of Satisfactory Completion ____________________

Instructor's Signature ____________________

PROCEDURE 26-3: ADULT CPR WITH AN AED

Name: ____________________ Date: ____________________

STEPS	S	U	COMMENTS
1. First determine unresponsiveness by gently tapping or shaking the person. Shout, "Are you OK?" If there is no response, the person is considered unresponsive.			
2. Activate the emergency response system and have someone get the AED.			
3. Position the person on his back. Logroll the person to avoid twisting the spine. Place the person on a flat hard surface, if available, with his arms alongside his body.			
4. The health care provider only should take no more than 10 seconds to check for a carotid pulse to see if the heart is beating. If no heartbeat is detected, proceed to chest compressions.			
5. Depress the chest at least 2" (5 cm) with each chest compression and with chest compression recoil/relaxation times approximately equal. Allow the chest to completely recoil after each compression. Perform 30 chest compressions at a rate of at least 100 compressions per minute. a. Count out loud: "1 and 2 and 3 and 4 . . .," continuing to 30.			
6. If the person is not breathing, give two rescue breaths. Each rescue breath should be delivered over 1 second with sufficient tidal volume to produce visible chest rise, being careful not to overinflate the lungs. Allow the chest to deflate before delivering the second breath. If the chest does not rise with the first rescue breath, reposition the head by performing the head-tilt/chin-lift maneuver again, and then give a second rescue breath. Use your bag-valve-mask device, pocket face-breathing mask, or barrier device on the patient's mouth, if available.			
7. Continue CPR with cycles of 30 compressions and 2 breaths until the AED arrives.			
8. Attach AED to patient as soon as possible with little interruption in CPR.			

9. Prepare to use the AED on the adult patient. a. Place the AED next to the patient and turn it on. b. Attach the AED pads to the patient's chest, following the directions on the pads. c. Allow the AED to analyze the patient's heart rhythm. Do not touch or move the patient during this time. d. Follow the AED voice prompts. e. If the AED states that a shock is advised, ensure that everyone is clear of the patient and not touching the patient in any way. f. Press the SHOCK button when the voice prompts you to do so. g. After the shock is delivered, follow the voice prompt to either continue CPR or stop CPR if the AED determines a sustainable heart rhythm.			
10. Continue to assess patient, providing CPR and using the AED as voice prompted, until emergency assistance arrives.			
11. Wash your hands.			
12. Document and report the results to the EMS crew and your supervisor.			

Charting:

____

____

____

____

Date of Satisfactory Completion ______________________

Instructor's Signature ______________________

PROCEDURE 26-4: CHILD CPR WITH ONE RESCUER

Name: ______________________ Date: ______________________

STEPS	S	U	COMMENTS
1. Determine unresponsiveness by gently tapping the victim and asking loudly, "Are you OK?" Call the child's name if you know it. If there is no response, the child is considered unresponsive. Shout for help.			
2. Have an available bystander activate the EMS system by calling 911. If you are the lone rescuer and you witnessed the sudden collapse of the child, activate the EMS and get the AED. If the child was found unresponsive, begin CPR immediately.			
3. Position the child on his back. Logroll the child to avoid twisting the spine. For best results, place the child on a firm surface with his arms alongside his body.			
4. The health care provider only should take no more than 10 seconds to check for a carotid or femoral pulse to see if the heart is beating. If no heartbeat is detected, proceed to chest compressions.			
5. Give 30 chest compressions. Compress the lower half of the sternum with the heel of one or both hands, depending on the size of the child. Push at a rate of at least 100 compressions per minute. Allow complete chest recoil after each compression.			
6. Open the airway using the head-tilt/chin-lift method for both the injured or noninjured child and give 2 breaths. Each breath should last 1 second. Watch for the chest to rise as you ventilate, and allow the chest to deflate completely between breaths. Use your bag-valve-mask device, pocket face-breathing mask, or barrier device on the child's mouth, if available.			
7. After giving 2 breaths, immediately give 30 compressions.			
8. The lone rescuer should continue this cycle of 30 compressions and 2 breaths for approximately 2 minutes (about 5 cycles) before leaving the child to activate the emergency response system and obtain an AED if one is nearby.			
9. Return to the child quickly and recheck the child's condition.			

10. If the child does not have a heartbeat and is not breathing, continue CPR until help arrives using a 30:2 compression to ventilation ratio.			
11. Wash your hands.			
12. Document and report the results to the EMS crew and your supervisor.			

Charting:

Date of Satisfactory Completion ______________________

Instructor's Signature ______________________

PROCEDURE 26-5: CHILD CPR WITH TWO RESCUERS

Name: ____________________ Date: ____________________

STEPS	S	U	COMMENTS
1. Determine unresponsiveness by gently tapping the child and ask loudly, "Are you OK?" Call the child's name if you know it. If there is no response, the child is considered unresponsive. Shout for help.			
2. The first responder should begin one-person CPR while the second rescuer calls for help, activating the EMS, and gets the AED.			
3. Position the child on his back. Logroll the child to avoid twisting the spine. For best results, place the child on a firm surface with his arms alongside his body.			
4. The health care provider only should take no more than 10 seconds to check for a carotid or femoral pulse to see if the heart is beating. If no heartbeat is detected, proceed to chest compressions.			
5. The first rescuer begins 15 chest compressions by compressing the lower half of the sternum with the heel of one or both hands, depending on the size of the child. Push at a rate of at least 100 compressions per minute. Allow complete chest recoil after each compression.			
6. The second rescuer opens the airway using the head-tilt/chin-lift method for both the injured or noninjured child and gives 2 breaths. Each breath should last 1 second. Watch for the chest to rise as you ventilate, and allow the chest to deflate completely between breaths. Use your bag-valve-mask device, pocket face-breathing mask, or barrier device on the child's mouth, if available.			
7. Continue this cycle of 15 compressions followed by 2 ventilations a. The rescuer giving compressions counts out loud: "1 and 2 and 3 and 4 . . .," continuing to 15. b. The rescuer providing rescue breathing opens the airway and gives two breaths. c. Repeat the cycle of 15 compressions followed by 2 breaths.			
8. Rescue personnel should switch between providing compressions and ventilations every 5 cycles of 15 compressions and 2 breaths to prevent fatigue.			

9. Continue two-rescuer CPR until help arrives to relieve you or the child resumes breathing and has a heartbeat.			
10. Wash your hands.			
11. Document and report the results to the EMS crew and your supervisor.			

Charting:

____

____

____

____

Date of Satisfactory Completion ____________________

Instructor's Signature ____________________

PROCEDURE 26-6: CHILD CPR WITH AN AED

Name: ______________________ Date: ______________________

STEPS	S	U	COMMENTS
1. Determine unresponsiveness by gently tapping the child and ask loudly, "Are you OK?" Call the child's name if you know it. If there is no response, the child is considered unresponsive. Shout for help.			
2. The first responder should begin one-person CPR while the second rescuer activates the EMS and gets the AED.			
3. Position the child on his back. Logroll the child to avoid twisting the spine. For best results, place the child on a firm surface with his arms alongside his body.			
4. The health care provider only should take no more than 10 seconds to check for a carotid or femoral pulse to see if the heart is beating. If no heartbeat is detected, proceed to chest compressions.			
5. Give 30 chest compressions. Compress the lower half of the sternum with the heel of one or both hands, depending on the size of the child. Push at a rate of at least 100 compressions per minute. Allow complete chest recoil after each compression.			
6. Open the airway using the head-tilt/chin-lift method for both the injured or noninjured child and give 2 breaths. Each breath should last 1 second. Watch for the chest to rise as you ventilate, and allow the chest to deflate completely between breaths. Use your bag-valve-mask device, pocket face-breathing mask, or barrier device on the child's mouth, if available.			
7. If the child does not have a pulse and is not breathing, continue CPR. Attach the AED as soon as possible with minimal interruptions in chest compressions.			
8. Prepare to use the AED on the child a. Place the AED next to the child and turn it on. b. Attach the AED pediatric pads to the child's chest following the directions on the pads. c. Allow the AED to analyze the child's heart rhythm. Do not touch or move the child during this time. d. Follow the AED voice prompts. e. If the AED states that a shock is advised, ensure that everyone is clear of the child and not touching the patient in any way.			

f. Press the SHOCK button when the voice prompts you to do so. g. After the shock is delivered, follow the voice prompt to continue CPR or stop CPR if the AED determines a sustainable heart rhythm.			
9. Continue to assess child, providing CPR and using the AED as voice prompted, until emergency assistance arrives.			
10. Wash your hands.			
11. Document and report the results to the EMS crew and your supervisor.			

Charting:

____

____

____

____

Date of Satisfactory Completion ______________

Instructor's Signature ______________

PROCEDURE 26-7: INFANT CPR WITH ONE RESCUER

Name: ____________________ Date: ____________________

STEPS	S	U	COMMENTS
1. Determine unresponsiveness by gently tapping the foot of the infant and stroking the infant shouting, "Are you OK?" Call the infant's name if you know it. If there is no response, the infant is considered unresponsive. Shout for help.			
2. If the infant was found unresponsive, begin CPR immediately.			
3. Position the infant on his back or support the infant on rescuer's arms. For best results, place the infant on a firm surface with his arms alongside his body.			
4. The health care provider only should take no more than 10 seconds to check for a brachial pulse on the arm nearest to the rescuer to see if the heart is beating. If no heartbeat is detected, proceed to chest compressions.			
5. Give 30 chest compressions. Compress the sternum at a depth of 1½", using two fingers placed just below an imaginary line drawn between the infant's nipples. Do not compress over the xiphoid or ribs. Gently compress the chest at a rate of at least 100 compressions per minute. Allow complete chest recoil after each compression.			
6. After 30 compressions, gently open the airway using the head-tilt/chin-lift method. Cover the infant's mouth and nose with your mouth. Prepare to give two rescue breaths. Use the strength of your cheeks to deliver gentle puffs of air into the infant. Each breath should last 1 second. Watch for the chest to rise as you ventilate and allow the chest to deflate completely between breaths. If you have difficulty making an effective seal around the infant's mouth and nose, try either mouth-to-mouth while pinching the nose closed or mouth-to-nose while closing the mouth. If the infant's chest still does not rise, examine the mouth to make sure no foreign material is inside. If an object can be seen, sweep it out with your finger.			
7. Give 2 breaths after each 30 compressions.			
8. The lone rescuer should continue this cycle of 30 compressions and 2 breaths for approximately 2 minutes (about 5 cycles) before leaving the infant to activate the emergency response system.			
9. Return to the infant quickly and recheck the infant's condition.			

10. If the infant does not have a heartbeat and is not breathing, continue CPR using a 30:2 compression to ventilation ratio until help arrives or the infant shows signs of life.			
11. Wash your hands.			
12. Document and report the results to the EMS crew and your supervisor.			

Charting:

____

____

____

____

Date of Satisfactory Completion ____________________

Instructor's Signature ____________________

PROCEDURE 26-8: INFANT CPR WITH TWO RESCUERS

Name: ____________________ Date: ____________________

STEPS	S	U	COMMENTS
1. Determine unresponsiveness by gently tapping the foot of the infant and stroking the infant while shouting, "Are you OK?" Call the infant's name if you know it. If there is no response, the infant is considered unresponsive.			
2. Activate the emergency response system and begin CPR immediately.			
3. Position the infant on his back.			
4. The health care provider only should take no more than 10 seconds to check for a brachial pulse on the arm nearest to the rescuer to see if the heart is beating. If no heartbeat is detected, proceed to chest compressions.			
5. The first rescuer gives 15 chest compressions using the two thumb-encircling hands to perform the chest-compression technique. Encircle the infant's chest with both hands, spreading your fingers around the thorax and placing your thumbs together over the lower third of the sternum. If you cannot physically encircle the infant's chest, compress the chest using the two-finger technique placed just below an imaginary line drawn between the infant's nipples. Compress the sternum at a rate of at least 100 compressions per minute and depth of 1½". Be careful not to compress over the xiphoid or ribs. Allow complete chest recoil after each compression.			
6. After 15 compressions, the second rescuer gently opens the airway using the head-tilt/chin-lift method and covers the infant's mouth and nose with his mouth. Using the strength of his cheeks, 2 breaths are delivered to the infant using gentle puffs. Each breath should last 1 second. Watch for the chest to rise as the breaths are delivered. Allow the chest to deflate completely between breaths. If you experience difficulty making an effective seal around the infant's mouth and nose, try either mouth-to-mouth while pinching the nose closed or mouth-to-nose while closing the mouth. If the infant's chest still does not rise, examine the mouth to make sure no foreign material is inside. If an object can be seen, the rescuer should sweep it out using his finger and reattempt to ventilate the infant.			
7. After the second rescuer gives the infant 2 breaths, the first rescuer follows with 15 compressions.			

8. The rescuers should switch positions with minimal interruption in CPR every 2 minutes (about 5 cycles) to avoid fatigue.			
9. If the infant does not have a heartbeat and is not breathing, continue CPR using a 15:2 compression-to-ventilation ratio until help arrives or the infant shows signs of life.			
10. Wash your hands.			
11. Document and report the results to the EMS crew and your supervisor.			

Charting:

____

____

____

____

Date of Satisfactory Completion ____________________

Instructor's Signature ____________________

PROCEDURE 26-9: RELIEVING CHOKING IN THE RESPONSIVE (CONSCIOUS) OR UNRESPONSIVE (UNCONSCIOUS) ADULT OR CHILD (OLDER THAN 1 YEAR)

Name: ______________________ Date: ______________________

STEPS	S	U	COMMENTS
1. Determine if there is a partial or complete airway obstruction. Ask, "Are you choking?" If the person is able to breathe, speak, or cough effectively, do not interfere. Offer assistance if the person cannot speak or make a sound. Some states require that the rescuer ask for permission before touching the victim.			
2. Stand behind the person and put your arms around the waist allowing the person's arms to hang free.			
3. Make a fist with one hand and place the thumb side of your hand on the abdomen between the umbilicus ("belly button") and the sternum.			
4. Grasp this hand with your other hand and press it into the abdomen with a quick upward movement to deliver an abdominal thrust.			
5. Be sure each abdominal thrust is a separate movement. Check the patient after five abdominal thrusts.			
6. Repeat and continue these steps until the object is dislodged successfully.			
7. If a choking patient becomes unresponsive and unconscious while you are performing emergency interventions, lower the person to the floor and continue providing care.			
8. Determine unresponsiveness by gently tapping the person and asking, "Are you OK?"			
9. If there is no response, call for help or send someone to activate EMS (dial 911).			
10. Position the head and neck to open the airway using the head-tilt/chin-lift method. Tilt the head back with one hand while you lift the chin with the other.			
11. Place your cheek near the victim's face and listen and look to feel air movement against your cheek.			
12. Attempt to ventilate the victim with two quick breaths. If unsuccessful, reposition the head and try to give the breaths again.			
13. Straddle the victim's legs while on your knees.			
14. Position one hand on top of the other and give three to five firm upward thrusts in the upper abdomen, above the umbilicus but below the sternum.			

15. Move to the patient's head and look in the mouth to see if you can visualize and remove the obstructing object.			
16. If not, repeat and continue abdominal thrusts until the object is dislodged.			
17. Once the object is removed, ventilate or do CPR if necessary.			
18. Stay with the patient until breathing has been restored and patient is no longer in distress.			
19. If EMS responders arrived, report your observations and actions to them.			
20. Wash your hands.			
21. Document and report your observations and actions to your supervisor.			

Charting:

___

___

___

___

Date of Satisfactory Completion ___

Instructor's Signature ___

PROCEDURE 26-10: RELIEVING CHOKING IN THE INFANT (YOUNGER THAN 1 YEAR)

Name: ____________________ Date: ____________________

STEPS	S	U	COMMENTS
1. Confirm obstruction. Check if the infant is cyanotic (blue), cannot make sounds, breathe, or cry.			
2. Hold the infant on your arm in a head-down position. Support the infant's head by cupping his face in your hand, being careful not to cover the mouth.			
3. Give five back blows, reposition infant on your other arm, cupping the head in your hand, and give five chest thrusts.			
4. Inspect the mouth and remove the object if visualized.			
5. Repeat five back blows and five chest thrusts until the object is expelled and your interventions are successful.			
6. If the infant becomes unconscious, start CPR following the infant CPR guidelines.			
7. If infant resumes breathing, place in the recovery position and monitor vital signs.			
8. Wash your hands.			
9. Document and report the results to the EMS crew and your supervisor.			

Charting:

____

____

____

____

Date of Satisfactory Completion ____________________

Instructor's Signature ____________________

Warm and Cold Applications

27

Key Terms Review

Match the key terms in the right column with the definitions in the left column by placing the letter of each correct answer in the space provided.

_____ **1.** 98.6°F or 37.0°C.

_____ **2.** A higher than normal body temperature.

_____ **3.** A lower than normal body temperature.

_____ **4.** A reaction of the tissues to disease or injury; there is usually pain, heat, redness, and swelling of the body part.

_____ **5.** Bluish or darkened color to the skin that occurs when there is not enough oxygen in the blood.

_____ **6.** A warm or cold application in which no water touches the skin.

_____ **7.** Alternating; stopping and beginning again.

_____ **8.** Limited to one place or part; affecting, involving, or pertaining to a definite area.

_____ **9.** A warm or cold application applied to a specific area or small part of the body.

_____ **10.** Affecting, involving, or pertaining to the whole body.

_____ **11.** A warm or cold application applied to the entire body.

_____ **12.** A bath in which the patient sits in a specially designed chair tub or regular bathtub with the hips and buttocks in the water.

Terms

A. Dilate
B. Constrict
C. Compress
D. Normal body temperature
E. Hypothermia
F. Hyperthermia
G. Cyanosis
H. Inflammation
I. Dry application
J. Localized application
K. Generalized application
L. Moist application
M. Soak
N. Sitz bath
O. Generalized
P. Localized
Q. Intermittent

_____13. A warm or cold application in which water touches the body.

_____14. Immerse the body or body part completely in water.

_____15. Folded piece of cloth used to apply pressure, moisture, heat, cold, or medication to a specific part of the body.

_____16. Get narrower.

_____17. Get bigger; expand.

MULTIPLE-CHOICE QUESTIONS

Circle the letter next to the word or statement that best completes the sentence or answers the question.

1. Heat may be applied to an area of the body to
   a. improve the patient's appearance.
   b. improve the appearance of the skin.
   c. speed up the healing process by increasing the circulation.
   d. speed up the healing process by decreasing the circulation.
2. Heat may be applied to the body to
   a. increase the pain to a joint.
   b. decrease the circulation.
   c. reduce the patient's weight.
   d. reduce the pain caused by inflammation and congestion.
3. Cold applications cause the blood vessels to constrict, which helps
   a. prevent or reduce swelling.
   b. prevent or reduce weight.
   c. improve cyanosis.
   d. increase bleeding.
4. Blood flow to a body part becomes slower when
   a. cold is applied.
   b. cold is reduced.
   c. heat is applied.
   d. heat is increased.
5. Which is an example of a dry warm application?
   a. sitz bath
   b. Soak
   c. Compress
   d. Heating pad
6. An Aquamatic Hydro-Thermal K-pad™ is a type of _________ application.
   a. moist
   b. dry
   c. steam
   d. dry–moist
7. The part of the patient's skin that is receiving a warm application treatment must be inspected often for redness and discoloration because
   a. the patient may not have feeling in the body area because of a disease process and may not realize there is a problem.
   b. this indicates the treatment is complete.
   c. your immediate supervisor wants you to do this.
   d. it makes the patient think you are doing a good job.
8. When performing cold treatment using an ice pack, the nursing assistant should stop treatment if cyanosis and _______ are noted in the skin.
   a. blanching
   b. goose-bumps
   c. tattoos
   d. body piercings
9. *Localized application* means that a treatment is
   a. given to any patient on the unit who wants it.
   b. applied every day for no more than 20 minutes at a time.

c. placed on a certain smaller spot on the body.

d. done on the entire body.

10. When offering warm or cold therapy, the nursing assistant should

a. always fill ice bags to the top with water.

b. leave the treatment on as long as it takes for edema to be reduced.

c. place the person in Trendelenberg position for comfort.

d. check for leaks and clean up spills immediately to prevent accidents.

11. How many minutes should an ice pack be left on the patient's arm?

a. 5 minutes

b. 20 minutes or more

c. 15–20 minutes

d. 10 minutes

12. What temperature should a hot compress be?

a. 92–100°F

b. 100–106°F

c. 80–95°F

d. 80–93°F

13. What is the purpose of placing a towel on the floor in front of a sitz bath?

a. To provide warmth to the patient's feet

b. To catch any overflow of water that might escape

c. To prevent falls from occurring

d. To make sure no bacteria get onto the sitz bath container.

14. Ms. Kline is to have a sitz bath. The nursing assistant should

a. submerge her arm in the water for approximately 15–20 minutes.

b. scrub the area with soap during the procedure.

c. ask her to do it herself.

d. assist her onto the toilet and show her how to work the stopcock.

15. Which of the following devices requires electricity in order for the procedure to work?

a. Aquamatic Hydro-Thermal K-pad™

b. Cold compress

c. Hot compress

d. Hot water bottle

16. How often should skin be checked for any problems when cold or warm therapy is being administered?

a. Every 5 minutes

b. Every 10 minutes

c. Between 10 and 20 minutes

d. After the therapy is stopped

17. If warm and cold therapy is done correctly,

a. tissue damage may result.

b. healing will occur.

c. swelling will increase blood flow.

d. discomfort will increase.

18. A *compress* is an example of a

a. dry heat application.

b. ice pack.

c. moist application.

d. soak.

19. If shivering occurs while warm or cold therapy is being done, the nursing assistant should

a. leave the compress on the person's extremity for the full time prescribed.

b. stop the treatment and report the complaint.

c. turn on the air conditioner in the room.

d. take the bed blanket off the patient immediately.

20. A nursing assistant can avoid accidents by

a. working with wet hands around electrical appliances.

b. applying a compress without checking the temperature of the water.

c. using nonsterile compresses when an eye infection occurs.

d. cleaning up spills as soon as they occur.

21. A warm and ________ compress may be placed on the eye to prevent an infection from occurring to this area.

a. then cold

b. then hot

c. sterile
d. aseptic

22. When a patient complains he feels _____ and _____, the cold therapy should be stopped.
a. good; refreshed
b. bad; rested
c. strong; warm
d. weak; cold

23. A nursing assistant should cover a hot moist compress with a(n) _____ to keep the temperature of the application warm for a longer period of time.
a. ice pack
b. flannel covering
c. glove
d. article of clothing the patient owns

24. A commercial heat pack may need to be _____ in order for it to work correctly.
a. warmed
b. cooled
c. left on longer than 45 minutes
d. placed in a basin

25. The sitz bath overflow opening should be placed
a. in the toilet bowl.
b. outside the toilet.
c. toward the front of the toilet.
d. toward the back of the toilet.

TRUE OR FALSE QUESTIONS

Determine whether each question is true or false. In the space provided, write "T" for true and "F" for false. If the statement is false, rewrite it on the line provided to make it a true statement.

_____ 1. When cyanosis, blanching, or a white appearance to the skin occurs, the nursing assistant should stop the cold soak and report her findings to the supervisor.

____

_____ 2. Make sure your hands are dry before touching any electrical appliances.

____

_____ 3. When applying an ice bag, placing water in the bag may reduce the ice's sharp edges.

____

_____ 4. The nursing assistant should use pins to secure the Aquamatic Hydro-Thermal K-pad™ in place.

____

_____ 5. Some commercial ice packs must be hit to activate them.

____

_____ 6. When a warm compress is applied, constriction to the blood vessels occurs.

____

_____ 7. When left out in the cold, a higher than normal body temperature (hyperthermia) can occur.

____

_____ 8. Hyperthermia can occur on a hot summer day.

____

_____ 9. During heat therapy, dilation occurs and waste products in the blood are more easily carried away and removed from the body.

____

_____ 10. Sometimes, cold therapy is applied to the entire body.

____

FILL-IN-THE-BLANK QUESTIONS

Provide the meaning of the following abbreviations.

1. F ____________________
2. C ____________________
3. ID ____________________

EXERCISE 27-1

Objective: To recognize and correctly spell words related to warm and cold applications.

Directions: Unscramble the words in the following word list.

1. NOITAMMALFNI ____________________
2. CLAOLZIDE ____________________
3. OMSTI ____________________
4. OASK ____________________
5. MOCRSEPS ____________________
6. ETHA ____________________
7. CANYSOIS ____________________
8. DCLO ____________________

EXERCISE 27-2

Objective: To apply what you have learned about warm and cold applications.

Directions: Read the following riddles carefully before writing the correct answer on the blank line.

1. I describe how something can get smaller or narrower. What am I? (*Hint:* My alternate definition is legally binding.)

   ____

2. This is a treatment that patients report as warm and soothing. What is it? (*Hint:* To walk, a person stands. To drive a car, he ____________.)

   ____

3. This cold application can cool a warm head. What is it? (*Hint:* There is also one of these at the North and South poles.)

   ____

EXERCISE 27-3

Directions: Draw a line and match the correct Fahrenheit temperature ranges in the first column to the correct Celsius temperature ranges in the second column.

Fahrenheit	**Celsius**
50–65° F	28–34°C
80–93° F	19–27°C
98–106°F	35–37°C
93–98°F	10–18° C
65–80° F	38–41°C

EXERCISE 27-4

Directions: Select from the list of procedures the letter of the procedure that best answers each question. Write the correct letter(s) on the blank line next to the question. There may be more than one letter used for each question.

A. Sitz bath

B. Aquamatic Hydro-Thermal K-pad™

C. Commercial heat pack

D. Warm or cold soak

E. Warm or cold compress

_____ **1.** Which procedure(s) might allow a patient to help with the application?

_____ **2.** In which procedure(s) should the nursing assistant observe for complications such as shivering and pain?

_____ **3.** Which procedure(s) is done primarily in the bathroom?

_____ **4.** Which procedure(s) involves keeping tubing at the bed level?

_____ **5.** Which procedure(s) requires a nursing assistant to wrap the treatment to keep temperature constant?

THE NURSING ASSISTANT IN ACTION

1. Your supervisor asks you to set up the Aquamatic Hydro-Thermal K-pad™ at the patient's bedside. You have never done this before and are unsure how to work the equipment. What should you do?

2. A sitz bath has been ordered for a woman who recently had an episiotomy. You gather the equipment and enter the bathroom but are unsure how to proceed. What should you do?

3. A patient refuses the heat treatment that has been ordered, stating, "Just leave me alone. I am in so much pain that nothing will help stop my aches and pains." What should you do?

4. You are to administer a warm compress to a patient's eye. What should you do?

5. A warm foot soak has been ordered for a diabetic patient. He has never had this done before. What should you do?

LEARNING ACTIVITIES

1. Using the Internet, find information about Aircast® Cryo/Cuff Therapy. Become familiar with how to use this equipment in case you must use this equipment in your facility.
2. Copy the information provided in Table 27-3 in the textbook on page 643 onto a small index card or perhaps post this inside a cabinet door in an area where staff prepares treatments frequently to help you remember the temperatures associated with each term. The next time you are asked to perform a procedure, you will have this information readily available.

PROCEDURE CHECKLISTS

PROCEDURE 27-1: APPLYING A WARM COMPRESS (MOIST HEAT APPLICATIONS)

Name: ____________________ Date: ____________________

STEPS	S	U	COMMENTS
1. Assemble equipment a. Disposable bed protector b. Basin c. Pitcher of water (98°F, 37°C) d. Washcloth, towel, or gauze pads e. Large sheet of plastic f. Bath towel g. Bath blanket h. Disposable gloves, if any potential exists for exposure to body fluids			
2. Wash your hands and apply gloves if indicated.			
3. Identify the patient by checking the ID bracelet.			
4. Inform the patient that you are going to apply a warm compress and where.			
5. Provide privacy and comfort for the patient.			
6. Raise the bed to a comfortable working position.			
7. Help the patient into a comfortable position. Have the body area exposed for application of a warm compress.			
8. Place a disposable bed protector under the body area that is to be given the warm compress.			
9. Fill the pitcher with warm water, then pour water into the basin.			
10. Dip the compress into the water and wring it out thoroughly.			
11. Apply the compress gently to the proper area.			
12. Cover the wet compress by wrapping the entire area with a large towel or blue pad.			
13. Cover the entire area, compress, and towel with a waterproof pad or blue pad to keep the compress warm.			
14. If the patient is cold, cover him with a blanket.			

15. Change the compress and remoisten it as necessary to keep it warm. Sometimes a patient is able to apply the compress himself. If your supervisor gives you permission for this, position and assist the patient as necessary.			
16. Check the skin under the application every 5 minutes. If the skin appears red, remove the compress. Cover the area with a towel, report these findings to your supervisor, and follow the policy of your agency regarding skin documentation.			
17. A warm compress is usually applied for 15–20 minutes; however, follow instructions give to you by your supervisor as to how long the warm compress is to be applied.			
18. After the treatment is completed, remove the compress and pat the area dry with a towel.			
19. Make the patient comfortable and replace the call light.			
20. Lower the bed to a position of safety.			
21. Raise the side rail when ordered or indicated.			
22. Clean standard equipment and put in its proper place. Discard disposable equipment and gloves.			
23. Wash your hands.			
24. Report to your supervisor • The time the warm compress was started • How long the compress was in place • The area of application • How the patient tolerated the procedure • Any unusual or abnormal observations			

Charting:

____

____

____

____

Date of Satisfactory Completion ____________________

Instructor's Signature ____________________

PROCEDURE 27-2: APPLYING A WARM SOAK

Name: ____________________ Date: ____________________

STEPS	S	U	COMMENTS
1. Assemble equipment a. Basin, foot tub, or arm basin b. Disposable bed protector c. Bath towel d. Bath blanket e. Disposable gloves, if any potential exists for exposure to body fluids			
2. Wash your hands and apply gloves if indicated.			
3. Identify the patient by checking the ID bracelet.			
4. Explain to the patient that you are going to apply a warm soak and where.			
5. Provide privacy and comfort for the patient.			
6. Raise the bed to a comfortable working position.			
7. Help the patient into a safe and comfortable position.			
8. Fill the basin one-half full with warm water.			
9. Place a disposable bed protector under the body area that is to receive the soak.			
10. Place the basin in a position so the patient's arm, hand, leg, or foot can be dipped into the basin easily.			
11. Place the patient's arm, hand, leg, or foot into the basin of water gradually.			
12. Check the temperature of the water every 5 minutes. When you must change the water, take the patient's arm, hand, foot, or leg out of the basin. Wrap it with a bath blanket or bath towel to keep it warm.			
13. If the patient says he is feeling weak or cold, stop the treatment. Cover the patient with extra blankets and report this to your immediate supervisor.			
14. Check the skin every 5 minutes. If the skin appears red, remove the compress. Cover the area with a towel, report these findings to your supervisor, and follow the policy of your agency regarding skin documentation.			
15. When the treatment is finished, dry the patient's arm or leg by patting it gently with a towel.			
16. Make the patient comfortable and replace the call light.			

17. Lower the bed to a position of safety.			
18. Raise the side rails when ordered or indicated.			
19. Clean equipment and put it in its proper place. Discard disposable equipment and gloves, if used.			
20. Wash your hands.			
21. Report to your supervisor • The time the warm soak was started • The length of treatment • The area of application • How the patient tolerated the procedure • Any abnormal or unusual observations			

Charting:

____

____

____

____

Date of Satisfactory Completion ____________________

Instructor's Signature ____________________

PROCEDURE 27-3: APPLYING A COMMERCIAL UNIT HEAT PACK

Name: ____________________ Date: ____________________

STEPS	S	U	COMMENTS
1. Assemble equipment a. Commercial unit, single-use heat pack that has been warmed following the manufacturer's instructions b. Disposable bed protectors c. Bath blanket d. Disposable gloves, if any potential exists for exposure to body fluids			
2. Wash your hands and apply gloves, if indicated.			
3. Identify the patient by checking the ID bracelet.			
4. Inform the patient you are going to apply a warm pack and where.			
5. Provide privacy and comfort for the patient.			
6. Raise the bed to a comfortable working position.			
7. Help the patient into a safe and comfortable position. Expose the area to be treated.			
8. Place the bed protector under the body part that is to receive the warm pack.			
9. Place the moist, warm pack on the proper body area.			
10. Cover the pack with a waterproof pad or blue pad to keep the pack warm.			
11. Check the skin under the application every 5 minutes. If the skin appears red, remove the compress. Cover the area with a towel, report these findings to your supervisor, and follow the policy of your agency regarding skin documentation.			
12. Follow instructions of your supervisor as to the length of the application. Replace with a new warm pack as necessary.			
13. When the treatment is finished, discard disposable equipment and gloves, if used.			
14. Make the patient comfortable and replace the call light.			
15. Lower the bed to a position of safety.			
16. Raise the side rails if ordered or indicated.			

17. Wash your hands.			
18. Report to your supervisor • The time the warm pack was applied • The length of treatment • The area of application • How the patient tolerated the procedure • Any abnormal or unusual observations			

Charting:

____

____

____

____

Date of Satisfactory Completion ____________________

Instructor's Signature ____________________

PROCEDURE 27-4: APPLYING AN AQUAMATIC® HYDRO-THERMAL (K-PAD)

Name: ______________________ Date: ______________________

STEPS	S	U	COMMENTS
1. Assemble equipment a. Aquamatic® Hydro-Thermal (K-pad) and control unit; select the appropriate size for its intended use b. Cover for pad (pillowcase, flannel cover, or cover from manufacturer) c. Disposable gloves, if any potential exists for exposure to body fluids			
2. Wash your hands and apply gloves, if indicated.			
3. Identify the patient by checking the ID bracelet.			
4. Inform the patient that you are going to apply a K-pad and where.			
5. Provide privacy and comfort for the patient.			
6. Raise the bed to a comfortable working position.			
7. Help the patient into a safe and comfortable position. Expose the area to be treated.			
8. Inspect the K-pad for leaks and make sure the cord and plug are in safe working condition.			
9. Plug the cord into an electrical outlet.			
10. Place the pad in the cover; *do not use pins.*			
11. Place the container on the bedside table. Arrange the tubing at the level of the bed. Do not allow the tubing to hang below the bed.			
12. Gently apply the pad in its cover on the proper dry body area.			
13. Check the skin under the pad. If the skin appears red, remove the pad. Cover the area with a towel, report these findings to your supervisor, and follow the policy of your agency regarding skin documentation.			
14. Follow the instructions of your supervisor as to how frequently to check the skin and the length of the application.			
15. When the treatment is finished, return the equipment to its proper place.			
16. Make the patient comfortable and replace the call light.			
17. Lower the bed to a position of safety.			

18. Raise the side rails if ordered or indicated.			
19. Wash your hands.			
20. Report to your supervisor • The time the K-pad was applied • The length of treatment • The area of application • How the patient tolerated the procedure • Any abnormal or unusual observations			

Charting:

____

____

____

____

Date of Satisfactory Completion ____________________

Instructor's Signature ____________________

PROCEDURE 27-5: USING A DISPOSABLE SITZ BATH

Name: ______________________ Date: ______________________

STEPS	S	U	COMMENTS
1. Assemble equipment: a. Disposable sitz basin b. Water bag c. Tubing and stopcock (clamp) d. Plastic laundry bag e. Bath towels f. Pitcher of warm water g. Gloves, if any potential exists for exposure to body fluids			
2. Wash your hands and apply gloves as indicated.			
3. Identify the patient by checking the ID bracelet.			
4. Inform the patient that you are going to give him a sitz bath.			
5. Provide privacy and comfort for the patient.			
6. Raise the toilet seat.			
7. Put the sitz basin into the toilet bowl. Be sure that the opening for overflow is toward the front of the toilet.			
8. Check the temperature of the bathwater to be sure it is about 90°F to 100°F.			
9. Pour the water into the basin, filling it half full.			
10. Close the stopcock on the tubing. Fill the water bag with water from the pitcher. Close the bag.			
11. Hang the water container 12" higher than the sitz basin.			
12. Help the patient to put on slippers and robe.			
13. Help the patient into the bathroom.			
14. Help the patient remove his robe and pajamas and sit down into the sitz basin. Be sure the patient can reach the signal cord.			
15. Place the tubing inside the basin with the opening of the tube under the water level. The tube fits into a little groove in the front of the basin.			
16. Open the stopcock and adjust the flow if necessary.			
17. Have the patient sit in the sitz bath with water running in for 10–20 minutes, as ordered or instructed by your supervisor.			
18. Cover the patient's shoulders with a bath blanket if he indicates he is cold.			

19. If the patient says he feels weak or faint, stop the treatment. Turn on the call light if you need assistance getting the patient out of the bathroom.			
20. When the treatment is finished, remove the tubing. Help the patient out of the sitz bath.			
21. Pat the patient's body gently with a towel to dry and assist the patient to redress.			
22. Help the patient back to bed.			
23. Make the patient comfortable and replace the call light.			
24. Lower the bed to a position of safety.			
25. Raise the side rails when ordered or indicated.			
26. Clean equipment and return it to its proper place. Discard disposable equipment.			
27. Bag and dispose of the dirty towels in the laundry hamper.			
28. Wash your hands.			
29. Report to your supervisor • The time the sitz bath was started • The length of time the patient was in the sitz bath • How the patient tolerated the procedure • Any abnormal or unusual observations			

Charting:

____

____

____

____

Date of Satisfactory Completion ____________

Instructor's Signature ____________

PROCEDURE 27-6: USING A PORTABLE CHAIR-TYPE OR BUILT-IN SITZ BATH

Name: ____________________ Date: ____________________

STEPS	S	U	COMMENTS
1. Assemble your equipment a. Portable chair with built-in sitz bath b. Bath towels c. Bath blanket d. Bath thermometer e. Plastic laundry bag f. Disposable gloves			
2. Wash your hands and apply gloves.			
3. Identify the patient by checking the ID bracelet.			
4. Inform the patient that you are going to give him a sitz bath.			
5. Provide privacy and comfort for the patient.			
6. Bring the sitz bath into the patient's room, or help the patient into the bathroom with the chair-type sitz bath.			
7. Fill it half full with water. Check the temperature to be sure it is about 90°F to 100°F.			
8. Place a towel on the seat and on the front edge of the sitz bath..			
9. Help the patient undress, except for gown and slippers.			
10. Help the patient sit down in the sitz bath. Hold his gown up so it does not get wet.			
11. Cover the patient's shoulders with a bath blanket if she complains of being cold.			
12. Continue the treatment for 10–20 minutes, or as directed by your supervisor.			
13. Check the patient every 5 minutes.			
14. If the patient feels weak or faint, stop the treatment. Turn on the call light for help getting the patient out of the tub. Let the water out of the tub.			
15. When the treatment is finished, help the patient out of the tub.			
16. Pat his body gently with a towel to dry and assist the patient to redress.			
17. Help the patient back into bed.			

18. Make the patient comfortable and replace the call light.			
19. Lower the bed to a position of safety.			
20. Raise the side rails when ordered or indicated.			
21. Clean the sitz tub with a disinfectant cleaner			
22. Put the portable, chair-type tub back into its proper place.			
23. Bag and dispose of dirty towels in the laundry hamper.			
24. Dispose of gloves. Wash your hands.			
25. Report to your supervisor • The time the sitz bath was started • The length of time the patient was in the sitz bath • How the patient tolerated the procedure • Any abnormal or unusual observations			

Charting:

____

____

____

____

Date of Satisfactory Completion ____________________

Instructor's Signature ____________________

PROCEDURE 27-7: APPLYING A COLD COMPRESS

Name: ______________________ Date: ______________________

STEPS	S	U	COMMENTS
1. Assemble equipment a. Disposable bed protector b. Basin c. Washcloth, towel, or gauze pads (compress) d. Bath towel e. Bath blanket f. Pitcher of cold water (ice cubes, if directed by your supervisor) g. Disposable gloves, if any potential exists for exposure to body fluids			
2. Wash your hands and apply gloves if indicated.			
3. Identify the patient by checking the ID bracelet.			
4. Inform the patient that you are going to apply a cold compress and where.			
5. Provide privacy for the patient.			
6. Raise the bed to a comfortable working position.			
7. Help the patient into a comfortable and safe position. Expose the area to be treated.			
8. Place a disposable bed protector under the body area to be given the cold compress.			
9. Put cold water in the basin (ice if ordered).			
10. Dip the compress into the water and wring it out completely.			
11. Apply the compress gently to the proper area of the patient's body as quickly as possible to prevent temperature changes in the compress from prolonged exposure to the environment or your hands.			
12. If the patient is cold or chilly, cover him with a blanket. Do not cover the compress or the area being treated.			
13. Change the compress and remoisten it, as necessary, to keep it cold. Sometimes a patient is able to apply the compress himself. If your supervisor gives permission for this, position and assist the patient as necessary.			
14. Check the skin under the application every 5 minutes. If the skin appears to be blue, blanched, or white, remove the compress. Cover the area with a towel or blanket and report to your supervisor.			

15. A cold compress is usually applied for 15–20 minutes. Follow instructions of your supervisor.			
16. When the treatment is finished, remove the compress and gently pat the area dry with a towel.			
17. Make the patient comfortable and replace the call light.			
18. Lower the bed to a position of safety.			
19. Raise the side rails if ordered or indicated.			
20. Clean equipment and return to its proper place. Discard disposable equipment.			
21. Wash your hands.			
22. Report to your supervisor • The time the cold compress was started • How long it remained in place • The area of application • How the patient tolerated the procedure • Any abnormal or unusual observations			

Charting:

____

____

____

____

Date of Satisfactory Completion ____________________

Instructor's Signature ____________________

PROCEDURE 27-8: APPLYING A COLD SOAK

Name: ____________________ Date: ____________________

STEPS	S	U	COMMENTS
1. Assemble equipment a. Basin, foot tub, or arm basin b. Disposable bed protector c. Washcloth, towel, or gauze pads (compress) d. Bath towel e. Bath blanket f. Disposable gloves, if any potential exists for exposure to body fluids			
2. Wash your hands and apply gloves if indicated.			
3. Identify the patient by checking the ID bracelet.			
4. Inform the patient that you are going to apply a cold soak and where.			
5. Provide privacy and comfort for the patient.			
6. Raise the bed to a comfortable working position.			
7. Help the patient into a safe and comfortable position. Expose the area to be treated.			
8. Place a disposable bed protector under the body area to receive the cold soak.			
9. Fill the basin half full with cold water.			
10. Place the basin in a position so that the patient's arm, leg, foot, or hand can be dipped into the basin easily.			
11. Gradually place the patient's arm or leg into the water.			
12. When you have to change the water, take the patient's arm, leg, foot, or hand out of the basin. Wrap it with a bath towel or bath blanket for comfort.			
13. If the patient says she feels weak or cold, stop the treatment. Cover the patient with extra blankets and report to your supervisor.			
14. Check the skin every 5 minutes. If skin appears blue, blanched, or white, stop the treatment and report to your supervisor.			
15. When the treatment is finished, dry the patient's arm or leg by gently patting with a towel.			
16. Make the patient comfortable and replace the call light.			

17. Lower the bed to a position of safety.			
18. Raise the side rails if ordered or indicated.			
19. Clean equipment and return to its proper place. Discard disposable equipment and gloves, if used.			
20. Wash your hands.			
21. Report to your supervisor • The time the cold soak was started • The length of treatment • The area of application • How the patient tolerated the procedure • Any abnormal or unusual observations			

Charting:

____

____

____

____

Date of Satisfactory Completion ______________________

Instructor's Signature ______________________

PROCEDURE 27-9: APPLYING AN ICE BAG OR DRY COLD APPLICATION

Name: ____________________ Date: ____________________

STEPS	S	U	COMMENTS
1. Assemble equipment a. Ice pack b. Flannel cover, or whatever cover is used in your institution c. Ice in a clean container d. Bath blanket e. Disposable gloves, if any potential exists for exposure to body fluids			
2. Wash hands and apply gloves if indicated.			
3. Identify the patient by checking the ID bracelet.			
4. Inform the patient you are going to apply an ice pack and where.			
5. Provide privacy and comfort for the patient.			
6. Raise the bed to a comfortable working position.			
7. Help the patient into a safe and comfortable position. Expose the area to be treated.			
8. Pour cold water over the ice to melt the sharp edges.			
9. Fill the ice pack one-half full of ice.			
10. Squeeze the sides of the ice pack to force air out of it.			
11. Fasten the top tightly.			
12. Dry the outside of the ice pack with a paper towel.			
13. Invert the ice pack to test for leaking.			
14. Place the ice pack into the type of cover used in your institution.			
15. Apply the ice pack to the proper area of the patient's body.			
16. If the patient is cold or chilly, cover him with a blanket. Do not cover the ice pack or area being treated.			
17. Follow the instructions of your supervisor as to the length of application. Replace ice as necessary.			
18. Check the skin under the application every 10 minutes. If the skin appears to be blue, blanched, or white, remove the ice bag. Cover the area with a towel and report to your supervisor.			

19. Clean equipment and put it in its proper place. Discard disposable equipment and gloves, if used.			
20. Make the patient comfortable and replace the call light.			
21. Lower the bed to a position of safety for the patient.			
22. Raise the side rails when ordered or indicated.			
23. Wash your hands.			
24. Report to your supervisor • The time the ice pack was applied • The length of treatment • The area of application • How the patient tolerated the procedure • Any abnormal or unusual observations			

Charting:

____

____

____

____

Date of Satisfactory Completion ______________

Instructor's Signature ______________

PROCEDURE 27-10: APPLYING A COMMERCIAL UNIT COLD PACK

Name: ______________________ Date: ______________________

STEPS	S	U	COMMENTS
1. Assemble equipment a. Commercial unit, single-use cold pack b. Cold pack cover used in your institution c. Bath blanket d. Disposable gloves, if any potential exists for exposure to body fluids			
2. Wash hands and apply gloves if indicated.			
3. Identify the patient by checking the ID bracelet.			
4. Inform the patient that you are going to apply a cold pack and where.			
5. Provide privacy and comfort for the patient.			
6. Raise the bed to a comfortable working position.			
7. Help the patient into a safe and comfortable position. Expose the area to be treated.			
8. Place the flannel cover (or your institution's cover) on the cold pack.			
9. Hit or squeeze the cold pack to activate it according to the manufacturer's directions.			
10. Apply the pack to the proper area of the patient's body.			
11. Check the skin under the application every 10 minutes. If the skin appears blue, blanched, or white, remove the pack and cover the area with a blanket. Report to your supervisor.			
12. Follow instructions of your supervisor as to the length of application. Replace with a new cold pack as necessary.			
13. Discard disposable equipment and gloves, if used.			
14. Make the patient comfortable and replace the call light.			
15. Lower the bed to a position of safety for the patient.			
16. Raise the side rails when ordered or indicated.			
17. Wash your hands.			

18. Report to your supervisor • The time the cold pack was applied • The length of treatment • Area of application • How the patient tolerated the procedure • Any abnormal or unusual observations			

Charting:

____

____

____

____

Date of Satisfactory Completion ____________________

Instructor's Signature ____________________

28

Care of the Surgical Patient

Key Terms Review

Match the key terms in the right column with the definitions in the left column by placing the letter of each correct answer in the space provided.

_____ **1.** Causes the loss of sensation in the entire body.

_____ **2.** Causes the loss of sensation in an area of the body.

_____ **3.** Causes a loss of feeling in a large area of the body, usually from the umbilicus ("belly button") down, including the legs and feet.

_____ **4.** Loss of feeling or sensation in a part or all of the body.

_____ **5.** A drug used to produce loss of feeling.

_____ **6.** The registered nurse who assists the anesthesiologist.

_____ **7.** The medical doctor who administers the anesthetic to the patient in the operating room.

_____ **8.** Performed to save life or limb.

_____ **9.** Chosen and not vital for health.

_____ **10.** To urinate; pass water.

_____ **11.** Material (vomitus, food, or liquids) inhaled into the lungs.

_____ **12.** An unexpected condition, such as the development of another illness in a patient who is already sick.

_____ **13.** Cannot eat or drink anything at all; usually 8 hours before surgery or a procedure requiring general anesthesia.

Terms

A. Anesthesia
B. Anesthetic
C. Anesthesiologist
D. Anesthetist
E. Preoperative
F. Postoperative
G. Skin prep
H. Unconscious
I. NPO (nothing by mouth)
J. Local anesthetics
K. General anesthetic
L. Spinal anesthetic
M. Elective surgery
N. Emergency surgery
O. Complication
P. Aspirate
Q. Void

_____ **14.** Unaware of the environment; occurs during sleep and in temporary episodes ranging from fainting or stupor to coma.

_____ **15.** After surgery.

_____ **16.** Before surgery.

_____ **17.** Clipping or shaving the area of the body where an operation is to be performed in preparation for surgery.

MULTIPLE-CHOICE QUESTIONS

Circle the letter next to the word or statement that best completes the sentence or answers the question.

1. The nursing assistant is helping a patient with deep-breathing exercises. She explains what she wants the patient to do. She pulls the curtain around the bed and offers the bedpan. What should she do next?
   a. Place the pillow on the patient's abdomen for support.
   b. Dangle the patient's legs over the side of the bed, if allowed.
   c. Encourage the patient to breathe 10 times in slowly and deeply.
   d. Collect a specimen if needed.

2. If the patient is not permitted to dangle his legs, what should the nursing assistant do?
   a. Place the patient in as much of a sitting position as possible.
   b. Do the exercises with the patient lying down.
   c. Prop the patient up with the pillows.
   d. Turn the patient's head to the side and encourage him to breathe deeply.

3. The nursing assistant placed a pillow on the patient's abdomen and asked him to breathe deeply 10 times. What should the nursing assistant do while the patient breathes?
   a. Take care of another patient.
   b. Count his pulse.
   c. Count the respirations out loud to the patient.
   d. Take his blood pressure.

4. Preoperative patient education includes which of the following?
   a. Deep-breathing and coughing exercises
   b. Head and neck exercises
   c. Staying as still as possible so bleeding does not occur
   d. Self-surgical procedures

5. Part of the nursing assistant's job is to make the patient who is going to have surgery feel
   a. lively and happy.
   b. sad and dejected.
   c. as calm and relaxed as possible.
   d. nervous and upset.

6. The preoperative patient may be worried about
   a. financial concerns.
   b. family concerns.
   c. the possibility of death or serious complications.
   d. all of the above.

7. One way to help reduce the patient's fears is to
   a. give him extra time and attention.
   b. ignore his childish behavior.
   c. report his fears to your team members while at lunch.
   d. tell him not to worry.

8. Preventing chest complications following surgery includes
   a. watching the patient for symptoms of respiratory infection before surgery.
   b. washing the chest with soap.
   c. shaving the chest regularly.
   d. wearing gloves at all times when doing the prep.

9. *NPO* means
a. non promote.
b. night procedures only.
c. nothing by mouth.
d. non-permanent only.

10. Hair on the body is a breeding place for
a. microorganisms.
b. blood clots.
c. knots.
d. tangles.

11. It is important to measure the patient's ___________ immediately after she returns to her unit after surgery.
a. feet
b. IQ
c. height and weight
d. vital signs

12. If the patient is unconscious and vomits,
a. rinse out his mouth
b. raise the side rails immediately
c. turn his head to one side and clear his mouth
d. place the patient in Trendelenburg position.

13. ______ surgery is performed to aid in confirming a suspected diagnosis.
a. Emergency
b. Urgent
c. Scheduled
d. Exploratory

14. Scheduled surgery may be
a. performed to correct a non-life-threatening situation.
b. done when the patient requests it.
c. an out-of-pocket expense for the patient and not covered by insurance.
d. all of the above.

15. A *colostomy* means that
a. a surgical opening was created in the colon to allow feces to drain into a bag.
b. the colon was removed after a surgical cut was made.
c. part of the colon was removed and reconstructed.
d. the entire small and large intestine was removed because of damage.

16. Zeus and DaVinci are two examples of
a. Greek gods.
b. well-known doctors who perform surgery frequently.
c. laser surgery techniques.
d. types of surgical robotic instruments.

17. Which statement would alert you that the patient is afraid of surgery?
a. "Can my mother bring me ice cream after I have my tonsils removed?"
b. "I miss my dog so much. Can she come for a visit while I am recovering?"
c. "After my breasts are removed, I am sure my husband will not want to be intimate with me anymore."
d. "I have faith that my surgeon will remove all of the skin cancer."

18. It is the responsibility of the ________ to complete the patient's preoperative checklist on the unit.
a. nurse
b. nursing assistant
c. anesthesiologist
d. surgeon

19. Before surgery can occur, consent that the patient understands the risks of the surgery
a. must be signed by the patient.
b. can be witnessed by a nursing assistant.
c. might be obtained by the nurse.
d. does not have to be obtained at all.

20. The chance that blood clots occur in the legs after surgery
a. can lessen by providing preoperative education about performing leg and foot exercises.
b. can increase when the patient performs deep-breathing exercises preoperatively.
c. stays the same when NPO is initiated.
d. decreases by encouraging the patient to rest and stay in bed.

21. When performing a skin prep the night before surgery, a nursing assistant should report
   a. scratches on the patient's skin.
   b. soap left on the skin.
   c. she changed the linens because they got soaked.
   d. she used a surgical razor.

22. When performing a surgical skin prep for _____ surgery, sometimes a _______ is prescribed.
   a. scrotal; douche
   b. vaginal; douche
   c. arm; massage
   d. back; massage

23. When clipping hair during a surgical skin prep, the nursing assistant should
   a. wipe the cut hair onto the floor so it does not cling to the bed linens and patient's skin.
   b. wash off the solution used thoroughly to avoid infection.
   c. clip hair in the direction it grows.
   d. place the used clipper head into the garbage once the prep is finished.

24. When a patient comes back to his room after surgery, the nursing assistant should
   a. keep the side rails down.
   b. place the height of the bed in the lowest position.
   c. remove the IV pole so it does not get in the way.
   d. offer the patient something to eat.

25. If a patient returns from the OR with a urinary drainage bag, the nursing assistant should
   a. clamp it to prevent urine from leaking.
   b. tie it to the side rails to promote drainage.
   c. hang it to the bed frame.
   d. get a specimen immediately.

TRUE OR FALSE QUESTIONS

Determine whether each question is true or false. In the space provided, write "T" for true and "F" for false. If the statement is false, rewrite it on the line provided to make it a true statement.

_____ **1.** A sign should be posted at the nurse's station if the patient is NPO.

____

_____ **2.** If a patient appears to be unconscious, he cannot hear what you are saying.

____

_____ **3.** It is very important that the patient void adequately within a certain period of time after surgery.

____

_____ **4.** Spinal anesthesia means the patient can be numb from the umbilicus (belly button) down toward the toes.

____

_____ **5.** Should a patient be afraid to breathe deeply after surgery, the nursing assistant should encourage him to rest.

____

_____ **6.** Some supplies a nursing assistant should bring to the bedside when teaching a patient how to deep breathe are a pillow, a specimen container, and tissues.

____

_____ **7.** A nursing assistant does not need to wear gloves when helping a patient perform breathing exercises.

____

_____ **8.** A patient can aspirate on his own vomit or saliva.

____

_____ 9. A nursing assistant should report to the nurse the color, secretions, and consistency of the secretions expelled by the patient during deep-breathing exercises.

____

_____ 10. Certified nurse anesthetists can administer anesthesia.

____

FILL-IN-THE-BLANK QUESTIONS

Provide the meaning of the following abbreviations.

1. NPO ______________________________
2. OR ______________________________
3. -plasty ______________________________
4. -otomy ______________________________
5. -ostomy ______________________________
6. RN ______________________________
7. IV ______________________________
8. ID ______________________________
9. I&O ______________________________
10. MD ______________________________
11. PCA ______________________________

EXERCISE 28-1

Objective: To apply what you have learned about care of the surgical patient.

Directions: Read the following riddles carefully before writing the correct answer on the blank line.

1. I carry the patient to surgery. What am I? (*Hint:* After sitting for a long period of time, you may become this.)

   ____

2. These must be measured before any surgery. What are they? (*Hint:* This also describes a stop sign at a busy intersection.)

   ____

3. This function must return to an adequate level after surgery. What is it? (*Hint:* Another name for an empty space.)

   ____

EXERCISE 28-2

Objective: To apply what you have learned about preoperative documentation.

Directions: Read the following situation description and then document the findings on the sample preoperative checklist that follows.

It is 7 AM, and you have just arrived at work. The nurse gives you the preoperative checklist for Tom Green. She tells you that he is scheduled to have surgery in 2 hours, explains the care you are to give him, and that she would like you to fill out the portion of the checklist labeled "Morning of Surgery."

After greeting Mr. Green and introducing yourself, you measure his vital signs, height, and weight. His temperature is 100.2°F, pulse is 68 beats per minute, respirations are 16 times per minute, blood pressure is 120/80, he weighs 186 pounds, and his height is 5 feet 11 inches.

He is able to bathe himself and brush his own teeth. You obtain a urine sample and send it to the lab. After his bath, he dresses in a clean hospital gown. There is no urinary drainage bag. You ask him if he is allergic or sensitive to any drugs and he answers, "None." He has no false teeth, prosthesis, nail polish, sanitary belts, makeup, hairpieces, or hairpins. He removes his wedding ring and his contact lenses, which he gives to his wife to take home.

The nurse comes in at 8 AM to give him his preoperative medications; the side rails are up. At 8:30 AM, the transportation attendant arrives and takes the patient to the operating room by stretcher.

Sample Preoperative Checklist Completed by Nursing Assistant

EVENING BEFORE SURGERY

Patient's Name: ______________________________

Identify the patient by checking his identification bracelet:	Yes ______	No ______	
Skin prep done by ______________ at ______ P.M.			
Skin prep checked by ____________ at ______ P.M.			
Food restrictions, if any, explained to the patient:	Yes ______	No ______	
"NPO AFTER MIDNIGHT" sign put on patient's bed and explained to the patient:	Yes ______	No ______	
Enema administered by __________ at ______ P.M.			

MORNING OF SURGERY:

Bath?	Yes ______	No ______	N/A ______
Oral hygiene?	Yes ______	No ______	N/A ______
False teeth (dentures) and removable bridges removed?	Yes ______	No ______	N/A ______
Jewelry and pierced earrings removed? __________	Yes ______	No ______	N/A ______
Hairpiece, wig, hairpins removed?	Yes ______	No ______	N/A ______
Lipstick, makeup, and false eyelashes removed?	Yes ______	No ______	N/A ______
Sanitary belt removed?	Yes ______	No ______	N/A ______
Nail polish removed?	Yes ______	No ______	N/A ______
Eyeglasses and contact lenses removed?	Yes ______	No ______	N/A ______
Prostheses (artificial hearing aid, eye, leg, arm, and so forth) removed?	Yes ______	No ______	N/A ______
All clothing removed except clean hospital gown?	Yes ______	No ______	N/A ______
Patient allergic or sensitive to drugs?	Yes ______	No ______	N/A ______
Preop urine specimen obtained and sent to lab?	Yes ______	No ______	N/A ______
Urinary drainage bag emptied?	Yes ______	No ______	N/A ______
Side rails in up position?	Yes ______	No ______	N/A ______

Temperature ______ Pulse ______ Respiration ______

Blood pressure ______ Weight ______ lbs. Height ______ ft. ______ in.

Time patient leaves for the operating room: ________

Observations: ______________________________

Signature: ______________________________

EXERCISE 28-3

Objective: To recognize appropriate tasks in preparing the postoperative patient's unit.

Directions: Circle the letters of all the tasks the nursing assistant should do to prepare the patient's unit to receive the patient after surgery.

A. Bring the IV pole to the bedside.
B. Attach a urine drainage bag to the bed frame.
C. Strip the linen from the bed.
D. Make the operating room or surgical bed.
E. Mop the floor.
F. Place tissues and emesis basin only on the bedside table.
G. Remove the drinking water.
H. Place a clean gown at the foot of the bed.

EXERCISE 28-4

Objective: To recognize appropriate actions to take for the preoperative patient.

Directions: Decide which of the following actions is the most appropriate for the situation descriptions. Put the letter for that action in the space next to the situation. More than one letter may be appropriate for each situation.

Actions

A. Listen and show interest in what the patient says.
B. Report this to your immediate supervisor.
C. Check or record this information on the preoperative checklist.

Situations

_____ **1.** You notice the patient is sneezing, sniffling, or coughing.
_____ **2.** After you post the NPO sign and explain it to the patient.
_____ **3.** After administering an enema the evening before surgery and noting the results.
_____ **4.** The patient wants to talk a lot.
_____ **5.** The patient expresses concern for his family.
_____ **6.** The patient's temperature rises the evening before surgery.
_____ **7.** The patient begins to talk about the possibility of death or serious complications.

_____ 8. You prepared the patient's skin as instructed at 7:30 PM.

_____ 9. On the morning of surgery, you helped the patient remove false teeth, jewelry, hairpins, and nail polish.

_____ 10. The patient complains of chest pains.

_____ 11. After weighing and measuring the patient

_____ 12. After obtaining a urine specimen

EXERCISE 28-5

Objective: To recognize appropriate actions to take for the postoperative patient.

Directions: Decide which of the following actions is the most appropriate for the situation descriptions. Put the letter for that action in the space next to the situation.

Actions

A. Signal for the nurse immediately.

B. Turn the patient.

C. Change the patient's gown and bed linens.

Situations

_____ 1. You notice that a patient is bleeding and the blood is bright red. What should you do?

_____ 2. A patient has been in the same position for 2 hours. What should you do?

_____ 3. The gown and linens of a postoperative patient have become wet. What should you do?

_____ 4. You just noticed a rise in the blood pressure of a postoperative patient. What should you do?

_____ 5. The patient's lips and fingernails are turning very pale or blue. What should you do?

_____ 6. You have just measured the patient's vital signs, and her pulse is less than 60. What should you do?

_____ 7. A postoperative patient has gotten himself into an uncomfortable position.

THE NURSING ASSISTANT IN ACTION

1. While giving Mr. Jones a backrub as part of his PM care the night before his open-heart surgery, you notice he is unusually nervous and his back muscles are really tight. He tells you in whispered tones, "I am so nervous about tomorrow's surgery. I did not plan for this and have not done anything to prepare should I die. Last night, I had such an awful dream that I would not wake up from surgery." What should you do?

____

____

____

____

2. A very quiet and stoic patient tells you he is not in pain when you ask. However, you notice he is sweating and when he moves he holds his hand over his bandage and grits his teeth. What should you do?

____

____

____

____

3. A child has a temper tantrum when the doctor comes into the room to talk to the parents to explain that it will be just a few minutes until a surgical theater will be available and the surgical team can get ready to perform the emergency appendectomy on the child. What should you do?

____

____

____

____

4. You are assigned to perform a surgical prep on a 15-year-old boy who presented in the Emergency Room with testicular torsion after falling off his all-terrain vehicle (ATV). He will have his testicle removed. What should you do to help prepare him for surgery?

____

____

____

____

5. A patient recently had a hysterectomy. While assisting her to walk in the hallway, she tells you, "I feel very weird and my head is spinning." You notice her skin color is pale and she is sweating. There is a huge clot of blood on the floor and blood is all over her indwelling catheter tubing and legs. What should you do?

____

____

____

____

LEARNING ACTIVITIES

1. Many patients are admitted for surgery and discharged home quickly after the procedure occurs. Brainstorm with a friend to create a checklist or "cheat sheet" the patient might be given to help him remember all the things that are important to do when he is recovering. If computer software is available, create a pamphlet containing key information about this information that the patient can refer to that will support his recovery once he is discharged.
2. Using the methods mentioned in the textbook, practice deep-breathing exercises. Note what was difficult and whether the technique was easy for you to perform. Use this experience when teaching a patient to perform deep-breathing exercises.

PROCEDURE CHECKLISTS

PROCEDURE 28-1: CLIPPING A PATIENT IN PREPARATION FOR SURGERY

Name: ____________________ Date: ____________________

STEPS	S	U	COMMENTS
1. Assemble equipment a. Disposable prep kit (if used) b. Electric clipper c. Disposable clipper heads (may need more than one) d. Washcloths and towels e. Basin of warm water f. Bath blanket g. Disposable gloves h. Clean linens			
2. Wash your hands and put on gloves.			
3. Identify the patient by checking the ID bracelet.			
4. Inform the patient that you are going to clip the hair on his skin in preparation for surgery.			
5. Provide privacy and comfort for the patient.			
6. Raise the bed to a comfortable working position.			
7. Place the bath blanket over the bedspread and top sheet. Ask the patient to hold the blanket in place. Fan-fold the top sheets to the foot of the bed. Do this from underneath the blanket without exposing the patient.			
8. Adjust the bedside light so that the area is well lit.			
9. Attach the clipper head to the clipper.			
10. Clip hair in the area of the prep. Clip in the direction in which the hair grows. If hair begins to pull or clipping becomes difficult, change the clipper head.			
11. When the area is completely clipped, use a towel or washcloth to brush the hair onto the bed.			
12. Prepare the prep kit solution or antimicrobial soap solution. Place several washcloths or sponges in the solution.			
13. Scrub the area as ordered or as directed by your supervisor. Rub gently, thoroughly soaking the area. Be careful not to rub so hard that it causes skin irritation.			

14. Most antimicrobial surgical soaps should not be rinsed. Follow the directions of your supervisor.			
15. Allow scrub to air dry.			
16. Change linens under the patient and place soiled linens in the laundry hamper.			
17. Clean your equipment and return it to its proper place. Discard disposable equipment. Discard clipper heads per your facility policy; do not place in garbage.			
18. Make the patient comfortable and replace the call light.			
19. Lower the bed to a position of safety.			
20. Raise the side rails when ordered or indicated.			
21. Dispose of gloves and wash your hands.			
22. Report to your supervisor • The time you performed the clip and prep • How the patient tolerated the procedure • Any abnormal or unusual observations			

Charting:

____

____

____

____

Date of Satisfactory Completion ____________________

Instructor's Signature ____________________

PROCEDURE 28-2: ASSISTING A PATIENT WITH COUGHING AND DEEP-BREATHING EXERCISES

Name: ______________________ Date: ______________________

STEPS	S	U	COMMENTS
1. Assemble equipment a. Pillow or folded bath blanket b. Specimen container, if a sputum specimen is ordered c. Tissues d. Disposable gloves			
2. Report to the patient's nurse that you are ready to start deep-breathing exercises.			
3. Wash your hands and put on gloves.			
4. Identify the patient by checking the ID bracelet.			
5. Inform the patient that you are going to help her with deep-breathing exercises.			
6. Provide privacy and comfort for the patient.			
7. Raise the bed to a comfortable working position.			
8. Offer the patient a bedpan or urinal.			
9. Dangle the patient's legs over the side of the bed, if allowed. If not, place the patient in as much of a sitting position as possible.			
10. If your patient had abdominal surgery, place the pillow or folded bath blanket on the patient's abdomen for support. Ask the patient to hold the pillow across the abdomen to splint the incision.			
11. Ask her to breathe deeply 10 times. (Explain: "Breathe slowly and evenly through your nose until your chest is fully expanded. Hold your breath 2–3 seconds and then exhale through your mouth. Continue exhaling until your chest is deflated. Repeat.") Use an incentive spirometer, if ordered.			
12. Count the respirations out loud to the patient as she inhales and exhales. If the patient cannot breathe deeply, ask her to cough. Coughing is just another way of breathing deeply.			
13. Ask the patient to feel her abdomen as she breathes to encourage deeper breathing.			
14. Tell the patient to cough up all loose secretions into the tissues, if a specimen is not necessary, or into a specimen container, if you have been instructed to collect a specimen.			

15. Assist the patient into a position of comfort and safety in bed.			
16. If a specimen has been collected, label it and send it to the laboratory with the appropriate request slip.			
17. Discard disposable equipment.			
18. Dispose of gloves and wash your hands.			
19. Replace the pillow under the patient's head.			
20. Lower the bed to a position of safety and replace the call light.			
21. Raise the side rails if ordered or indicated.			
22. Report to your supervisor • That you helped the patient with coughing and deep-breathing exercises • The number of breathing exercises • The color, amount, and consistency of the secretions the patient was able to cough up • If a specimen was collected and sent to the laboratory • How the patient tolerated the procedure • Any abnormal or unusual observations			

Charting:

____

____

____

____

Date of Satisfactory Completion ______________

Instructor's Signature ______________

29

Special Procedures

Key Terms Review

Match the key terms in the right column with the definitions in the left column by placing the letter of each correct answer in the space provided.

_____ **1.** Inflammation of a vein.

_____ **2.** Inflammation and blood clots in a vein.

_____ **3.** Designed to promote blood to flow and to prevent the formation of blood clots in the bloodstream.

_____ **4.** The administration of fluids, nutrients, or medication into a vein.

_____ **5.** Occurs when an IV solution runs into nearby tissue instead of into a vein.

_____ **6.** A type of bandage applied to a large body area (abdomen or chest) to secure a dressing in place or to put pressure on or support a body part.

_____ **7.** Stretchable bandage used to create localized pressure and support; also called ACE™ bandage.

Terms

A. Thrombophlebitis

B. Phlebitis

C. Antiembolism stockings

D. Intravenous (IV) therapy

E. Infiltration

F. Elastic bandage

G. Binder

MULTIPLE-CHOICE QUESTIONS

Circle the letter next to the word or statement that best completes the sentence or answers the question.

1. Binders are used with patients to help
   a. relieve diarrhea.
   b. constrict body parts.
   c. secure blood clots to prevent movement.
   d. secure a dressing in place.

2. An IV located in a patient's arm
   a. drains urine out of the patient's bladder and into a collection bag.
   b. should always deliver fluid to the patient fast.
   c. is used on occasion to deliver blood to the patient.
   d. removes excess fluids from the body.

3. Medications, ________, and ________ can be administered through an IV.
   a. blood; urine
   b. glucose solutions; nourishments
   c. solid food; liquids
   d. bleach; water

4. The IV catheter
   a. helps change chemical make-up in the blood.
   b. keeps a metal needle inside the arm while an IV is infusing.
   c. is a hollow plastic tube that remains in the vein.
   d. drains urine away from the body.

5. The _______ on the IV tubing allows a certain number of drips per minute to enter the vein.
   a. clamp
   b. catheter
   c. solution bag
   d. drip chamber

6. Mrs. Jones needs to ambulate from her bed to the bathroom. She calls for assistance because she has an IV in her left arm. The nursing assistant
   a. keeps the IV below the level of the patient's waist while the transfer occurs.
   b. wraps her hand tightly around the drip chamber so it does not get damaged during the transfer.
   c. moves any furniture out of the pathway so the IV pole can move freely.
   d. folds the tubing to prevent blood from backing up while the transfer occurs.

7. Miss Ford complains that her IV is burning and she can feel the burn moving up her arm. The nursing assistant should
   a. call the doctor immediately.
   b. discontinue the IV right away.
   c. open the drip chamber all the way.
   d. check the skin around the site and report the complaint and observations to the nurse.

8. When infiltration occurs, the
   a. skin around the IV site may appear swollen.
   b. IV pump should never again be used.
   c. patient will complain of a tingling sensation in his lips.
   d. tubing should be disconnected immediately from the pump by the nurse assistant.

9. When assisting a patient who has an IV in her arm to remove her gown, the nursing assistant
   a. places the old gown on the floor while the new gown is offered.
   b. only changes the old gown when it becomes wet.
   c. removes the old gown from the patient's arm that has the IV in it first and then removes it from the arm that is free of the IV.
   d. removes the old gown from the arm that is free from the IV first and then removes it from the arm that has the IV in it.

10. Binders are made primarily of
    a. latex
    b. cotton.
    c. gauze
    d. plastic.

11. A binder may be applied to a woman's _____ who just delivered a baby via Cesarean section.
a. abdomen
b. scrotum
c. arms
d. legs

12. Usually when a binder is placed properly, the patient
a. experiences more pain.
b. is more comfortable.
c. will have decubitus ulcers.
d. may ask for an increase in pain medication.

13. A single T binder may be ordered after a patient has a(n)______.
a. hemorrhoidectomy
b. abdominal surgery
c. Cesarean section
d. all of the above.

14. Breast binders can
a. decrease the amount of bruising.
b. increase swelling.
c. increase the chance of hematomas occurring.
d. all of the above.

15. Antiembolism stockings are used
a. on the abdomen to prevent hematomas from occurring.
b. to prevent thrombophlebitis.
c. because they help arterial blood return to the heart.
d. on the upper extremities.

16. In order to ensure that the antiembolism stocking fits securely, the _____ ______ the leg.
a. doctor assesses
b. nursing assistant massages
c. nursing assistant measures
d. nurse measures

17. Antiembolism stockings should always be
a. placed on a patient while he is sitting in a chair.
b. pulled up to his groin area.
c. left on wrinkled and clean.
d. applied while the patient is lying in bed.

18. Antiembolism stockings must be removed and reapplied every ___ hours or as ordered by a doctor.
a. 2
b. 8
c. 12
d. 24

19. ACE™ bandages are used
a. to hold a dressing in place.
b. increase blood return to the heart.
c. decrease edema.
d. all of the above.

20. If a bandage is wrapped too tightly, the patient may complain that
a. his fingers feel numb.
b. he cannot move his fingers.
c. the bandage is causing him pain.
d. all of the above.

21. A patient has a sprained ankle. Which type of binder is the best choice to offer comfort and support to the injured area?
a. Antiembolism stockings
b. Warm compression
c. Cold soak
d. ACE™ bandage

22. Inflammation of a vein is called
a. phlebitis
b. thrombophlebitis
c. pulmonary emboli
d. cerebral emboli

23. Which is the correct position when applying a bandage?
a. Keep the joint bent.
b. Start at the top of the extremity and work toward the fingers.
c. Start at the toes and work up the leg.
d. Cover the finger or toes.

24. Blood in a vein flows
a. back to the heart
b. away from the heart
c. towards the kidneys
d. to the outside of the body.

25. Which is a sign or symptom that something is not right with the IV?

a. The patient complains he is very comfortable and wants to rest.

b. The site looks swollen and is cool to touch.

c. The site has a little bit of dried blood where the catheter was inserted.

d. The patient is moving his arm and is able to cut all his food with ease.

TRUE OR FALSE QUESTIONS

Determine whether each question is true or false. In the space provided, write "T" for true and "F" for false. If the statement is false, rewrite it on the line provided to make it a true statement.

_____ **1.** Inflammation of a vein is called *infiltration.*

____

_____ **2.** Bandages and stockings that provide support may be elastic.

____

_____ **3.** The IV container should always be held below the IV site.

____

_____ **4.** The amount of IV fluid that can flow into the patient's body is controlled and monitored by the nursing assistant.

____

_____ **5.** Secure the ACE™ bandage with glue.

____

_____ **6.** You should apply a single T binder to a sprain or strained joint.

____

_____ **7.** It is part of the nursing assistant's job to wash the antiembolism stockings out should they become soiled.

____

_____ **8.** Antiembolism stockings come in a variety of lengths and widths.

____

_____ **9.** Swelling and bleeding around an IV site should be reported immediately by the nursing assistant to the nurse.

____

_____ **10.** The doctor orders the type of IV solution that must be infused into the patient.

____

FILL-IN-THE-BLANK QUESTIONS

Provide the meaning of the following abbreviations.

1. IV _______________

2. ACE™ _______________

3. ID _______________

EXERCISE 29-1

Objective: To apply what you have learned about special procedures that nursing assistants may perform while caring for patients.

Directions: Look carefully at the items shown in Figure 29-1. Label each one with the number of the correct word(s) from the following word list.

Word List

1. T binder (female)
2. Elastic bandage
3. Breast binder
4. T binder (male)
5. Straight abdominal binder
6. Antiembolism elastic stocking
7. IV infusion
8. IV solution
9. IV drip chamber
10. IV tubing
11. IV insertion site
12. IV clamp
13. IV pump or controller
14. Skin near IV site
15. IV pole

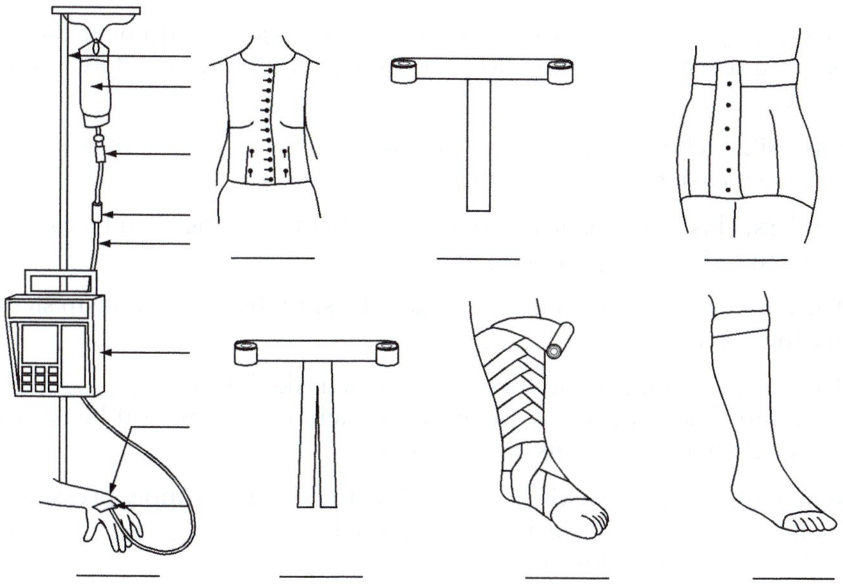

FIGURE 29-1

EXERCISE 29-2

Objective: To be able to recognize important safety measures related to performing special procedures.

Directions: Select the correct word(s) from the following word list to complete the following sentences.

Word List

overlap	kinked
circulation	one-half
Velcro®	hour
size	flow rate
infiltration	interrupting

1. You must provide care for the patient or change his position without __________ the flow of the IV solution.
2. Make sure the IV tubing is not ______________ and that the patient is not lying on the tubing.
3. Nursing assistants do not independently adjust the ________________ using the IV clamp or electronic controller.
4. A(n) ____________ of the IV solution can cause the skin near the site to become painful or swollen. Report this condition immediately to the nurse.
5. If possible, choose a patient gown with ____________ to make changing the gown easier for the patient.
6. Binders, elastic bandages, and antiembolism stockings can be too tight and can reduce the patient's ____________.
7. The patient's legs must be measured to be sure the antiembolism stockings are the correct ____________.
8. The patient's fingers and toes should be checked each ____________ for pain, numbness, cyanosis, paleness, or lack of movement if he is wearing an elastic bandage on his arms or legs.
9. When applying an elastic bandage, it is important to apply pressure evenly and with each turn to overlap the bandage ____________ the width of the one before it.
10. If more than one bandage is used, ____________ them to prevent slipping or uneven pressure on the body part.

EXERCISE 29-3

Select from the following list of procedures the letter of the procedure that best answers each question. Write the correct letter(s) on the blank line next to the question.

A. Changing a gown

B. Checking an IV site

C. Placing a binder

D. Applying a bandage

E. Applying antiembolism stockings

_____ 1. Which procedure(s) could a patient do for himself if taught first?

_____ 2. In which procedure(s) should the nursing assistant observe for pain and swelling?

_____ 3. Which procedure(s) involves making sure the patient is comfortable?

_____ 4. Which procedure(s) is nursing assistant allowed to perform?

THE NURSING ASSISTANT IN ACTION

1. Mrs. Smith had a bilateral radical mastectomy (removal of both breasts) 8 hours ago and arrived to your floor wearing a breast binder. You check Mrs. Smith's breast binder and find that the binder and bed linens are soaked with fresh, bright-red blood. What should you do?

____

____

____

____

2. Mrs. Hyde is walking in the hallway when you notice her antiembolism stockings have fallen to her ankles. You ask Mrs. Hyde to return to her room with you so you can adjust them correctly. She adamantly refuses to go with you and says, "These things make my legs sore. They are so tight. They are more comfortable just where they are and at least keep my feet warm." What should you do?

____

____

____

____

3. Mr. Calhoun recently had surgery and a scrotal binder was applied. You check the binder only to find he repositioned it so it is not supporting his bandage. You explain you would like to help him readjust/reapply the bandage the correct way. He grunts and tells you, "Oh yeah, you pretty little thing. You can help me; but, readjusting that thing is not what I had in mind." What should you do?

____

____

____

____

4. You are assisting a patient with bathing when she complains that her IV is causing her so much pain. You check her right arm and notice quite a lot of swelling where the catheter enters the skin. Along with edema, her skin is cool. What should you do?

____

____

____

____

5. The nurse applied an ACE™ to a patient's left forearm. You enter his room to give him fresh water and notice his fingers are cyanotic (blue); however, he is sleeping comfortably. What should you do?

____

____

____

____

LEARNING ACTIVITIES

1. Working with a classmate or friend, practice applying an ACE™ bandage to each other. Give feedback to each other about the technique used, how tight or loose it felt, and what questions you should ask to assess comfort level.
2. If you have access to a pair of antiembolism stockings, try putting a pair on and wearing them for 8 hours. Remember the technique used when applying them and when taking them off. Discuss with classmates how you felt wearing them.

PROCEDURE CHECKLISTS

PROCEDURE 29-1: CHANGING THE GOWN OF A PATIENT RECEIVING IV THERAPY

Name: ____________________ Date: ____________________

STEPS	S	U	COMMENTS
1. Assemble equipment a. Clean gown b. Disposable gloves, if the potential exists for exposure to body fluids			
2. Wash hands and apply gloves as applicable.			
3. Identify the patient by checking the ID bracelet.			
4. Inform the patient that you are going to change his gown.			
5. Place a clean gown and laundry bag on the chair near the bed.			
6. Adjust the bed to a comfortable working height.			
7. Untie the patient's gown.			
8. Remove the arm without the IV from the sleeve.			
9. Remove the gown from the arm with the IV carefully, considering the tubing and bag of fluid as part of the arm. Move the sleeve down the arm, over the tubing, and up to the IV bag.			
10. Remove the container or bag from the hook, being careful not to lower the IV bag below the area on the patient's arm where the catheter is inserted.			
11. Slip the gown over the IV bag and return the IV bag to its hook.			
12. Place the soiled gown in the laundry bag.			
13. Considering the IV bag and tubing as part of the patient's arm, lift the bag from the hook carefully, without allowing it to drop below the area on the patient's arm where the catheter is inserted.			
14. Slip the sleeve of the gown over the IV bag quickly.			
15. Place the IV bag on the hook.			
16. Slip the gown down the IV tubing and then over the patient's arm.			
17. Slip the gown over the other arm without the IV.			
18. Tie the back straps for patient comfort.			
19. Make sure IV fluid is running. Consult the nurse for any concerns.			

20. Make the patient comfortable and replace the call light.			
21. Lower the bed to a position of safety.			
22. Raise the side rails when ordered or indicated.			
23. Remove gloves and wash your hands.			
24. Report to your supervisor a. That you replaced the patient's gown with a clean one b. Any unusual observations			

Charting:

____

____

____

____

Date of Satisfactory Completion ____________________

Instructor's Signature ____________________

PROCEDURE 29-2: APPLYING ELASTIC BANDAGES

Name: ____________________ Date: ____________________

STEPS	S	U	COMMENTS
1. Assemble equipment a. Elastic bandages b. Clips or tape c. Disposable gloves, if the potential exists for exposure to body fluids			
2. Wash hands and put on gloves if applicable.			
3. Identify the patient by checking the ID bracelet.			
4. Explain to the patient that you are going to wrap his leg or arm (or whatever area is to be wrapped) with an elastic bandage.			
5. Provide privacy and comfort for the patient.			
6. Adjust the bed to a comfortable working height.			
7. Expose the area that is to be wrapped.			
8. Extend the part of the body to be bandaged. Support the patient's heel or wrist.			
9. Stand directly in front of the patient or facing the part to be bandaged.			
10. Hold the bandage with the loose end coming off the bottom of the roll.			
11. Anchor the bandage by two circular turns around the body part at its smallest point (usually the ankle or wrist).			
12. Apply the bandage in the same direction as venous circulation, that is, toward the heart.			
13. Roll the bandage smoothly and wrap it firmly, but not too tightly.			
14. Exert even pressure. Keep the bandage smooth and evenly applied to cover the part of the body being bandaged.			
15. If possible, leave fingers or toes exposed for observation of circulatory changes.			
16. Continue wrapping upward with a spiral turn. Each turn should overlap the one before about one-half width of the bandage.			
17. After applying the bandage, secure the terminal end by taping or clipping it, or fastening with Velcro®.			
18. If more than one bandage is used, overlap them to prevent the bandages from slipping.			

19. To remove the bandage, unwind it gently. Gather it into a loose mass, passing the mass from hand to hand as the bandage is unwound, then roll the bandage smoothly so it is ready for the next application.			
20. Make the patient comfortable and replace the call light.			
21. Lower the bed to a position of safety.			
22. Raise the side rails if ordered or indicated.			
23. Dispose of gloves and wash your hands.			
24. Report to your supervisor • That you applied or removed the elastic bandages • The area of application • How the patient tolerated the procedure • Any abnormal or unusual observations			

Charting:

____

____

____

____

Date of Satisfactory Completion ____________________

Instructor's Signature ____________________

30

Patients with Special Needs: Cancer, Immune System Disorders, Mental Illness, and Substance Abuse

Key Terms Review

Match the key terms in the right column with the definitions in the left column by placing the letter of each correct answer in the space provided.

_____ **1.** Malignant neoplasms or tumors.

_____ **2.** The use of high doses of radiation, many times the dose used for x-ray exams, to treat cancer.

_____ **3.** A tumor that stays at its site of origin and does not usually regrow once removed.

_____ **4.** New growth; the words *tumor* and *neoplasm* are interchangeable.

_____ **5.** New growths that spread, invade, and destroy organs.

_____ **6.** The spreading of cancer cells through the systems of the body.

_____ **7.** The use of drugs to treat cancer.

_____ **8.** The immune system is not functioning normally.

_____ **9.** Removal of a small part of the breast.

_____ **10.** Removal of the entire breast.

_____ **11.** An individual's ability to identify who she is, where she is, and some information about time (e.g., month, year, time of day).

Terms

A. Mental illness

B. Mental health

C. Orientation

D. Substance abuse

E. Acquired immunodeficiency syndrome (AIDS)

F. Cancer

G. Neoplasm (tumor)

H. Benign tumor

I. Malignant (neoplasms)

J. Metastasis

K. Radiation therapy

L. Chemotherapy

M. Mastectomy

N. Lumpectomy

O. Immunocompromised

_____ **12.** The best adjustment an individual can make at a given time, based on internal and external resources.

_____ **13.** A number of chemical imbalances in the brain or genetically based brain diseases that interfere significantly with people's abilities to live and work.

_____ **14.** The excessive use of mood-altering illegal drugs, alcohol, prescription or over-the-counter medications, inhalants, tobacco, and solvents that results in negative changes to a person's life.

_____ **15.** A condition in humans caused by HIV in which the immune system begins to fail, leading to the development of life-threatening opportunistic infections.

MULTIPLE-CHOICE QUESTIONS

Circle the letter next to the word or statement that best completes the sentence or answers the question.

1. The nursing assistant can help mastectomy patients by

a. being calm and accepting of their responses.
b. encouraging them to be happy.
c. being absent from their unit as much as possible.
d. all of the above.

2. ____________ is a leading cause of death in the United States.

a. Alopecia
b. Dermatitis
c. Gastritis
d. Cancer

3. ___________ is the use of drugs to treat cancer.

a. Manipulation
b. Psychotherapy
c. Canceropathy
d. Chemotherapy

4. ___________ can be a(n) side effect of chemotherapy.

a. Nausea
b. Vomiting
c. Fatigue
d. All of the above

5. The cancer patient often undergoes surgical procedures that

a. may alter body functions.
b. are not useful.
c. may alter the form of the body.
d. both a and c.

6. Special cells the body produces to fight bacteria and viruses are

a. osteoclasts.
b. immunocells.
c. antibodies.
d. super cells.

7. An example of an immune-compromising condition is

a. myocardial infarction.
b. acne.
c. AIDS.
d. osteoporosis.

8. Another name for a tumor is a

a. neoplasm.
b. benign.
c. malignant.
d. cancer.

9. Substance abuse may be excessive use of ______ and ________.
   a. chocolate; coffee
   b. alcohol; food
   c. prescription drugs; food
   d. prescription drugs; controlled substances for pain relief

10. A leading cause of automobile accidents in the United States is
   a. drinking alcohol and driving.
   b. taking illegal drugs and driving.
   c. the use of a designated driver.
   d. both A and B.

11. Drinking alcohol during pregnancy can cause a pattern of birth defects referred to as
   a. drunk baby syndrome (DBS).
   b. sad results syndrome (SRS).
   c. fetal alcohol syndrome (FAS).
   d. fetal death syndrome (FDS).

12. In situations of substance abuse, the
   a. habit frees the user.
   b. substance enhances the user.
   c. user controls the substance.
   d. habit controls the user.

13. The medical diagnosis of depression
   a. is a mood disorder.
   b. affects 10% to 12% of older adults.
   c. has a negative social stigma attached to it.
   d. all of the above.

14. A strategy to prevent cancer is to
   a. continue to smoke.
   b. eat a diet high in fats and cholesterol.
   c. use sunscreen and reapply often.
   d. rest as often as you can and avoid exercising.

15. The memory device (*mnemonic*) used to remember the early warning signs of cancer is
   a. CAUTION
   b. STOP
   c. PREVENTION
   d. TREATMENT

16. The _____ a diagnosis is given, the _____ treatment can begin and the chance for a patient to recover from cancer can increase.
   a. later; later
   b. earlier; earlier
   c. later; earlier
   d. earlier; later

17. _____________ should be taught to any woman who has begun to menstruate (get her period).
   a. Yearly mammograms
   b. Mastectomies
   c. Lumpectomies
   d. Monthly self-breast examination

18. ________ means that a breast was removed.
   a. Lumpectomy
   b. Mastectomy
   c. Colostomy
   d. Prostatectomy

19. A man may experience ______ and ________ from having an enlarged prostate.
   a. difficulty urinating; breast tenderness
   b. impotence; incontinence of urine
   c. impotence; stronger erections
   d. incontinence of stool; improved urination

20. A cancer patient who has lost a lot of weight and has sores in her mouth may not want to eat. The nursing assistant
   a. should offer hot liquids and ice cubes to ease the pain.
   b. can brush the patient's teeth and ask her to rinse with mouthwash.
   c. could offer soft, cool foods or liquid drinks high in nutrients.
   d. must leave the patient alone to rest.

21. A patient is severely immunocompromised and is on isolation precautions. The nursing assistant should
   a. be extra careful to wash her hands frequently before and after entering this patient's room.
   b. tell the nurse supervisor when she is sick so she does not get the patient sick.

c. offer emotional support to the patient.
d. all of the above.

22. ________________ like encephalitis, meningitis, pneumonia, and tuberculosis can further decrease a person's immune system and possibly cause death.
a. Opportunistic infections
b. Opportunity infarctions
c. Brain damage
d. Thinking disorders

23. Mrs. Patrick recently buried her husband of 40 years after she cared for him when he was dying of cancer. She tells you she has trouble sleeping at night and then has no energy in the morning to get up and do anything. You know that she might be suffering from
a. suicidal thoughts.
b. depression.
c. schizophrenia.
d. menopause.

24. Schizophrenia
a. affects 5- to 12-year-olds.
b. is also called *multiple personality disorder*.
c. allows a person to think clearly and speak softly.
d. is considered a thinking disorder.

25. *Social low-risk drinking* is defined as no more than __ drink(s) per hour and no more than __ drink(s) per day.
a. 1; 2
b. 2; 1
c. 2; 4
d. 2; 8

TRUE OR FALSE QUESTIONS

Determine whether each question is true or false. In the space provided, write "T" for true and "F" for false. If the statement is false, rewrite it on the line provided to make it a true statement.

____ **1.** Breast cancer is one of the leading causes of death among women.

____

____ **2.** Normal cells are killed during radiation treatment along with cancer cells.

____

____ **3.** A nursing assistant is able to assess a patient is oriented when a patient can tell her his name, where he is and the month, year, and time of day.

____

____ **4.** Substance abuse occurs only to people living in poverty situations.

____

____ **5.** One community resource that helps people who are alcoholics is Alchoholics Anonymous (AA).

____

____ **6.** No vaccine exists to prevent HPV; therefore, a woman should use condoms when having sex to prevent disease from occurring.

____

____ **7.** Excessive drinking increases the risk of mouth, throat, esophageal, larynx, liver, and breast cancer.

____

____ **8.** A person should increase his diet in fiber so he should eat more rice and white bread.

____

____ **9.** Beer, hot dogs with sauerkraut, and pickles help ward off cancer.

____

____ **10.** Exposure to secondhand smoke can cause cancer.

____

FILL-IN-THE-BLANK QUESTIONS

Provide the meaning of the following abbreviations.

1. AIDS ____________________
2. HIV ____________________
3. SPF ____________________
4. OSHA ____________________
5. HPV ____________________
6. CAUTION ____________________
7. OIS ____________________
8. PCP ____________________
9. CDC ____________________
10. A + O × 3 ____________________
11. NHSDA ____________________
12. NIAAA ____________________
13. NSAASA ____________________
14. LSD ____________________
15. FAS ____________________
16. WHO ____________________
17. oz ____________________

EXERCISE 30-1

Objective: To recognize and correctly spell words related to the care of patients with special needs.

Directions: Unscramble the words in the following word list.

Word List

1. NCAREC ____________________
2. ASANEU ____________________
3. EBNGIN ____________________
4. ASDI ____________________
5. BSUANCSTE BUAES ____________________
6. TLAENM LILESNS ____________________
7. SISATSATEM ____________________
8. PLOASNEM ____________________

EXERCISE 30-2

Directions: Circle the words you found in Exercise 30-1 in the word search grid.

M	A	N	T	I	R	P	I	C	M	L	H	N	J	B
E	Y	C	Z	V	G	Q	V	K	E	S	N	E	A	F
T	Z	S	A	X	S	B	Y	U	N	J	S	O	K	G
A	H	C	A	N	C	E	R	Z	T	W	N	P	D	P
S	K	J	I	O	N	N	Y	P	A	O	A	L	I	R
T	I	Q	D	I	W	I	E	L	L	X	U	A	M	G
A	X	G	S	Z	B	G	D	C	I	K	S	S	P	A
S	Y	R	U	O	L	N	U	O	L	H	E	M	O	M
I	E	S	F	R	D	M	P	A	L	B	A	A	K	P
S	V	L	J	H	J	X	M	G	N	J	Q	R	T	B
D	S	U	B	S	T	A	N	C	E	A	B	U	S	E
O	N	L	C	P	U	K	S	Y	S	X	S	O	H	C
A	E	T	Q	H	J	Y	B	W	S	D	N	K	I	F

EXERCISE 30-3

Objective: To demonstrate your ability to recognize the signs and symptoms of malignant tumors.

Directions: Circle the words in the following word list that are the signs and symptoms of malignant tumors.

Word List

1. A sore that does not heal
2. Weight loss
3. Unusual bleeding
4. All lumps in the breast
5. A rash that reappears
6. Change in bowel habits
7. Changes in the appearance of a mole
8. Nausea and vomiting
9. Diarrhea for 3 days
10. Unaccountable weight loss
11. A feeling of tiredness that lasts
12. Hoarseness, coughing, difficulty breathing or swallowing
13. Difficulty swallowing

EXERCISE 30-4

Directions: Draw a line from the illnesses described in the first column to the possible community resource a person might seek support from in the second column.

Illness	**Community Resource**
Cocaine addiction	American Cancer Society
Alcohol abuse	Private psychiatrist
Melanoma	Alcoholics Anonymous
Depression	Narcotics Anonymous

THE NURSING ASSISTANT IN ACTION

1. You pass by a patient's room and overhear a colleague belittling a newly admitted 20-year-old male patient who is homosexual. Your colleague is preaching that the patient will go to the devil for the way he thinks and acts and tells him that sinners like him will get AIDS if he doesn't have it already. She tells him that he should be ashamed of himself and that she will pray for his salvation. What should you do?

____

____

____

____

2. You notice that the significant other of one of your surgical patients who left the floor an hour ago to have a mastectomy is crying in the unit's common meeting area. You sit down next to him and ask, "Can I help you in any way?" He holds his head in his hands and while sobbing tells you he is so worried about the outcome of his wife's diagnosis and about the way they will continue to interact with each other once she comes out of surgery and they return home. What should you do?

____

____

____

____

3. A wife accompanies her husband to his follow-up visit with the urologist at the office after his prostate was removed 6 weeks ago. While the patient is being seen by the doctor, the wife comes to the receptionist's window and asks to talk with someone in private. You ask her to come inside, and in whispered tones she explains to you that her husband is having a really difficult time with this and won't touch her or engage in intimate relations anymore. What should you do?

____

____

____

____

4. You are assigned to work the night shift when you notice that once again, your coworker is late. As the night progresses, you notice she goes to the staff locker room frequently. You enter the locker room to grab your snack for break and find her drinking from a flask she has stored in her locker. She quickly hides it and asks you, "Please don't tell on me. My husband got laid off. I have been having some family issues and this job is bringing me

down with all the recent deaths we have had on the floor. I really need this job. Be a good friend and don't tell." What should you do?

____

____

____

____

5. Mrs. Williams has been in the nursing home for a month now. You have noticed a decrease in her appetite; she does not want to eat in the dining room with her peers and has taken to sleeping most of the day. You think she may be experiencing depression. You encourage her to tell you what is wrong because you have noticed something is bothering her. She explains that there is no purpose for an old lady like herself. She has lost her home and all her things. She has seen her friends all pass away and even two of her children. No one comes to visit because their lives are so busy. She knows no one at this place and she cannot even have her pet live with her. What are some things you could do to help her?

____

____

____

____

LEARNING ACTIVITIES

1. Contact an organization that provides assistance and support to persons living with cancer. Find out what financial, social, and emotional resources they provide. Report your findings to your class.
2. Make an appointment with your own family physician if you are over the age of 40 for a physical and a breast check-up, whether you are a woman or a man. Although breast cancer is usually thought of as being a female issue, men have breast tissue and can get breast cancer as well. Schedule an appointment and discuss when you should have a mammography and a colonoscopy. If you are a man over the age of 50, make an appointment to have your prostate checked and have a colonoscopy if needed. As a health care provider, you should take the necessary precautions that you know can keep you healthy and save your life.

Neonatal and Pediatric Care

31

Key Terms Review

Match the key terms in the right column with the definitions in the left column by placing the letter of each correct answer in the space provided.

_____ **1.** Solid waste material discharged from the body through the rectum or anus; other names include *feces, excrement, bowel movement,* and *fecal matter.*

_____ **2.** To remove the foreskin of the penis by surgical procedure.

_____ **3.** Difficult and infrequent defecation, with passage of hard or dry fecal matter.

_____ **4.** Loss of body fluids.

_____ **5.** Washable or disposable covering applied to the perineal area for the purpose of containing stool or urine.

_____ **6.** Abnormally frequent discharge of fluid fecal material from the bowel.

_____ **7.** Inside the uterus or womb.

_____ **8.** Outside the uterus or womb.

_____ **9.** Long, flexible, rough organ that carries nourishment from the mother to the baby; it connects the unborn baby in the mother's uterus to the placenta.

_____ **10.** A baby age birth to 1 month; newborn.

_____ **11.** A baby age birth to 1 month; neonate.

_____ **12.** An unborn baby still in the mother's uterus.

Terms

A. Intrauterine
B. Extrauterine
C. Umbilical cord
D. Premature baby
E. Infant
F. Baby
G. Toddler
H. Pediatric patient
I. Preschooler
J. School-age child
K. Adolescent
L. Gestation
M. Fetus
N. Newborn
O. Neonate
P. Circumcise
Q. Dehydrate
R. Diaper
S. Diarrhea
T. Constipation
U. Stool

_____13. Pregnancy.

_____14. A baby age 1 month to 1 year.

_____15. Born before the completion of 37 weeks gestation.

_____16. All patients through 18 years of age, including infants, children, and adolescents.

_____17. Child from 3 to 6 years of age.

_____18. From 6 to 12 years of age.

_____19. Child from 1 to 3 years of age.

_____20. Child from 12 to 18 years of age.

_____21. Age birth to 1 year.

MULTIPLE-CHOICE QUESTIONS

Circle the letter next to the word or statement that best completes the sentence or answers the question.

1. An important part of any care given to infants and children is being careful of
- a. speed.
- b. fecal tolerance.
- c. safety measures.
- d. bowel and bladder training.

2. Most infants eat every _____________ hours, on average.
- a. 12
- b. 4
- c. 2
- d. 8

3. The nursing assistant supports the mother when she is breastfeeding by providing
- a. food and nourishment.
- b. fun and laughter.
- c. formula preparation.
- d. privacy and comfort.

4. When breastfeeding, the arm holding the baby should be
- a. supported by a pillow or folded blanket.
- b. wrapped in an ACE™ bandage.
- c. chilled in ice water.
- d. washed thoroughly before use.

5. If the mother is sleepy, do not
- a. disturb her while holding the infant.
- b. leave her alone while she is holding the baby.
- c. worry because she can sleep and breastfeed at the same time.
- d. give her the baby until she has slept 8 hours.

6. The _____________ should be notified if the mother appears to be having difficulty breastfeeding.
- a. father
- b. doctor
- c. nurse
- d. family

7. When performing infant care, it is important to prevent the spread of microorganisms by doing which of the following?
- a. Applying infection control measures
- b. Washing hands frequently
- c. Avoiding coughing and sneezing
- d. All of the above

8. If the breast tissue blocks the infant's nose when breastfeeding, the baby will stop feeding and let go of the breast; therefore,
   a. the mother should keep the breast tissue away from the infant's nose by pressing down on the breast in that area with her finger or thumb.
   b. the mother should be prepared for the infant to cry often during the time he is nursing.
   c. women with large breasts should bottle-feed.
   d. extend the feeding time by 15 minutes.

9. An important infant feeding skill for the nursing assistant to develop is
   a. changing the diaper.
   b. burping the baby.
   c. fast-food delivery.
   d. a taste for formula.

10. When burping the baby, gently rub and pat
   a. the infant's feet.
   b. the infant's stomach.
   c. the mother's back.
   d. the infant's back.

11. When changing the diaper, the nursing assistant should observe the stool for
   a. at least 5 minutes after changing the diaper.
   b. color, consistency, amount, and frequency.
   c. seeds and pits.
   d. microorganisms.

12. Cloth diapers are held in place with
   a. tabs.
   b. tape.
   c. safety pins.
   d. waterproof pants.

13. An infant with watery stools can become dehydrated
   a. in 2 days or less.
   b. in 2 hours.
   c. within 2 weeks.
   d. within 1 week.

14. When the baby has been circumcised, the nursing assistant should
   a. check with his immediate supervisor for care instructions.
   b. be gentle when changing diapers.
   c. be gentle when cleaning the area.
   d. all of the above.

15. Within 5 to 20 days the umbilical cord will
   a. turn green and develop an odor.
   b. turn red and bleed.
   c. grow 1 inch and turn black.
   d. dry, turn black, and eventually fall off.

16. In the home, it is important to
   a. never use heating pads on infants or children.
   b. never use blankets on babies.
   c. never use incubators.
   d. take the infant's temperature every day.

17. Keep all medications and cleaning solutions out of reach of
   a. the nurse.
   b. the child.
   c. the nursing assistant.
   d. the mother.

18. Before measuring the vital signs of children, it is important that the nursing assistant
   a. check the identification band first.
   b. use the right-size cuff for the blood pressure.
   c. inform the child what is going to be done.
   d. all of the above.

19. Good communication with the ___________ as well as the child is an important skill for the nursing assistant to develop.
   a. family pet
   b. parents
   c. child's playmates
   d. neighbors

20. It is important that the nursing assistant report to the immediate supervisor if the family seems to be worried about
   a. a problem with the child's illness.
   b. the child's response to care received.
   c. the care the child is receiving in the hospital.
   d. all of the above.

21. Safety must always be a concern of the nursing assistant because
   a. children are unpredictable and can be injured easily.
   b. it's a nice thing to be aware of.
   c. he or she will be blamed if a child is injured.
   d. the nursing assistant is unpredictable and could be injured easily.

22. Diarrhea may be caused from
   a. proper and frequent hand washing.
   b. cleaning and sterilizing equipment correctly.
   c. following directions precisely when mixing formula.
   d. bacteria or allergies.

23. To prevent air from entering a baby's stomach during feeding, the nursing assistant should
   a. hold the bottle straight.
   b. make sure the nipple is filled with milk by tipping the end of the bottle up.
   c. never fill the nipple with milk and keep the bottle flat.
   d. check the temperature and prop the bottle on a pillow.

24. ______ can be placed on a newborn's penis after circumcision occurs to prevent the area from sticking inside the diaper and causing pain.
   a. Petroleum jelly or ointment
   b. An absorbent pad
   c. A bandage
   d. A cool compress

25. When cleaning the eyes of a newborn, the nursing assistant should
   a. make the soapy water greater than 100°F.
   b. use a different cotton ball for each eye and wipe from the nose outward.
   c. use one cotton ball and wipe the eye outward toward the nose.
   d. never clean the eyes to prevent infection.

TRUE OR FALSE QUESTIONS

Determine whether each question is true or false. In the space provided, write "T" for true and "F" for false. If the statement is false, rewrite it on the line provided to make it a true statement.

_____ **1.** When feeding formula, the bottle may be propped if the caregiver is too busy to hold the infant.

____

_____ **2.** Microorganisms from spoiled formula or the contaminated hands of those who handle the infant can cause diarrhea.

____

_____ **3.** Diarrhea can be a serious and life-threatening condition for infants.

____

_____ **4.** While the umbilical cord is still attached, the baby should only be given sponge baths and not immersed in water.

____

_____ **5.** An infant who has not yet learned to roll over can be left lying on the couch.

____

_____ **6.** Providing good care for the child is worrisome to the family members.

____

_____ 7. The nursing assistant should allow the family to help in the care of the child, if possible.

____

_____ 8. A "football hold" is a common position for a newborn to be held while hair care is being offered.

____

_____ 9. A lubricated rectal thermometer should be inserted at least ½" into the rectum.

____

_____ 10. A nursing assistant should take a child's pulse and respiration first and then take the child's temperature last.

____

FILL-IN-THE-BLANK QUESTIONS

Provide the meaning of the following abbreviations.

1. mL _______________________________
2. lbs _______________________________
3. F _______________________________
4. C _______________________________
5. TA _______________________________
6. ID _______________________________
7. BP _______________________________
8. kg _______________________________

EXERCISE 31-1

Objective: To apply what you have learned about neonatal and pediatric care.

Directions: Read the following riddles carefully before writing the correct answers.

1. When feeding the infant you look forward to this happening. What is it? (*Hint:* If done in public by an adult, it is rude.)

   ____

2. You feed this to an infant. What is it? (*Hint:* Many mathematical calculations are solved with this.)

   ____

3. The appearance of this item can reveal much about the health of an infant. What is it? (*Hint:* You can stand on this to reach items that are too high for you.)

   ____

EXERCISE 31-2

Directions: Fill in the answers in the following boxes *below* that correspond to pediatric pulse, respiration, and blood pressure normal values.

Normal Values for	Pulse	Respirations	Blood Pressure
Newborns	120–160		
Infants		30–60	
Toddlers			90/55–105/70
Preschool-age child	80–140		
School-age child		18–30	
Adolescents			110/65–135/85

EXERCISE 31-3

Directions: Select from the following list of procedures the letter of the procedure that best answers each question. Write the correct letter(s) on the blank line next to the question. There may be more than one answer used for each question.

A. Circumcision cleaning

B. Giving a sponge bath

C. Giving a tub bath

D. Diapering

_____ **1.** Which procedure(s) should the nursing assistant never leave an infant unattended?

_____ **2.** In which procedure(s) should the nursing assistant observe for skin redness?

_____ **3.** Which procedure(s) may involve the use of rubbing alcohol?

_____ **4.** Which procedure(s) involves checking the water temperature?

EXERCISE 31-4

Directions: Select from the following list of procedures the letter of the procedure that best answers each question. Write the correct letter(s) on the blank line next to the question. There may be more than one answer used for each question.

A. Oral temperature

B. Rectal temperature

C. Tympanic temperature

D. Axillary temperature

_____ 1. Which procedure(s) requires the nursing assistant to clean the probe of the thermometer?

_____ 2. For which procedure(s) should the nursing assistant hold the thermometer until the temperature reading is obtained?

_____ 3. For which procedure(s) should a nursing assistant lubricate the probe?

_____ 4. Which procedure(s) is done in less than 3 seconds?

_____ 5. Which procedure(s) should be avoided if the child cannot understand verbal directions well?

THE NURSING ASSISTANT IN ACTION

1. You find a 35-year-old first-time mother crying in her room. You sit and ask her if there is anything you can do for her and if she wants to talk. She tells you, "I so wanted to breastfeed my newborn, but my breasts hurt and I cannot get the hang of getting the baby to latch on. I am a successful businesswoman and can run a company and manage 100 employees, but when it comes to breastfeeding, I feel like such a failure." What should you do?

____

____

____

2. You enter the room where an infant has been crying for the last 20 minutes only to find him placed face down in his bassinet and his 18-year-old mother listening to her music through earbuds. When she sees you, she pulls one earbud out and tells you, "I cannot stand this crying anymore! I keep feeding him and he just won't stop crying." What should you do?

____

____

____

3. A new mother who has been breastfeeding her baby for 6 weeks brings her baby to her wellness visit. You ask if everything is going well and she tells you she is concerned because her baby's stool is wet and has little seeds in it. She adds, "Why is the stool not formed? Hannah only has about two poops a day. I think something is wrong and I should take her to her pediatrician, don't you?" What should you do?

____

____

____

4. A 20-year-old female patient will be discharged with her newborn in 12 hours. She has not given the baby a bath yet, and tells you although she knows she has to bathe him and she wants to bathe him, she is scared to death of dropping the baby in the bathtub and hurting him. What should you do?

____

____

____

5. In a nearby hospital, an infant was abducted recently. The parents of the infant in your care tell you they are worried sick that this will happen here at this facility. What should you do?

____

____

____

LEARNING ACTIVITIES

1. Research the security and safety strategies your facility has implemented to ensure infant and children abductions are avoided. Become familiar with equipment used and policies in place to report any unusual observations or concerns.

2. If possible, contact a lactation specialist and ask if you can spend a day with her or participate in a workshop offered in your community on breastfeeding or parenting techniques. Discuss with classmates what you learned about the benefits of breastfeeding, techniques taught to help a new mother breastfeed, and any other parenting information that you found educational or beneficial that could encourage and support mothers whom you care for to breastfeed comfortably and successfully, as well as help them assume the role of "parent."

PROCEDURE CHECKLISTS

PROCEDURE 31-1: DIAPERING A BABY

Name: ______________________ Date: ______________________

STEPS	S	U	COMMENTS
1. Assemble equipment a. Disposable gloves b. Clean prefolded cloth diaper or disposable diaper c. Disposable baby wipes or cotton balls d. Baby soap e. Baby cream or powder f. Basin of warm water g. Waterproof changing pad h. Washcloth			
2. Wash your hands.			
3. Place baby on pad.			
4. Put on gloves.			
5. Unfasten tabs or pins on diaper.			
6. Remove as much feces as possible by wiping front to back.			
7. Remove diaper, fold to enclose feces, and set aside.			
8. Use disposable wipe or cotton balls with soap and water to clean from front to back. Use washcloth if there is a large amount of stool. Rinse well.			
9. Clean umbilical cord by wiping it with a disposable wipe or cotton ball moistened with soap and water. Ask your supervisor if a cotton ball moistened with alcohol should be used.			
10. Clean the circumcision gently with a disposable wipe or cotton ball moistened with soap and water.			
11. Place diaper under the baby by raising the baby's legs and sliding the diaper under the buttocks.			
12. Apply cream, lotion, or powder. If using powder, never shake it onto the baby, because fine particles can get into the baby's lungs. Instead, put powder on the palm of your hands and smooth onto the baby's skin.			
13. Cloth diapers must be folded before use. Fold so that there is more diaper thickness in the back for a female baby and more thickness in the front for a male baby.			

14. Bring the diaper up between the legs to cover the lower abdomen. If there is still an umbilical cord attached or it has not healed, make sure the diaper lies across the abdomen, but under the umbilical cord.			
15. Use the tabs to secure the edges of the diaper together at the hips: If pins are used, place the first and second fingers of your left hand between the skin and the diaper, holding the diaper edges in place with the thumb. Using the opposite hand, insert the pin sideways (not up and down) and close it.			
16. Apply waterproof pants over the cloth diaper.			
17. Place the baby in a crib or other safe place.			
18. Rinse feces from the cloth diaper in the toilet. Store in a prepared diaper pail or plastic bag. Throw disposable diaper in a covered trash can.			
19. Dispose of gloves and wash your hands.			
20. Document the urine, feces, appearance of the skin, and whether cream or powder was applied.			

Charting:

____

____

____

____

Date of Satisfactory Completion ____________________

Instructor's Signature ____________________

PROCEDURE 31-2: GIVING A BABY A SPONGE BATH

Name: ______________________ Date: ______________________

STEPS	S	U	COMMENTS
1. Assemble equipment on a table or countertop a. Bath basin or sink b. Two bath towels c. Cotton balls d. Washcloth e. Warm water f. Baby soap g. Baby shampoo (optional) h. Baby powder, lotion, or cream i. Diaper j. Clean clothes			
2. Wash your hands.			
3. Identify the baby.			
4. Place a towel on the counter next to the basin as you may want to lay the baby down to wash and dry him.			
5. Fill the basin with 2"–3" of warm water (100°F; 37.8°C). Use a tub thermometer to check the water temperature.			
6. Undress the baby. Wrap him in a towel or blanket. Fold the lower corner of the towel over the feet and legs. Fold the two side corners of the towel under the arms and over the chest, wrapping the baby. Bring the baby to the table or sink.			
7. Use a cotton ball moistened with warm water and squeezed out, gently wipe baby's eyes from the nose toward the ears. Use a clean cotton ball for each eye.			
8. To wash the hair, hold the baby in the football hold with the baby's head over the sink or basin. This frees your other arm to wet the hair, apply a small amount of shampoo, lather, and rinse.			
9. Dry the baby's head with a towel.			
10. Unwrap the baby and gently place him on the towel on a table. One of your hands should be holding the baby. Never let go, not even for a second.			
11. Wash the baby's body with the soap and your hands or the washcloth, being careful to wash in the folds of the skin.			

12. If the baby is female, always wash the genital area from front to back.			
13. Rinse the baby thoroughly with warm water.			
14. Dry the baby well, being careful to dry in the folds in the skin.			
15. Lightly apply powder, lotion, or cream to the baby, whichever is the preference of the mother or the instructions of the nurse.			
16. Diaper and dress the baby.			
17. Place the baby in his crib and raise the crib side rails or allow the mother to hold him. Show the mother how to hold the baby in either the upright position or the cradle position.			
18. Clean the counter, sink, equipment, and supplies and return them to their proper place.			
19. Wash your hands.			
20. Report to your supervisor • The time you gave the baby a sponge bath. • Any abnormal or unusual observations			

Charting:

____

____

____

____

Date of Satisfactory Completion ____________________

Instructor's Signature ____________________

PROCEDURE 31-4: MEASURING A CHILD'S PULSE RATE

Name: ____________________ Date: ____________________

STEPS	S	U	COMMENTS
1. Assemble equipment a. Stethoscope and aseptic swabs b. Watch with a second hand c. Pen			
2. Wash your hands.			
3. Identify the child by checking the ID bracelet.			
4. Explain to the child or caregiver what you are going to do.			
5. Place the diaphragm of the stethoscope over the heart.			
6. Count the beats for 1 minute.			
7. Immediately record the full-minute count.			
8. Clean the earplugs of the stethoscope.			
9. Wash your hands.			

Charting:

____

____

____

____

Date of Satisfactory Completion ____________________

Instructor's Signature ____________________

PROCEDURE 31-5: MEASURING A CHILD'S RESPIRATORY RATE

Name: ____________________ Date: ____________________

STEPS	S	U	COMMENTS
1. Assemble equipment a. Watch with a second hand b. Pen			
2. Wash your hands.			
3. Identify the patient by checking the ID bracelet.			
4. Do not tell the child that you are going to count respirations. If the child is sleeping, count respirations before he wakes up.			
5. For infants and toddlers, *watch the stomach and chest.*			
6. For children over 4 years old, *watch the chest.*			
7. Count the number of times the stomach and/or chest rises during 1 minute.			
8. Immediately record the full-minute count.			
9. Wash your hands.			

Charting:

____

____

____

____

Date of Satisfactory Completion ____________________

Instructor's Signature ____________________

PROCEDURE 31-6: MEASURING A CHILD'S BLOOD PRESSURE

Name: ______________________ Date: ______________________

STEPS	S	U	COMMENTS
1. Assemble equipment a. Blood pressure cuff (correct cuff for size of the child) b. Stethoscope c. Watch with a second hand d. Pen			
2. Wash your hands.			
3. Identify the patient by checking the ID bracelet.			
4. Tell the child what you are going to do, explaining that she might feel a gentle squeeze on his arm.			
5. Wrap the cuff securely on the arm above the elbow area.			
6. Feel for the brachial pulse on the inner aspect of the elbow below the cuff.			
7. Place the stethoscope in your ears and the diaphragm over the area where you felt the pulse.			
8. Pump up the cuff until the pulse is no longer felt. If it is a manual blood pressure cuff, release the valve until you can hear the systolic and diastolic sounds. Count the beats for 1 minute. Many devices are automatic and pump up the cuff, release the valve, and display the results.			
9. Immediately record the results.			
10. Clean the earplugs of the stethoscope and return equipment to its proper place.			
11. Wash your hands.			

Charting:

____

____

____

____

Date of Satisfactory Completion ______________________

Instructor's Signature ______________________

PROCEDURE 31-7: WEIGHING A BABY

Name: ______________________ Date: ______________________

STEPS	S	U	COMMENTS
1. Assemble equipment a. Baby scale (calibrated) b. Pen			
2. Wash your hands.			
3. Identify the patient by checking the ID bracelet.			
4. Tell the baby and parent what you are going to do.			
5. Remove the baby's clothing.			
6. Position the baby in the center of the scale tray.			
7. Weigh the baby in kilograms, to the nearest 0.01 kg.			
8. Immediately record the results.			
9. Replace the baby's diaper and dress the baby.			
10. Return the infant to its parent or to the crib for safety.			
11. Clean the scale with an antiseptic wipe. Return equipment to its proper place.			
12. Wash your hands.			

Charting:

____

____

____

____

Date of Satisfactory Completion ______________________

Instructor's Signature ______________________

Home Health Care

32

Key Terms Review

Match the key terms in the right column with the definitions in the left column by placing the letter of each correct answer in the space provided.

_____ **1.** The care provided to acutely ill clients or those with a worsening illness with the goal of teaching the clients to become independent in self-care and functional ability.

_____ **2.** Health care services provided in the client's home.

_____ **3.** The care of clients with terminal conditions who are expected to live 6 months or less.

_____ **4.** The care of chronically ill clients who are unable to care for themselves and live alone or have limited family support.

_____ **5.** A period of care with increasing physical activity to allow the client's return to pre- injury or pre-illness activity and functioning levels.

_____ **6.** A group brought together by shared needs, interests, and mutual concern for the well-being of all its members.

_____ **7.** Most often, a nursing assistant assigned to work in a client's home.

_____ **8.** The family member or significant other who is taking the major responsibility for the care of the client.

_____ **9.** Getting all of one's duties completed in an organized fashion within a set work period.

Terms

A. Sterilize

B. Microorganism

C. Infection control

D. Formula

E. Bedbound

F. Flammable

G. Advance directive

H. Short-term intermittent skilled nursing care

I. Long-term supportive care

J. Home health care

K. Hospice care

L. Rehabilitative care

M. Caregiver

N. Family unit

O. Home health aide

P. Responsibility

Q. Time/travel record

R. Efficiency

S. Punctuality

_____10. Arriving at one's planned destination on time.

_____11. A duty or obligation; that for which one is accountable.

_____12. Record or log describing how time is spent in a client's home or account of travel time to and from the client's home or running errands.

_____13. Destroying all microorganisms.

_____14. A living thing so small it cannot be seen with the naked eye, but only through a microscope.

_____15. A liquid food prescribed for an infant containing most required nutrients.

_____16. Restraining or curbing the spread of microorganisms.

_____17. Capable of burning quickly and easily.

_____18. A document of an individual's wishes at the end of life; living will.

_____19. Unable to get out of bed.

MULTIPLE-CHOICE QUESTIONS

Circle the letter next to the word or statement that best completes the sentence or answers the question.

1. A personal quality not necessary for a nursing assistant to acquire is
   a. the ability to be a self-starter.
   b. dependability and punctuality.
   c. an ethical approach to patient care.
   d. musical ability.

2. By not discussing the patient's condition with your own family, you show
   a. respect for the privacy of your patient.
   b. respect for the confidentiality of the patient.
   c. a lack of interest in your patient.
   d. both a and b

3. In your role as a home health care aide, it is important to maximize your time by
   a. balancing time and money.
   b. balancing patient preferences with travel distances.
   c. driving at high speeds, when necessary, to be on time.
   d. working in an organized fashion and getting your job done so that you can be on time for the next patient.

4. If you are delayed __________, you must call the patient to set a new arrival time.
   a. more than 30 minutes
   b. more than 45 minutes
   c. more than 2 days
   d. for any amount of time

5. As a member of the health care team, you are expected to maintain __________ in the home.
   a. the *status quo*
   a. a sense of humor
   c. complete silence
   d. a professional attitude

6. While working in the home, you are part of the health care team, but an important difference is that you usually do not have another member of the team
   a. to whom you can refer problems.
   b. to whom you can speak if you have questions.
   c. physically present in the home with you while you care for the patient.
   d. to act as a supervisor.

7. An example of demonstrating honesty and accuracy when handling the patient's money is to
a. attach all receipts to the shopping list.
b. mix it with your own money.
c. simply tell the patient what you have spent, because you know she has a good memory.
d. keep the loose change for yourself.

8. The discharge planning process requires communication with the home health care team, which includes the nurse, home health aide, and the _____.
a. patient.
b. banker.
c. clergy.
d. neighbor.

9. It is important that all team members understand what the __________ are for each patient's plan of care.
a. outcome prices
b. outcome goals
c. outcome costs
d. insurance benefits

10. The home health aide must be alert to prevent accidents in the patient's home by ________ unsafe conditions.
a. creating, berating, and aggregating
b. improvising, supervising, and relating
c. maintaining, prolonging, and inventing
d. eliminating, preventing, and correcting

11. When all the outcome goals have been met, the patient
a. receives the bill.
b. is cured.
c. is hospitalized.
d. is discharged from home care services.

12. If you are not sure how long a baby's formula has been in the refrigerator,
a. taste it yourself.
b. boil it for 10 minutes.
c. leave it in there for another time.
d. discard it and make fresh formula.

13. There are several different kinds of formulas, but in all cases it is important to
a. wash your hands, as well as the containers before opening them.
b. read the instructions for preparation.
c. shake all containers of liquid and concentrated formulas before opening.
d. do all of the above.

14. Once formula is prepared, it must be
a. fed to the infant immediately.
b. fed to the infant after boiling for 10 minutes.
c. kept refrigerated until ready to use.
d. kept at room temperature.

15. ________ is an inexpensive disinfectant found in most homes that can be used to clean sinks, bathtubs, and toilets.
a. Isopropyl alcohol
b. A mixture of vinegar and oil
c. Baking soda and vinegar
d. Laundry bleach

16. When preparing food for the patient, remember to consider
a. your likes and dislikes.
b. the cultural and religious preferences of the patient.
c. special dietary restrictions the patient may have.
d. both b and c.

17. It is very important to arrange your visit during the mealtime hours if part of your duties are to
a. eat three meals a day.
b. bathe the patient only.
c. do the laundry.
d. prepare a meal and record the amount eaten.

18. To be a *self-starter* means to be able to
a. carry out duties with much assistance.
b. accomplish only tasks you started yourself.
c. work independently and effectively.
d. start working only when by yourself.

19. If a patient has no toothpaste or denture cleaner, you may use ________________ in its place.

a. salt
b. hand soap
c. baking soda
d. vinegar

20. When you show respect for the cultural beliefs and customs of the patient and his family, you

a. make them feel valued as individuals.
b. will make them like you.
c. will change their daily habits.
d. will make them happy.

21. The goal of rehabilitation is to

a. help the family regain their strength so they can take care of the client.
b. help the client relearn skills he may have lost through illness or injury.
c. stay with the client until he dies.
d. clean soiled linens and do light housekeeping chores when necessary.

22. Usually, hospice services are provided

a. for more than 2 years.
b. in the client's home.
c. by a team of doctors who come to the bedside on a daily basis.
d. from physical therapists who help the client return to his normal functioning.

23. A __________ can be sent to a client's home when direct hands-on care is not necessary.

a. homemaker
b. registered nurse
c. licensed practical nurse
d. person from the clergy

24. Home health aides

a. work under the supervision of a speech language pathologist.
b. must complete a special training course in some states.
c. always work with a partner in the home.
d. never assist the client when performing activities of daily living.

25. One duty a home health aide is allowed to perform is

a. administer medications that are to be taken by injection.
b. irrigate a colostomy.
c. change a non-sterile dressing.
d. insert a urinary catheter.

TRUE OR FALSE QUESTIONS

Determine whether each question is true or false. In the space provided, write "T" for true and "F" for false. If the statement is false, rewrite it on the line provided to make it a true statement.

_____ **1.** The number one complaint of home health care aides is lack of punctuality by the patient.

____

_____ **2.** In most cases, the goal of patient care in the home is to promote increasing dependence of the client on the home health aide.

____

_____ **3.** The home health aide is responsible for making the first home evaluation and developing the plan of care to be followed by caregivers.

____

_____ **4.** The use of boiled and then cooled water to make formula is important because boiling kills the microorganisms in the water. These microorganisms may make the baby sick.

____

_____ 5. The home health aide may have housekeeping responsibilities in addition to care of the patient.

____

_____ 6. Any unused baby formula should be frozen so the mother can use this at a later time.

____

_____ 7. Powdered baby formula mixes best with warm sterile water, not completely cooled sterile water.

____

_____ 8. Concentrated baby formula should be diluted with tap water before feeding the infant.

____

_____ 9. When washing baby nipples, the nursing assistant should squirt hot soapy water through the nipple to decrease the chance that formula has dried.

____

_____ 10. It is not necessary to sterilize the tongs that pick up the sterile bottles and other sterile baby feeding equipment.

____

FILL-IN-THE-BLANK QUESTIONS

Provide the meaning of the following abbreviations.

1. OASIS __________________________________
2. RN __________________________________
3. LPN __________________________________
4. LVN __________________________________

EXERCISE 32-1

Objective: To recognize and correctly spell words related to home health care.

Directions: Unscramble the words in the following word list.

Word List

1. EBD-BNDUO __________________________________
2. FYAILM NTIU __________________________________
3. NOGL RMTE __________________________________
4. EARCVEGIR __________________________________
5. MREENGCYE __________________________________
6. MOEH LEHTHA __________________________________
7. EIAD __________________________________
8. EGRAHCSID __________________________________

EXERCISE 32-2

Directions: Find the words from Exercise 32-1 in the following word search puzzle.

B	E	D	B	O	U	N	D	C	E	P	B	E	D	X
A	L	E	S	G	Z	W	G	L	M	T	R	A	C	D
P	F	T	R	Z	A	C	A	B	E	S	V	X	D	L
G	A	B	X	T	L	Q	G	J	R	B	H	W	S	N
X	M	W	N	U	S	I	C	P	G	I	T	B	I	G
K	I	X	V	D	A	O	A	J	E	A	L	E	N	T
S	L	O	N	G	T	E	R	M	N	V	A	I	D	E
Q	Y	E	S	F	Y	Z	E	L	C	B	E	Y	C	X
L	U	I	R	T	Z	Y	G	E	Y	C	H	L	D	V
B	N	T	C	O	A	H	I	B	B	R	E	M	J	U
C	I	L	A	D	R	M	V	D	I	O	M	E	C	L
S	T	F	M	X	S	D	E	G	T	X	O	A	G	D
O	D	S	W	F	L	Z	R	D	B	C	H	F	S	O
D	I	S	C	H	A	R	G	E	O	A	S	T	W	P

EXERCISE 32-3

Objective: To be able to recognize the variety of important duties you will perform as a home health nursing assistant.

Directions: Place the correct letters next to the matching phrase. More than one set of letters may be selected for some of the phrases. Answers may vary.

ADL—activities of daily living
PMT—positioning, moving, transporting the patient
C—communication
CE—care of the environment
SKC—skin care
IC—infection control
SP—special procedures
N—nutrition
SPC—specimen care
PC—personal care
VS—vital signs

_____ **1.** Informing the patient of procedures you perform

_____ **2.** Washing the bathtub before and after use

_____ **3.** Recording intake and output

_____ **4.** Washing the dishes used to prepare the meals

_____ **5.** Keeping the patient's skin clean and dry

_____ **6.** Making the patient's bed and changing the linen as needed

_____ **7.** Changing simple dressings and applying non-medicated ointment

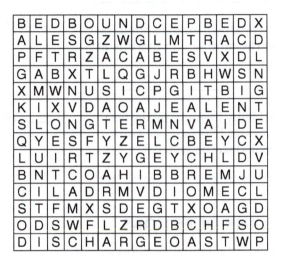

_____ **8.** Transporting the patient to the doctor's office

_____ **9.** Assisting the patient to use a bedside commode

_____ **10.** Applying an elastic bandage to the patient's leg

_____ **11.** Shopping for the patient's groceries

_____ **12.** Helping the patient brush his teeth and get dressed

_____ **13.** Taking the patient's temperature, pulse, respirations, and blood pressure

_____ **14.** Positioning the patient in the bed

_____ **15.** Using good handwashing skills and wearing disposable gloves

_____ **16.** Performing range-of-motion exercises

_____ **17.** Making an accurate record of duties performed for the patient

_____ **18.** Washing the patient's clothing and linens

_____ **19.** Cooking and preparing nutritious meals for the patient

_____ **20.** Applying a binder to the patient

_____ **21.** Offering in-between and mealtime nourishment

_____ **22.** Cleaning patient equipment

EXERCISE 32-4

Objective: To demonstrate appropriate responses to family situations.

Directions: Read the following situation descriptions and then choose the appropriate responses to the questions.

1. You are assigned to provide home care 3 hours a day for a patient who is terminally ill with advanced lung cancer. She and her husband smoke heavily each time you are there. You are a nonsmoker and do not like being exposed to the smoke. Although the doctor has encouraged the family to not smoke, they choose to continue. What should you do?

A. You continue to inform them about the dangers of smoking.

B. You repeatedly inform them of your dislike of smoking.

C. You tell them, "It's me or the cigarettes! Make your choice!"

D. You arrange to have the husband leave the room when he smokes, and you leave the room when the patient smokes.

2. You are uneasy around your home care patient's pet, a large dog. Each time you visit the home, he follows you around, growling occasionally, and watches you closely as you care for the patient. What should you do?

A. Bring the dog a bone to occupy him each time you visit.

B. Take him by the collar and put him outside.

C. Explain how you feel to the patient, and ask that the dog be put in another room or outside when you visit.

D. Ignore the dog and pretend it doesn't bother you.

3. The family members begin to argue with each other about whose turn it is to do the laundry for your patient. What should you do?
   A. Because you know who should be doing the laundry, you point this out to the group.
   B. Offer to do the laundry for the family.
   C. Continue to care for the patient and do not get involved in the argument.
   D. Ask the family to stop arguing.

4. When working at a patient's home, you observe that it is very dusty, dirty, and cluttered. What should you do?
   A. You decide to be nice and stay late one day to clean the entire house so that it meets your standards.
   B. You offer to clean up the mess for pay.
   C. You ignore the condition of the house and focus on the patient.
   D. You call up some of the patient's relatives and ask them to clean the house before your next visit.

5. You notice that the locked security grates over all the windows would not allow escape in case of a fire. What should you do?
   A. Talk to the family about a plan of escape in case of fire.
   B. Bring this situation to the attention of your supervisor immediately.
   C. Talk to the family about the danger posed by the grates on the windows.
   D. All of the above.

THE NURSING ASSISTANT IN ACTION

1. Your hospice client is in immense pain. He is on a morphine drip, and his family asks you if there is anything else you can do for him. His wife pulls you aside and asks you to call your supervisor to see if the nurse can increase the pain medication so all this can end soon. What should you do?

   ____

   ____

   ____

2. You notice many scatter rugs in your client's bathroom and kitchen. The wife has not had time to clear boxes in the hallway that were to go to the attic after the holidays. It is very difficult for you and the client to ambulate throughout the house without navigating around the clutter. You fear the scatter rugs may cause an accident when he ambulates with his walker. What should you do?

   ____

   ____

   ____

3. A new mom who is mentally challenged requires some help from a home health aide in learning how to take care of her new infant. She heads to the refrigerator and opens a can of ready-to-feed formula, pours it into a bottle that she opened from a new box bought at the store this morning and gets ready to feed the infant while you are there. What should you do?

___

___

___

4. While providing care for a new client, you notice that there are no cleaning supplies in the bathroom or the rest of the house to scrub the toilet and tub correctly before offering care. What should you do?

___

___

___

5. You call your last client of the day and tell him you will be a late. You were supposed to shop for him and prepare a dinner meal, but, because you were running so late, you did not go shopping. You see he has a can of chicken broth; some random leftover vegetables; some fresh, dried pasta; 2 slices of cheese; 2 slices of bread; butter; and a variety of herbs and spices. What should you do?

___

___

___

LEARNING ACTIVITIES

1. Create a small book containing simple recipes that you can keep with you whenever you visit clients' homes and find you must cook for them as part of your responsibilities.
2. Practice fire safety in your own home and the home of your clients by checking to see if there is a fire extinguisher and fire or carbon monoxide detectors and if they are all working properly. If you or the client you are caring for does not have proper fire safety devices, then update your own and suggest to the family they buy and install these devices correctly.

PROCEDURE CHECKLISTS

PROCEDURE 32-1: STERILIZING TAP WATER

Name: ______________________ Date: ______________________

STEPS	S	U	COMMENTS
1. Wash your hands.			
2. Assemble your equipment a. Saucepan and cover b. Water c. Timer, watch, or clock			
3. Fill the saucepan two-thirds full with water and place on burner. When the water comes to a full boil, begin timing. Allow the water to remain at a full boil for 20 minutes in a covered pan.			
4. Allow the water to cool before using it to mix the formula.			
5. Empty the water out of the saucepan, clean, and put it away.			

Charting:

____

____

____

____

Date of Satisfactory Completion ______________________

Instructor's Signature ______________________

PROCEDURE 32-2: STERILIZING BOTTLES

Name: ______________________ Date: ______________________

STEPS	S	U	COMMENTS
1. Wash your hands.			
2. Assemble your equipment a. Bottles b. Nipples, caps, and jar c. Bottle brush d. Dishwashing detergent e. Hot water from the tap f. Large pan with cover or a special sterilizing pan for baby bottles g. Small towel h. Tap water i. Timer, watch, or clock j. Tongs			
3. Scrub bottles, nipples, and caps with hot, soapy water. Use the bottle brush to clean inside the bottles. Always squirt hot, soapy water through the holes in the nipples to clean out any dried-on formula.			
4. Rinse thoroughly with hot water.			
5. Stand the washed bottles in a circle around the inside of the pan.			
6. Place the caps and nipples into the clean, empty jar and place it into the center of the pan.			
7. Pour water into and around the bottles and into the jar with the nipples until two-thirds of each bottle is under water. Place the tongs upright in the pan to sterilize them.			
8. Cover the pan and place on the stove.			
9. When the water comes to a full boil, begin timing. Allow the water to remain at a full boil for 20 minutes.			
10. Using the sterile tongs, remove the nipples and caps in the jar 10–15 minutes after the full boil began. With the nipples still inside the jar, stand the jar on the table to cool.			

11. Take the cover off the pan and allow it to cool.			
12. Remove the sterile bottles from the pan with sterile tongs.			
13. Empty the water out of the pan. The pan is now sterilized and can be used for mixing the formula, if needed.			

Charting:

____

____

____

____

Date of Satisfactory Completion ______________________

Instructor's Signature ______________________

33

The Older Adult Resident and Long-Term Care

Key Terms Review

Match the key terms in the right column with the definitions in the left column by placing the letter of each correct answer in the space provided.

_____ **1.** Care given to help residents attain or maintain their highest level of function and independence.

_____ **2.** Care that addresses the physical, social, spiritual, and psychological needs of residents.

_____ **3.** Involved with or caused by disease.

_____ **4.** Pertaining to an older person.

_____ **5.** Health care provided for older adults, usually age 65 and older.

_____ **6.** An acute and reversible condition characterized by mental changes.

_____ **7.** A syndrome of progressive cognitive decline characterized by memory loss and eventual loss of ability to care for self.

_____ **8.** Inability to remember, recognize, or describe people, places, times; confused perception of reality.

_____ **9.** Repeating of words or phrases said by another person.

_____ **10.** Also known as pocketing of food or medications (between the cheek and teeth).

_____ **11.** Difficulty swallowing, usually requiring evaluation by a speech therapist to prescribe a certain diet and method of feeding.

Terms

A. Sundown syndrome
B. Validation therapy
C. Reality orientation
D. Dysphagia
E. Pouching
F. Echolalia
G. Dangling position
H. Vertigo
I. Pathology
J. Holistic care
K. Restorative care
L. Geriatric
M. Geriatric care
N. Disoriented
O. Delirium
P. Dementia

_____12. Extreme dizziness.

_____13. Sitting up on the edge of the bed with the feet hanging down loosely.

_____14. A state of increased confusion and disorientation that usually occurs in persons with cognitive dysfunction as evening approaches.

_____15. A way of communicating with confused residents in which the caregiver follows the resident's lead and responds to the resident's feelings.

_____16. Reminding residents of the time, date, and name of the caregiver.

MULTIPLE-CHOICE QUESTIONS

Circle the letter next to the word or statement that best completes the sentence or answers the question.

1. Which of the following is an example of meeting the older adult patient's psychosocial needs?
   a. Providing meaningful activities in which he can participate
   b. Encouraging him to do as much as he is able
   c. Showing respect for him as an individual
   d. All of the above
2. The nursing assistant can help to keep the patient oriented by
   a. displaying a clock and calendar where the patient can see them easily.
   b. referencing daily events, such as, "It will be lunchtime soon."
   c. telling the patient where she is.
   d. all of the above.
3. Patients who are disoriented
   a. have clear recall of events that recently happened.
   b. may be quite lucid.
   c. may have difficulty remembering people, places, and times.
   d. should always be physically restrained.
4. In persons with cognitive dysfunction, __________ is a state of confusion and disorientation that may occur as evening approaches.
   a. moonbeaming
   b. stargazing
   c. sunstroke
   d. sundowning
5. An important responsibility of the health care team members is to provide safety for the older adult by
   a. exposing him to 8 hours of sunlight a day.
   b. making sure the patient is in a full sitting (dangling) position and not dizzy before standing up after lying in bed.
   c. keeping the patient in a room furthest from the nurses' station so others are not annoyed by his behavior.
   d. rushing the patient to complete simple tasks.
6. To make mealtime a positive experience, the nursing assistant should
   a. remove patient's dentures.
   b. place the tray in her room and give the patient privacy.

c. rush the feeding.
d. identify the foods and tell patients with visual impairments where to find them on the tray.

7. Because the nursing assistant must reposition and turn the non-ambulatory patient many times each day,
a. she should not worry about good body mechanics.
b. she should not ask your team members to help you.
c. she should use a pull (turn) sheet properly to prevent damage to the patient's fragile skin.
d. reddened areas on the patient's skin should be expected.

8. The patient should be repositioned
a. every 2 hours.
b. every 2 hours or whenever necessary to keep her in good body alignment and promote good circulation.
c. only when awake.
d. only when she asks to be moved.

9. A serious problem that can develop in bedbound patients who do not move around is
a. constipation.
b. muscle growth and increased strength.
c. an increased interest in food.
d. a dangerous increase in time spent watching television.

10. As the nursing assistant cares for the older adult, she should remember to treat the patient
a. with dignity and respect.
b. as you would want to be treated.
c. with kindness and gentleness.
d. all of the above.

11. A specialty within health care that relates to the care of older adults is
a. pediatrics.
b. energetics.
c. orthopedics.
d. geriatrics.

12. The Patient's Bill of Rights includes
a. assigning a doctor without the patient's input.
b. prompt response to reasonable requests.
c. sharing patient's medical information with all family members.
d. unreasonable treatment of caregivers.

13. According to the Omnibus Budget Reconciliation Act (OBRA), long-term care facilities must
a. provide free care.
b. inform the patient of his rights.
c. discharge the patient within 7 days.
d. bathe a patient each day even if he refuses.

14. During the aging process, a decrease in body fat and changes in the circulatory system can contribute to
a. the patient feeling cold.
b. increased sweating.
c. drier skin.
d. edema.

15. The ________ system is responsible for the way a person metabolizes food and the time it takes for a wound to heal.
a. circulatory
b. endocrine
c. respiratory
d. urinary

16. Changes in the gastrointestinal system during the aging process can lead to
a. an increase in the amount of saliva produced.
b. swallowing difficulties.
c. a patient wanting to eat more food than usual.
d. a faster metabolism.

17. Delirium is ________, whereas dementia is ________.
a. permanent; irreversible.
b. reversible; irreversible.
c. a slow onset; fast and progressive.
d. a normal part of aging; a disease that affects all older persons.

18. Miss Jones forgets where she placed her keys to her car; but, after searching for them and retracing her footsteps, she finds them within minutes. This is

a. normal and does not necessarily mean she has mild dementia.
b. a sign that Miss Jones is entering the moderate stage of dementia.
c. indicative of the most severe stage of Alzheimer's disease.
d. a sign that Miss Jones needs a home health care aide to watch her.

19. Mr. Williams, a 90-year-old male, becomes increasingly agitated each time he asks when his mother will come to pick him up. He begins to scream out, "When is my mother coming for me to take me home? You cannot keep me here all day!" The nursing assistant should

a. politely ask Mr. Williams to keep his voice down because he is disturbing other patients.
b. ignore his remarks because this is how he is all day long.
c. ask another nursing assistant to take him to his room.
d. Say, "You must miss your mother." Then ask him about his mother and the times he spent with her.

20. A sign that a patient is entering the terminal end of Alzheimer's disease is when he

a. begins to have trouble balancing his check book.
b. uses his knife to pick up peas and carrots.
c. wanders at night.
d. no longer can walk, forgets to eat, and has limited speech.

21. _________ is a common disease and disorder associated with old age and is the result of the breakdown of cells in the *macula*, an area on the retina of the eye, and causes loss of central vision.

a. Glaucoma
b. Retinal detachment
c. Macular degeneration
d. Blindness

22. A nursing assistant can apply _______ to a patient's dry, flaky skin to prevent problems from occurring.

a. cooking oil
b. lotion
c. cortisone cream
d. topical medication

23. When caring for a bedbound patient, the nursing assistant should

a. involve family members to care for the patient as much as they can.
b. encourage the patient to drink fluids frequently.
c. perform ROM at least once a shift.
d. all of the above.

24. When coughing, gurgling, or pouching is noticed when feeding a patient, the nursing assistant should _________.

a. ask the patient to swallow twice and then continue to feed.
b. offer fluids to help wash the food down.
c. rub the patient's neck firmly to stimulate swallowing.
d. stop feeding the patient and get the nurse.

25. One method to use when encouraging independence during feeding is to

a. orient a person who has difficulty seeing well to the food on his plate by using the "clock method" (e.g., chicken at 12 o'clock, potatoes at 3 o'clock, salad at 7 o'clock).
b. open all containers, cut food into small bites, pull the curtain for privacy, and leave the patient to eat quietly.
c. move the patient to the common dining room and have him sit with people he has never met.
d. put food on a spoon and play "choo-choo train," encouraging him to open his mouth.

TRUE OR FALSE QUESTIONS

Determine whether each question is true or false. In the space provided, write "T" for true and "F" for false. If the statement is false, rewrite it on the line provided to make it a true statement.

_____ 1. The spiritual needs of the patient can be met by involving the minister, priest, rabbi, or other spiritual leader in the plan of care.

____

_____ 2. Keeping lights on in a room can reduce disorientation.

____

_____ 3. An unsteady patient may be permitted to ambulate by himself if he is provided a walker or cane.

____

_____ 4. The walker and the patient's feet should be moving at the same time to ensure safety for the older adult when ambulating.

____

_____ 5. It is not the responsibility of the nursing assistant to be aware of what kind of special diet the patient may be required to follow.

____

_____ 6. Pillows should be placed behind the knees if the patient is going to be sitting for an extended period of time.

____

_____ 7. Providing daily hygiene to the bedbound patient helps the patient feel better and more relaxed.

____

_____ 8. Every person residing in a nursing home should be aware of his rights as outlined in the American Constitution and be able to refuse treatment should he desire to do so.

____

_____ 9. One way to increase the social aspect during mealtime is to sit with the patient and talk about things that interest her.

____

_____ 10. Giving the patient choices about what clothes to wear, what food he would like to eat next on his plate and allowing him to choose a morning or nighttime bath schedule are ways a nursing assistant can make a patient feel in control.

____

FILL-IN-THE-BLANK QUESTIONS

Provide the meaning of the following abbreviations.

1. AD _______________
2. CVA _______________
3. CHF _______________
4. COPD _______________
5. ADL _______________
6. ROM _______________
7. ID _______________
8. OBRA _______________

EXERCISE 33-1

Objective: To recognize common physical changes in older adults as they age.

Directions: Place the correct letters representing a system change next to the matching physical change.

System Change

SKS—skeletal system
CVS—cardiovascular system
US—urinary system
RS—respiratory system
ES—endocrine system
NS—nervous system
GS—gastrointestinal system
IS—integumentary system
MS—muscular system
MH—mental health

Physical Change

_____ **1.** Decreased ability to heal
_____ **2.** Decreased bladder tone (incontinence)
_____ **3.** Shorter memory; forgetfulness
_____ **4.** Decreasing strength
_____ **5.** Decreased muscle mass and tone
_____ **6.** Decreased lung capacity
_____ **7.** Increased pigmentation ("age spots")
_____ **8.** Increased incidence of depression
_____ **9.** Changes in sleeping patterns
_____ **10.** Decreased appetite
_____ **11.** Increased incidence of diabetes
_____ **12.** Decreased cardiac output
_____ **13.** Decreased kidney function
_____ **14.** Bones become brittle
_____ **15.** Decreased elasticity of ear drum

EXERCISE 33-2

Directions: Place a V or a RO on the line provided next to the following question for the best method to use in the scenario provided.

V—Validation Therapy
RO—Reality Orientation

_____ **1.** A 90-year-old resident wants to go home to an address he used to live when he was 9 years old.

_____ **2.** A 78-year-old man insists that his mother will miss him and he needs to leave right now to catch the bus because school is over.

_____ **3.** You enter a room in the morning and the resident asks is it morning or night.

_____ **4.** A resident asks you if this is the day his sister planned to visit with his niece.

_____ **5.** For the third time today, an 82-year-old patient begins to worry about what her mother will do to her when she finds out she broke the lamp in the living room.

EXERCISE 33-3

Directions: Using the following word bank, fill in the following boxes in relationship to feeding a resident.

Word Bank

Sit resident upright in the bed or a chair.
Offer foods and fluids separately.
Sit eye level with the patient.
Make sure dentures fit correctly.
Seat resident with peers who have common interests.
Clean the patient privately if spills occur.
Open all containers and cut food into small bites.
Offer foods the resident enjoys.
Offer food at a slow pace.
Offer choices and allow resident to decide what to eat next.

Methods to implement to ensure safety when feeding	Methods to implement to increase socialization or independence during feeding

EXERCISE 33-4

Directions: Complete the following crossword puzzle using the clues provided.

Across

3. Things look fuzzy (aging eye issue)
6. An umbrella term for forgetfulness
7. Yo-lay-e-hoo (repetitious language)
8. In the evening, his personality changes
9. Difficulty swallowing

Down

1. Today is Monday, October 24, 2012
2. Go where the person is in his reality.
4. "I feel blue."
5. The middle is missing (aging eye issue)

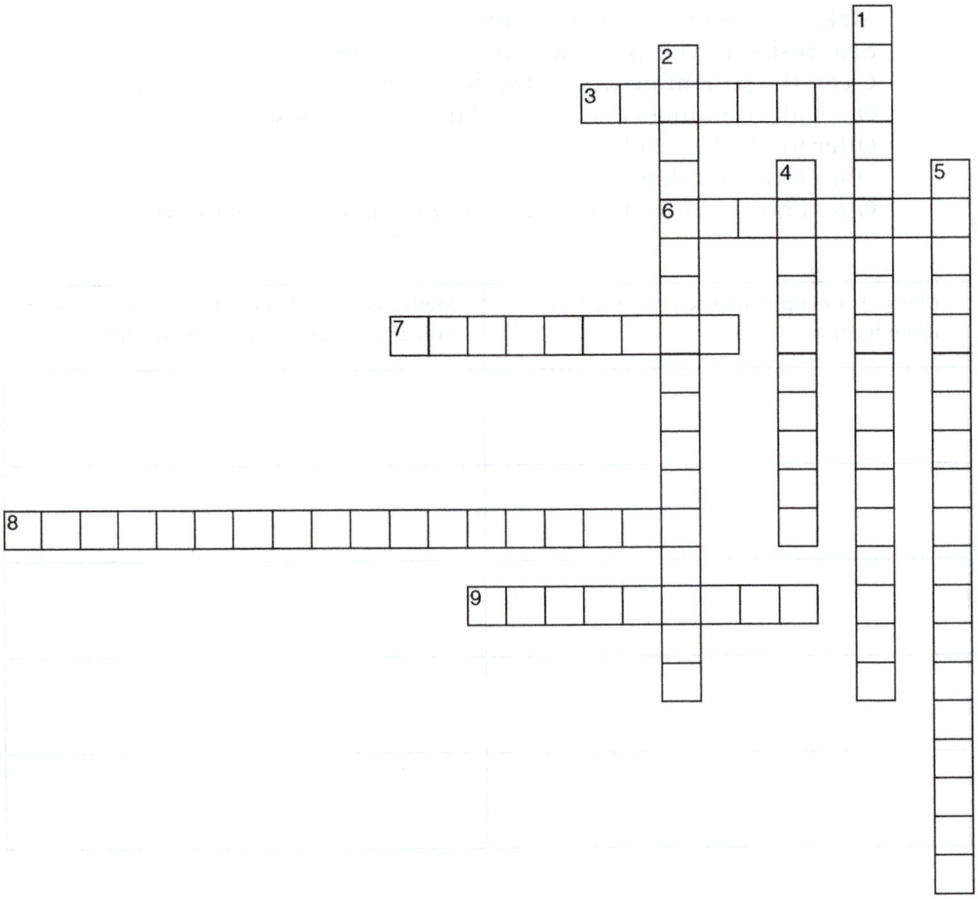

THE NURSING ASSISTANT IN ACTION

1. An 88-year-old woman was recently admitted to the nursing home where you work. Her children moved her to where they live some 200 miles away from her home so they could take care of her. She knows no one. Besides bringing some clothing, she has a few photo albums and her crocheting supplies. What should you do to help her adjust and encourage her to socialize?

____

____

____

____

____

2. Mr. Jones wanders throughout the day and into other residents' rooms. Sometimes he comes out wearing other residents' clothing and carrying objects that do not belong to him. His peers have had enough of this behavior. What should you do?

____

____

____

____

____

3. Mrs. Cathell has moderate Alzheimer's disease. You see her coming down the hallway swaying and flailing her arms, singing a raucous tune and taking off articles of clothing one by one. You approach her in her bra and underwear and she sings, "I am hot, hot, hot!" What should you do?

____

____

____

____

____

4. You are asked to assist a recreational therapist with an activity for a group of Alzheimer's residents in the art room. Larry is sitting at the end of the table repeating, "Mama, mama, mama." Nick, who has moderate Alzheimer's, cannot stand it anymore, gets up, and begins to strangle Larry, screaming to him, "I am not your mama. Cut it out!" What should you do?

____

____

____

____

____

5. You find that a resident, fully dressed and looking quite dapper, has walked off the locked Alzheimer's unit and into the parking lot with a visitor who mistook her for a visitor as well. What should you do?

____

____

____

____

____

LEARNING ACTIVITIES

1. Visit a locked Alzheimer's unit in a nearby facility. Ask if you can have a tour, and note all the technology and architectural components incorporated into the design used to help ensure the patient is safe. If possible, ask the employees about some methods they use when working with combative or difficult patients. Discuss you findings with your peers.
2. Make a list of a week's worth of clothing and accessories, two pieces of furniture you cannot live without, and items you might place in a box that could help you remember things that are important to you. Now consider leaving your home and family and being admitted into a nursing home. The only things you can take with you are those items on your list. You may or may not have a roommate. What are some feelings you may have about this exercise? What coping mechanisms do you have in place to help you stay positive about this move into your new "home"? With a peer, discuss ways you can help a new resident feel comfortable and supported as he adjusts to his new environment.

34

Rehabilitation and Return to Self-Care

Key Terms Review

Match the key terms in the right column with the definitions in the left column by placing the letter of each correct answer in the space provided.

_____ **1.** Ability to move.

_____ **2.** Producing, involving, or participating in an activity or movement.

_____ **3.** Bending movement that decreases the angle between two body parts.

_____ **4.** The motion that occurs when one body part is bent toward another body part.

_____ **5.** A straightening movement that increases the angle between two body parts.

_____ **6.** A motion where a body part is moved away from the midline of the body.

_____ **7.** A motion where a body part is moved toward the midline of the body.

_____ **8.** A motion that occurs when a body part turns on its axis.

_____ **9.** Making movable; putting into action.

_____ **10.** Exercises that move each muscle and joint through its full range of motion and help patients exercise the muscles and joints.

_____ **11.** Not active, but acted upon; enduring with effort or resistance.

Terms

A. Holistic
B. Restorative care
C. Rehabilitation
D. Subacute care
E. Physical therapist
F. Rehabilitation nurse
G. Occupational therapist
H. Prosthetics
I. Orthotics
J. Incontinence
K. Ventilator
L. Motivation
M. Psychological
N. Psychosocial
O. Fatigue
P. Apathy
Q. Depression
R. Unilateral neglect
S. Residual limb

_____12. Intended to meet the needs of the whole patient; based on the belief that human beings function as complete units and cannot be treated effectively part by part.

_____13. The process by which people who have been disabled by injury or sickness are helped to recover as much of their original abilities as possible for the activities of daily living.

_____14. Care given to help a patient attain and maintain the highest level of function and independence.

_____15. Ongoing medical, nursing, rehabilitative, or dietary care provided to patients who need a lower level of care than an acute care (i.e., hospital) setting provides.

_____16. A nurse with special training in the causes and treatment of disabilities; may be certified in this specialty.

_____17. Person trained to assist the patient with activities related to motion.

_____18. Person trained to assist the patient with performing activities of daily living.

_____19. Involving aspects of the mind, such as feelings and thoughts.

_____20. Involving aspects of living together in a group of people.

_____21. Reason, desire, need, or purpose that causes a person to do something.

_____22. Pain felt in the area where an arm or leg has been amputated.

_____23. A lack of feeling or interest in things.

_____24. Low spirits that may cause a change in activity.

_____25. A feeling of tiredness or weariness.

_____26. The portion of the arm or leg remaining after amputation; the stump.

_____27. Failure of a patient disabled on one side of the body to dress, bathe, or otherwise care for that side because the patient forgets that side exists.

_____28. The science concerned with making and fitting prosthetic devices, and devices that support or correct the function of a limb or the torso.

_____29. Artificial limbs or substitutes for missing body parts.

_____30. Machine that mechanically breathes for and provides oxygen to sustain a patient unable to inhale and exhale on his own.

_____31. Inability to control the bowels or bladder; inability to control urination or defecation.

T. Phantom limb pain
U. Mobility
V. Active motion
W. Passive motion
X. Range-of-motion (ROM) exercises
Y. Mobilization
Z. Abduction
AA. Adduction
BB. Flexion
CC. Extension
DD. Deviation
EE. Rotation

MULTIPLE-CHOICE QUESTIONS

Circle the letter next to the word or statement that best completes the sentence or answers the question.

1. Rehabilitation takes time and patience, and it often may not
 a. do any good.
 b. bring about a complete return to normal.
 c. challenge the patient.
 d. involve the patient.

2. The nursing assistant helps the patient gain skill in
 a. becoming dependent.
 b. feeding only.
 c. dressing only.
 d. dressing, personal hygiene tasks, and feeding.

3. The patient's motivation can be very helpful in the rehabilitation process by
 a. keeping him uninformed.
 b. providing fear of the unknown.
 c. stopping his involvement in the process.
 d. getting him interested in his treatment.

4. An observation of the patient that should be reported to the occupational therapist is
 a. tiredness.
 b. complaint of pain.
 c. how he tolerated each procedure.
 d. all of the above.

5. Which is not a responsibility of the nursing assistant?
 a. Listening to the patient
 b. Maintaining a safe environment
 c. Medicating the patient
 d. Observing the patient

6. Patients should be encouraged to dress in
 a. a hospital gown.
 b. the middle of the night, if they are awake.
 c. the bathroom.
 d. street clothes to enhance their feelings of self-esteem.

7. When dressing the patient, dress the weakest or most involved _________ first.
 a. nursing assistant
 b. family member
 c. extremity
 d. visitor

8. Rehabilitative care helps a patient ___________ whereas restorative care helps the patient ___________.
 a. return to an increased level of functioning; keep a current level of independence.
 b. return to his family; go to a nursing home.
 c. learn how to perform all activities of daily living; rely on a nursing assistant to do everything for him.
 d. return to original functioning before the accident or trauma occurred; regain 100% of the skill that was lost.

9. Holistic care makes sure that the spiritual, emotional, socioeconomic, physical, and ________ needs of a patient are assessed.
 a. feeding
 b. psychological
 c. family
 d. immediate

10. One reason rehabilitation may be ordered by a doctor is because
 a. the patient had eyebrow lift surgery and is still a little swollen.
 b. the patient has shown he can cope with her injury well.
 c. the patient was left in one position too long over a long period of time and has muscle weakness.
 d. the stitches from a laceration on the arm got infected.

11. Rehabilitation should start
 a. as soon as the patient wakes up from surgery.
 b. when an acute illness passes.

c. when the patient has the ability to walk and talk.
d. only when the patient is motivated and ready.

12. Another medical term used to describe an artificial leg or arm is called a(n)
a. orthotic.
b. fake extremity.
c. prosthesis.
d. assistive device.

13. It is the nursing assistant's duty to
a. make sure the patient does all the exercises listed in the care plan even if the patient complains of pain.
b. take the cane away from the patient who is carrying it over their arm and not using it correctly.
c. shout "Stop!" at the patient who carries their walker above the ground.
d. understand what the patient can and cannot do before carrying out assignments.

14. How often should a nursing assistant reposition a patient who cannot move easily in bed?
a. Minimally every 2 hours, unless repositioning is needed more frequently.
b. Once a shift.
c. Only after getting the person on or off a bedpan.
d. 8 times in an 8-hour shift.

15. The cane should be placed on the
a. stronger side of the body.
b. weaker side of the body.
c. side rail of the bed when not in use.
d. doorknob when the patient is sleeping.

16. Walkers and canes can be cleaned with
a. undiluted bleach.
b. a damp cloth with mild soap.
c. antiseptic wipes.
d. both b and c.

17. The person responsible for planning trips, holiday and dance parties, crafts and games, along with guest speakers in a nursing home is the
a. recreational therapist.
b. respiratory therapist.
c. movement therapist.
d. choreographer.

18. A social worker's role is to
a. get patients involved in craft programs.
b. offer advice on how to use a walker, cane, or crutch.
c. rearrange a person's furniture so falls do not occur.
d. provide emotional counseling as needed.

19. A sign or symptom of depression is
a. the patient is willing to participate in programs each day.
b. when a patient refuses to leave his room or have visitors for the last week.
c. when a patient smiles and tells you, "I cannot wait to get out of here tomorrow."
d. found crying after just being told his dog died.

20. A nursing assistant can build a trusting relationship with her patient by
a. keeping all the secrets the patient tells her.
b. being honest and explaining to the patient that he probably will never walk again, no matter how hard he tries.
c. letting him eat and drink whenever and whatever he wants.
d. making sure his room is clean, he is well groomed, and is wearing his non-skid slippers when he walks.

21. Mrs. Jones recently had a stroke. She takes a long time getting dressed. The nursing assistant should
a. dress the affected side first for her.
b. tell her that she will help her.
c. report to the nurse the amount of time Mrs. Jones needed to dress.
d. allow for a little more time so Mrs. Jones can try to dress herself.

22. Miss Aiken frequently chokes when eating and drinking. The nursing assistant should
  a. make sure all her food is pureed.
  b. make sure to use a lot of thickening product when preparing her meals.
  c. fill the spoon only half way and remind Miss Aiken to chew slowly.
  d. sit Miss Aiken up in a chair and wash her hands.

23. If a patient who had his right leg amputated complains of burning and pain, the nursing assistant should
  a. rub his leg vigorously to see if the pain goes away.
  b. assess the area every few days and tell him, "It is nothing but phantom pain."
  c. check the residual limb for bruising, redness, or skin damage.
  d. reassure him that this is just his mind playing tricks on him.

24. During bladder retraining, the nursing assistant should
  a. clamp the urinary drainage tube for the entire shift.
  b. reassure the patient that it is normal to feel pain and discomfort when bladder retraining occurs.
  c. place a rectal suppository in the patient to promote evacuation.
  d. keep a log updated as to when the patient voids during the day or between toileting.

25. When providing eye care to a patient on a ventilator, it is important to
  a. remember to wipe each eye from the cheek toward the nose.
  b. report any edema noted around the eye.
  c. never use artificial tear solution, because this can cause drying.
  d. tape the eyes open so nursing staff can assess for dryness.

TRUE OR FALSE QUESTIONS

Determine whether each question is true or false. In the space provided, write "T" for true and "F" for false. If the statement is false, rewrite it on the line provided to make it a true statement.

_____ **1.** An example of the nursing assistant developing a helping relationship with the patient is to discourage him from participating in his plan of care.

____

_____ **2.** The nursing assistant should encourage the patient to do as many personal care tasks as she is capable of performing.

____

_____ **3.** Cultural and religious beliefs may play an important role in the rehabilitative process.

____

_____ **4.** Subacute care facilities cannot take care of patients using ventilators.

____

_____ **5.** A barber or a beautician can be asked to join the rehabilitation team.

____

_____ **6.** OBRA requires nursing homes to offer rehabilitation or restorative care programs to their residents either on site or through contracted services.

____

_____ **7.** It is the role of the speech language pathologist to teach the patient how to use a cane, walker, or crutches.

____

_____ **8.** Discouraging a diet high in fiber and fluids is essential for bowel retraining to be successful.

____

_____ 9. A patient who has sensory changes as the result of a stroke should be taught to turn the hot water on first when bathing and turn the cold water off first when bathing is finished.

____

_____ 10. When a patient learns to dress himself in rehabilitation, he dresses the weakest side first when putting on his pants or top. However, when undressing, he is taught to take the clothes off the side that is unaffected first.

____

FILL-IN-THE-BLANK QUESTIONS

Provide the meaning of the following abbreviations.

1. OBRA _______________
2. ROM _______________
3. NA _______________
4. ID _______________
5. AROM _______________
6. PROM _______________
7. AAROM _______________
8. SNF _______________
9. IV _______________

EXERCISE 34-1

Objective: To recognize and correctly spell words related to rehabilitative care.

Directions: Unscramble the words in the following word list.

Word List

1. CATIVE _______________
2. AVITONIMOT _______________
3. GENRA FO NOITOM _______________
4. SICOTROHT _______________
5. BIMOZLTAOINI _______________
6. SPASVIE _______________
7. CITSILOH _______________
8. IHERIABLTOATNI _______________

EXERCISE 34-2

Directions: Locate and circle the words found in Exercise 34-1 in the following word search.

A	L	E	R	T	U	Y	A	Z	C	M	H	C	F	O	H	B	C
I	C	Q	Z	K	S	D	T	D	I	T	G	K	P	W	S	R	I
M	O	T	I	V	A	T	I	O	N	S	I	Z	S	O	C	E	D
J	P	A	I	C	Z	X	H	V	A	X	B	R	Z	W	A	H	S
K	G	Z	W	V	O	B	Z	V	H	Z	V	L	Z	A	P	A	K
C	Z	D	D	F	E	I	Z	S	D	Z	K	Z	R	O	V	B	R
B	O	F	S	F	U	G	R	O	P	C	Y	B	E	C	T	I	B
H	P	J	C	T	M	K	F	M	D	Q	S	D	I	Z	I	L	G
R	A	N	G	E	O	F	M	O	T	I	O	N	X	E	Y	I	S
K	S	T	Q	H	B	G	T	R	R	L	R	G	B	A	Z	T	L
L	S	A	M	X	I	A	Y	J	Z	F	T	Y	Z	F	C	A	J
D	I	J	D	U	L	Q	B	X	F	O	H	I	P	Z	O	T	B
M	V	O	S	S	I	M	B	W	B	H	O	L	I	S	T	I	C
F	E	C	G	Y	Z	O	L	B	H	D	T	K	O	D	V	O	Z
I	Q	T	A	I	A	T	G	K	O	D	I	O	I	J	M	N	D
E	P	B	H	X	T	C	P	Z	V	E	C	M	Z	C	Q	I	M
J	K	T	Y	D	I	J	Q	E	T	W	S	H	X	R	T	F	B
G	R	W	Z	Y	O	Z	C	D	Z	G	X	Y	K	S	P	K	O
B	L	X	L	Z	N	S	F	Z	K	C	O	I	D	E	O	A	J

EXERCISE 34-3

Objective: To apply what you have learned about rehabilitation and return to self-care.

Directions: Read the following riddles carefully before writing the correct answer on the blank line.

1. If your patient expresses frequent feelings of excessive tiredness and weariness, he may be showing this common symptom of depression. (*Hint:* If you were in the military, you would wear this item.)

____

2. A stroke or trauma can cause this function of the hand to become weak. (*Hint:* This can also be a stagehand in a movie production.)

____

3. Before beginning bladder or bowel training, keep track of the current excretory pattern for 2–3 days by writing it in this item. (*Hint:* This is also a fallen tree without branches.)

____

EXERCISE 34-4

Objective: To recognize important aspects of holistic care and appropriate actions to be taken.

Directions: Place the correct letters next to the holistic need described in each situation. Then circle the best response to meet that need. More than one letter can be selected for each situation.

PH—physical needs
SOC—social needs
EC—economic needs
SP—spiritual needs
PSY—psychological needs
M—mental needs
EM—emotional needs

1. Your patient has been incontinent of urine since coming home from the hospital.

LETTERS: ________________ What should you do?

A. You complain of the increasing amount of work this is for you.
B. You encourage him to stay positive.
C. You start a log to establish a voiding or evacuation pattern.
D. Both B and C.

2. Your stroke patient takes a very long time to dress herself.

LETTERS: ________________ What should you do?

A. You notify the nurse.
B. You help her so that it only takes a few minutes.
C. You keep her in her pajamas until all other work is completed.
D. No matter how long it takes, you let her select her own clothing and do as much of the dressing as she can.

3. Although the patient appears to receive comfort from it, you find that on days when the minister comes to see the patient, you are forced to reorganize your patient care duties to accommodate his visit.

LETTERS: ________________ What should you do?

A. You speak positively of the visit both before and after it occurs.
B. You report the minister to the nurse.
C. You continue with your schedule while he is there.
D. You encourage the minister to come only on days when you are not there.

4. During range-of-motion exercises, the patient mentions that he can't sleep at night because he is worried about his increasing health care bill.

LETTERS: ________________ What should you do?

A. You notify the nurse, who can make a referral to the financial counselor.
B. You tell him not to worry so much, and just to concentrate on the exercises.

C. You tell him about your financial difficulties.
D. You tell your family about your patient's problem.

5. The child you are working with watches television all day. He will complete his rehabilitation program soon and go back to school.

LETTERS: ________________ What should you do?

A. You encourage him to do the homework left by the teacher.
B. You do nothing, because it is not related to patient care.
C. You call the minister to speak to the child.
D. You do the homework for him.

6. The elderly patient you care for has diminished speaking ability. He is understandable, but it takes him a long time to get his thoughts communicated. Today, he wants to talk about his deceased wife, since, because this would have been their 50th wedding anniversary.

LETTERS: ________________ What should you do?

A. Encourage him to talk about his wife, and spend as much time listening to him as you can spare.
B. Remind him that he shouldn't live in the past.
C. Refer him to the speech therapist.
D. Continue working and hope that he will take his nap soon.

7. Mrs. Green is in rehabilitation for hand and arm injuries she received in an automobile accident. Her family lives far away, and she cannot afford to telephone them regularly.

LETTERS: ________________ What should you do?

A. Tell her not to think about them.
B. Give her crafts such as basket-weaving to occupy her mind.
C. Offer to write short letters to her family for her, encouraging them to write.
D. Do nothing, this is not related to her well-being.

8. Your patient spends quite a long time in bed each day and is unable to move or change position without help.

LETTERS: ________________ What should you do?

A. Make sure she assists you as much as possible when repositioning her in bed.
B. Take the time to give her backrubs twice a day.
C. Put her body in good alignment when positioning her with pillows.
D. All of the above.

THE NURSING ASSISTANT IN ACTION

1. You are assigned to take care of a devout Christian. You go to check on her and find her rocking back and forth, sobbing while praying in her chair and whispering loudly, "God, why are you punishing me so? I tried to be all you wanted; a faithful wife, a good mother and a devoted follower. Now I have this broken body! Is this another test of my faith?" What should you do?

____

____

____

____

2. While helping a patient unpack her belongings in her bedside cabinet, you notice she has quite a lot of herbal supplements she has brought with her to the rehabilitation unit. One bottle contains St. John's Wort. You say to her, "My, I have never known anyone to have this many herbal remedies. What do you take them for?" She replies, "Oh, for a multitude of problems I have. If you ever need anything, come to me. I can help you with your aches and pains." What should you do?

____

____

____

____

3. You hear a patient screaming for someone to help him. You enter the room of a patient who had both legs amputated from a farming accident. He is lying on the floor holding his residual limbs and crying out in pain, "I had to go to the bathroom. I forgot where I was and that I did not have any legs. I stood up and fell to the floor. I think I injured myself." What should you do?

____

____

____

____

4. You notice that a Jewish man you are caring for has long curls near each ear. His hair is long, and his beard is very shaggy and unkempt. You enter the room with an electric razor and offer to shave him and get the barber to come to his room to cut his hair. He looks at you with glaring eyes and retorts, "Are you that stupid that you do not know what you are asking is wrong? Get out of my room. You have insulted me. Never come back!" What should you do?

____

____

____

____

5. You must change soiled bed linens for a patient with a ventilator. You explain to the patient what you are about to do. His eyes open wide and he starts waving you away from the bed, indicating you to leave the room. What should you do?

____

____

____

____

LEARNING ACTIVITIES

1. Gather a button-down shirt or a zip-up cover-up top like a sweatshirt. Pretend you cannot use your dominant arm. Try undressing yourself first with the clothes you are wearing. Then try to dress yourself with the new clothing article. What did you find was difficult to do? What strategies did you use to get your clothes off and then on? Remember what it was like for you to go through this exercise the next time you work with a patient who has problems using his arms or legs. Encourage the patient to be as independent as possible, but assist when you observe the patient is getting frustrated. Offer them tips to use that you found helpful.
2. If possible, borrow a walker, crutches, or even a wheelchair from your learning facility or a friend. For a period of time, try to use one of these assistive devices in the community. What activities were difficult for you to perform? What response did you get from other people with whom you may have come in contact? How did you feel, both emotionally and physically, by the time this exercise was over? Discuss these findings with a classmate or peer and become more sensitive to those patients who use these assistive devices.

PROCEDURE CHECKLISTS

PROCEDURE 34-1: ASSISTING WITH FEEDING

Name: ____________________ Date: ____________________

STEPS	S	U	COMMENTS
1. Provide an opportunity for the patient to go to the bathroom and take care of all personal needs.			
2. Help the patient with hand washing.			
3. If the patient is eating in bed, position the patient in the Fowler's or semi-Fowler's position. If the patient is to eat at a table, make sure the patient is properly positioned and aligned in the chair, with his feet supported.			
4. If the patient is on a feeding/dining program, obtain specific instructions from the rehabilitation nurse or therapist before you start feeding. The nurse or therapist will also have information about how much help each patient needs with feeding.			
5. Wash your own hands.			
6. Check the diet order and the patient's wristband to make sure you are with the correct patient and that he has the correct diet.			
7. If the patient can handle finger foods but cannot grip a spoon or hold a glass or cup, arrange the plate so the finger foods are in reach.			
8. Sit down at eye level to assist with meals.			
9. Offer choices about seasonings and beverages.			
10. When offering food on a spoon, touch the tip of the spoon on the patient's tongue and gently press down. Do not fill the spoon more than half full.			
11. Allow the patient time to taste, chew, and swallow. A straw should be used with fluids. If a patient doesn't drink a sufficient amount of fluids during the meal, tell the nurse so that additional fluids can be offered between meals.			
12. Focus your attention on the patient you are feeding. Be alert for signs of choking.			
13. Document or report the patient's progress and any unusual observations.			

Charting:

____

____

____

____

Date of Satisfactory Completion ____________________

Instructor's Signature ____________________

PROCEDURE 34-2: BOWEL AND BLADDER REHABILITATION AND TRAINING

Name: ______________________ Date: ______________________

STEPS	S	U	COMMENTS
1. Assemble your equipment a. Urinal, if appropriate b. Bedpan or bedside commode c. Container of warm water d. Towel			
2. Wash your hands.			
3. Knock on the door and identify yourself to the patient. Explain what you are going to do.			
4. Identify the patient by checking the ID bracelet.			
5. Ask visitors to step out of the room, if this is your hospital's policy.			
6. Tell the patient that you are going to assist with use of a bedpan, bedside commode, or toilet.			
7. Pull the curtain for privacy.			
8. Raise the bed to a comfortable working position.			
9. Place the patient on a bedpan or on the bedside commode, or walk the patient to the bathroom every 2 hours to stimulate evacuation of the bowel and bladder.			
10. If the patient has difficulty in voiding, turn the water faucet on in the sink to let the patient hear the sound of running water, which may help stimulate the patient to void. You may also pour warm water over the genital area into the bedpan to stimulate elimination.			
11. Dry the patient with toilet tissue when finished.			
12. Remove the bedpan or assist the patient back to bed from the bedside commode or toilet.			
13. Assist the patient to wash hands.			
14. Make the patient comfortable.			
15. Lower the bed to a position of safety for the patient.			
16. Pull the curtains back to the open position.			
17. Raise the side rails when ordered, indicated, and appropriate for patient safety.			
18. Place the call light within easy reach of the patient.			
19. Wash your hands.			

20. Report to your supervisor • That the patient was placed on the bedpan, commode, or toilet on a regular basis • The time this was done • Whether the patient urinated or had a bowel movement into the bedpan, commode, or toilet. Chart this on the Intake and Output record. • How the patient tolerated the procedure • Any abnormal or unusual observations			

Charting:

____

____

____

____

Date of Satisfactory Completion ______________

Instructor's Signature ______________

PROCEDURE 34-3: RANGE-OF-MOTION EXERCISES

Name: ______________________ Date: ______________________

STEPS	S	U	COMMENTS
1. Assemble your equipment a. Blanket b. Extra lighting, if needed			
2. Wash your hands.			
3. Knock on the door and identify yourself and your purpose.			
4. Identify the patient by checking the identification bracelet.			
5. Ask visitors to step out of the room, if this is your hospital's policy.			
6. Explain to the patient that you are going to help her exercise her muscles and joints while she is in bed.			
7. Pull the curtain around the bed for privacy.			
8. Raise the bed to a comfortable working position.			
9. Assist the patient to a supine position (on his back) with knees extended and arms at his side.			
10. Loosen the top sheets, but don't expose the patient.			
11. Raise the side rail on the far side of the bed.			
12. Hold the extremity to be exercised at the joint (e.g., the knee, wrist, elbow)			
13. Exercise each shoulder.			
14. Exercise each elbow.			
15. Exercise each wrist.			
16. Exercise each finger.			
17. Exercise each hip.			
18. Exercise each knee.			
19. Exercise each ankle.			
20. Exercise each toe.			
21. Make the patient comfortable.			
22. Replace the sheets if a blanket was used. Fold and return the blanket to its proper place.			
23. Lower the bed to a position of safety for the patient.			
24. Pull the curtains back to the open position.			

25. Raise the side rails where ordered or indicated.			
26. Place the call light within easy reach of the patient.			
27. Replace any extra lighting in its proper place after washing with an antiseptic or disinfectant solution.			
28. Wash your hands.			
29. Report to your supervisor • That you completed range-of-motion exercises with the patient • The time the exercises were done • How the patient tolerated the exercises • Any unusual or abnormal observations			

Charting:

____

____

____

____

Date of Satisfactory Completion ____________________

Instructor's Signature ____________________

35

The Terminally Ill Patient and Postmortem Care

Key Terms Review

Match the key terms in the right column with the definitions in the left column by placing the letter of each correct answer in the space provided.

_____ **1.** Prewritten instructions on withholding, or not giving, resuscitation and life-prolonging measures and equipment.

_____ **2.** A strong emotional response of displeasure, irritation, and resentment.

_____ **3.** Trying to make a deal to change the situation.

_____ **4.** Admitting, understanding, or facing the truth or reality of the situation (e.g., one's death).

_____ **5.** Refusal to admit the truth or face reality.

_____ **6.** A place for keeping dead bodies temporarily for identification, autopsy, retrieval by funeral home staff, and burial.

_____ **7.** Deceased, dead.

_____ **8.** After death.

_____ **9.** The natural stiffening of a body and limbs shortly after death.

_____ **10.** Program that allows a dying patient to stay at home or in a nonhospital environment and die there while receiving professionally supervised care.

_____ **11.** Care designed to comfort, instead of cure, the patient.

Terms

A. Depression
B. Advance directive
C. Denial
D. Anger
E. Bargaining
F. Acceptance
G. Expired
H. Postmortem
I. Morgue
J. Rigor mortis
K. Terminally ill
L. Palliative care
M. Hospice

_____ **12.** Having an illness that can be expected to cause death, usually within a predictable time.

_____ **13.** A state of sadness, grief, or low spirits that may cause change of activity.

MULTIPLE-CHOICE QUESTIONS

Circle the letter next to the word or statement that best completes the sentence or answers the question.

1. Members of the family should be _______________ if they wish to spend increased amounts of time with the terminally ill patient.
   a. discouraged
   b. encouraged
   c. denied
   d. rescheduled

2. The family may want to stay with the patient, even if she
   a. is unconscious.
   b. is receiving care from the nursing assistant.
   c. has died.
   d. all of the above.

3. The patient's family may ask many questions; therefore, it is important that the nursing assistant
   a. know all the answers.
   b. only answer five questions per day.
   c. tell them to ask the nurse.
   d. understand what kind of questions he is allowed to answer and which questions should be referred to the nurse.

4. When the patient is visited by the pastor, rabbi, minister, or other religious leader, the nursing assistant should
   a. include the visitors.
   b. provide suitable music.
   c. provide patient care.
   d. provide privacy for them.

5. Unconscious patients require more time
   a. and less thorough care.
   b. and as thorough care as conscious patients.
   c. and less work for the nursing assistant.
   d. but are more responsive than conscious patients.

6. The patient's family should be directed to the _______________ so that they do not neglect their nutritional needs if they have spent long periods of time at the hospital.
   a. chapel
   b. lounge
   c. nurse's station
   d. cafeteria

7. The body of the deceased person must be
   a. treated quickly before the family arrives.
   b. removed immediately and taken to the morgue.
   c. pronounced dead by the nurse.
   d. treated with respect.

8. After the patient has expired, _______________ care is given.
   a. catheter
   b. postoperative
   c. postpartum
   d. postmortem

9. The dentures must be
   a. placed in the mouth immediately after death.
   b. discarded.
   c. placed in a bag and labeled with the patient's time of death.
   d. cleaned and stored.

10. The body should be placed in a flat, _______________ position.
   a. posterior
   b. standing

c. dignified
d. sitting

11. At the direction of the ____________, turn off the oxygen and IV.
a. family
b. clergy
c. significant other
d. nurse or doctor

12. Follow the ______________ policy on care of the patient's belongings.
a. finders keepers
b. family
c. sticky finger
d. institution's specific

13. In most instances, jewelry, especially wedding rings,
a. is removed immediately.
b. is given to any relative present at the death.
c. is removed by relatives as soon as death occurs.
d. should be taped in place instead of being removed, until the surviving spouse or family makes the decision to remove it.

14. Postmortem care should be done before ________________ occurs.
a. procrastination
b. nursing assistant resistance
c. corpus delecti
d. rigor mortis

15. ____________ must be worn by the nursing assistant when providing postmortem care.
a. A bath blanket
b. Disposable shoe covers
c. Disposable gloves
d. A face mask

16. A sign that death is approaching is
a. the face becomes pink.
b. the muscles get stronger.
c. the pulse gets weaker.
d. urine output increases.

17. Straighten up the room and remove any ______________ before the family comes to view the body.
a. valuables
b. furniture
c. emergency equipment
d. all of the above

18. Turn off any ____________ over the bed when finished with postmortem care.
a. call lights
b. electric blankets
c. bright lights
d. fans

19. In Elizabeth Kübler-Ross' five stages of dying, she believes
a. every patient and family member must go through each stage before grieving can occur.
b. patients go through these stages in an orderly fashion.
c. most terminally ill patients experience similar emotional responses to their diagnosis.
d. a patient who knows for a long time that he is dying will never go through any of these stages.

20. Mrs. Jones is found praying. You overhear her ask God that if she makes a deal with him to stop smoking, he should let her stay alive just long enough so she can see her granddaughter get married in a few months. Having learned about Kübler-Ross' stages of dying, you know that Mrs. Jones is
a. bargaining for more time because she has lung cancer.
b. accepting of the fact that she will die in a few months.
c. denying that she has a terminal illness.
d. angry that she may not live long enough to see the wedding.

21. Mrs. White, a 90-year-old patient living with advanced bone cancer, tells you, "I have lived a long, full life and have seen many a thing in this world. Now I am ready to meet my Maker and be with my husband, my

parents, my sisters and brothers, and my three babies I buried a long time ago. This body serves no purpose to me anymore." You know that Mrs. White

a. has accepted her diagnosis and is ready to die.
b. is bargaining for more time to live and do the things she never got to do.
c. denying the fact that she will ever get well.
d. is angry and feels hopeless and has lost purpose.

22. When the heart and lungs are removed from the body for donation,

a. the brain must be checked first to make sure there is no electrical activity detected that can support life.
b. this is called *harvesting.*
c. the patient is kept on a ventilator while surgery is being performed.
d. all of the above.

23. A terminally ill patient uses his call bell approximately every 20 minutes and asks you to check on him or to get him things he needs. As a nursing assistant, you

a. ignore the call bell after the third time because he is seeking attention because he is dying.
b. know this is abnormal behavior for a dying patient and ask the nurse to get a psychological consult for him.
c. explain to him that you have other patients to take care of and for him to think of all the things he needs right now so he can stop bothering you.
d. get what he needs and offer to spend some time talking with him after you get back from your dinner break if he would like for that to happen.

24. Mrs. Sweetbriar needs a bed bath. She is in a coma. However, her daughter just arrived for a visit. The nursing assistant should

a. reschedule the bath for tomorrow morning because she is not that dirty and it can wait.
b. ask the daughter to leave and perform the bed bath right this minute.
c. involve the daughter by asking if she would want to help you give the bed bath or if she would prefer it happen later in the day.
d. offer the daughter a few minutes to visit and then tell her to and come back tonight so this task can be completed before break occurs.

25. The nursing assistant suspects death is approaching for the patient because she observes and reports to the nurse that the patient's

a. respirations are fast and regular.
b. jaw is tight and the eyelids are tightly closed.
c. eyes appear to stare into space and there is no eye blink.
d. hands and feet are warm to the touch.

TRUE OR FALSE QUESTIONS

Determine whether each question is true or false. In the space provided, write "T" for true and "F" for false. If the statement is false, rewrite it on the line provided to make it a true statement.

_____ **1.** You can demonstrate to members of the family that the patient is well cared for by leaving the room as soon as they arrive for a visit.

____

_____ **2.** It is important that the family realize that the patient's needs are being met, even though she is near death.

____

_____ **3.** You can help the patient's family most by maintaining a concerned and efficient approach to your work.

____

_____ **4.** An Advance Directive describes the type and extent of care the patient wants at the end of life.

____

_____ **5.** Every patient who is diagnosed with a terminal illness will have a Do Not Resuscitate (DNR) order written by the doctor.

____

_____ **6.** It is not abnormal for a dying person to carry on a conversation with someone who may be dead already.

____

_____ **7.** The nursing assistant must respect the patient's rights when he is dying and even after he is dead.

____

_____ **8.** The nursing assistant does not need to report any skin damage that occurred to the nostrils or the ears when oxygen is administered via nasal cannula because tissue damage is expected in a dying patient.

____

_____ **9.** Pain may lessen as death approaches because it is believed that there is a decrease in oxygen to the brain and a change in the way pain is perceived.

____

_____ **10.** When performing postmortem care, the patient should be placed in supine position with a pillow under his head to prevent pooling of blood in the face and neck.

____

FILL-IN-THE-BLANK QUESTIONS

Provide the meaning of the following abbreviations.

1. AIDS ______________________________
2. DNR ______________________________
3. PMC ______________________________
4. IV ______________________________

EXERCISE 35-1

Objective: To recognize and correctly spell words related to the care of terminally ill patients and providing postmortem care.

Directions: Unscramble the words in the following word list.

Word List

1. SHPOCIE ______
2. LILPAAVTIE ______
3. DINLEA ______
4. GNINIAGRAB ______
5. PRDEEISNSO ______
6. CEPCAATCNE ______
7. TIRIPSAUL NEDE ______

EXERCISE 35-2

Objective: To apply what you have learned about care of the terminally ill patient.

Directions: Read the following riddles carefully before writing the correct answer on the blank line.

1. If you ask me, I will tell you that I get more from the patients than I give. Who am I? (*Hint:* Rhymes with "very dear.")

   ______

2. I can provide cleanliness, moisture, and lubrication, and I taste good too. Who am I? (*Hint:* I'm not made of only cotton, like my cousin, "Q.")

   ______

3. If the patient can feel clean, comfortable, and cared for, she will die with this important characteristic. What is it? (*Hint:* Important aspect of being human.)

   ______

EXERCISE 35-3

Objective: To recognize the needs of terminally ill patients.

Directions: Place the correct letters with the matching phrases. More than one set of letters may be selected for each phrase.

PN—Personal Need
VN—Visual Need
CN—Communication Need
EN—Elimination Need
OHN—Oral Hygiene Need
SN—Spiritual Need
PON—Positioning Need
NN—Nutrition Need
OXN—Oxygen Therapy Need

_____ **1.** Check nostrils for dryness and behind the ears for redness of the skin, where the tubing may cause irritation.

_____ **2.** Learn your institution's policy concerning religious observances and requirements at the time of death.

_____ **3.** Use a glycerin applicator for the mouth.

_____ **4.** As the patient becomes weaker, she may require more of your help with bathing or toileting.

_____ **5.** Change the bedding whenever necessary to keep the skin dry.

_____ **6.** Change the patient's position at least every 2 hours.

_____ **7.** Speak to the patient, even though he may appear unconscious.

_____ **8.** Semisoft foods may be easier to swallow than liquids.

_____ **9.** Adjust the light in the room to suit the patient.

_____ **10.** Members of the nursing staff should stay calm and sympathetic when working with the patient, her family, and her significant others.

EXERCISE 35-4

Objective: To recognize the five stages of death and dying.

Directions: Place the correct letters with the matching statements.

D—Denial
A—Anger
B—Bargaining
DP—Depression
AC—Acceptance

_____ **1.** "I know now that I won't last long. Life is too short! There are so many things I wish I had done with my life. Do you have time to listen to me if I tell you a little story right now?"

_____ **2.** "This can't be happening! The tests must be wrong. I never smoked or drank in my life!"

_____ **3.** "Well, you sure are slow today! If you take much longer with this bath I'll be dead before you finish!"

_____ **4.** "I have prayed every day since I found out about this problem I have. I have told God that if I get through this I will devote the rest of my life to the poor and unfortunate."

_____ **5.** "I guess this is really going to happen to me. I don't feel like talking today. I would just like to listen to the music on the radio and rest. Please close the door and pull the window shades down for me."

THE NURSING ASSISTANT IN ACTION

1. A 20-year-old man was in a motorcycle accident and has been placed on a ventilator. His family has just been told that he will never regain consciousness and he has no brain activity. The nurse asks the family to take some time to think about whether they would consider donating his organs. His parents confide in you that although he checked off he wanted to be an organ donor on his driver's license, they cannot bear to think how he might look in the casket once all his organs are harvested. What should you do?

____

____

____

____

2. Hannah, a 16-year-old patient dying of cancer, asks you to stay with her for a little while. You sit next to her on her bed and hold her hand. She is frail and looks thin and tired. In a whispered voice, she asks you, "What do you think will happen to me when I am gone?" What should you do?

____

____

____

____

3. A young mother wants to stay in the room with her dying toddler. She asks you if she can sleep in the bed with her daughter so she can make sure the child knows she is there should she take a turn for the worse at night. What should you do?

____

____

____

____

4. A new nursing assistant is asked to perform postmortem care. You find her crying in the bathroom only to find out she is really scared to have to prepare the corpse for the morgue because this is her first time ever seeing a dead person. What should you do?

____

____

____

____

5. You walk by a room where an 85-year-old woman is sitting vigil at the bedside of her dying husband of 67 years. You enter to see if you can get her anything and find her lying next to him, caressing his hair and singing softly to him. She looks at you with watery eyes and tells you, "I think he is gone. I think he died while I held him and sang him our wedding song. Doesn't he look peaceful?" What should you do?

____

____

____

____

LEARNING ACTIVITIES

1. Take some time and decide whether being an organ donor is the right decision for you. If it is, make sure key people and friends know your decision. If you have a place where you keep your medical information safe, then place your written request in that file or locked box. Make sure your driver's license is updated and your decision is noted on it as well. Although this is a difficult thing for most people to talk about with their loved ones, the more your family and friends know what you want, the less guilt and anxiety they will endure if a tragedy happens to you and the decision is left in their hands.
2. If you have not already done so, consider seeking the advice of a lawyer about creating a Will and an Advanced Directive. This is an important way to make sure your family understands what it is you want to happen to you if you should become injured or become terminally ill and die. In addition, it allows you to make sure that your children, loved ones, assets, and estate are taken care of properly. Nowadays, you can prepay for your funeral at most funeral homes. If this interests you, make an appointment with a funeral director to find out your options of arranging your own funeral so your loved ones do not have this responsibility.

PROCEDURE CHECKLIST

PROCEDURE 35-1: GIVING POSTMORTEM CARE

Name: ______________________ Date: ______________________

STEPS	S	U	COMMENTS
1. Assemble your equipment a. Soap b. Washcloth c. Towels d. Washbasin with warm water e. Bed protectors f. Clean gown			
2. Wash your hands and put on gloves.			
3. Turn off oxygen, suction, or IVs at the nurse's or doctor's instructions.			
4. Raise the bed to a comfortable working position.			
5. Lower the head of the bed so the patient is lying flat with the pillow under the head. This keeps the blood from pooling in the face and neck.			
6. Replace dentures if they are not in the patient's mouth.			
7. Gently close the eyelids if they are open. If they do not remain closed, notify your supervisor before the family comes to be with the body.			
8. If the body is soiled with urine or feces, clean gently to remove odor. Place clean bed protectors under the body.			
9. Straighten the body in a dignified position.			
10. Cover the body with clean bed linen, but do not cover the head.			
11. Straighten the room and remove any emergency equipment.			
12. Turn off the bright light over the bed.			
13. Remove gloves and wash your hands.			
14. Provide privacy and support for the family's visit.			

Charting:

____

____

____

____

Date of Satisfactory Completion ______________________

Instructor's Signature ______________________

36

Beginning Your Career as a Nursing Assistant

Key Terms Review

Match the key terms in the right column with the definitions in the left column by placing the letter of each correct answer in the space provided.

_____ **1.** On-the-job training or classes provided to enhance or expand an employee's skills or abilities.

_____ **2.** A skill or ability that can be demonstrated.

_____ **3.** Formal classes, courses, or training programs to develop new knowledge or qualify one for career advancement.

_____ **4.** Assessment of one's ability or skill to perform a given task.

Terms

A. Evaluation

B. Continuing education

C. Competency

D. Staff development

MULTIPLE-CHOICE QUESTIONS

Circle the letter next to the word or statement that best completes the sentence or answers the question.

1. The Omnibus Budget Reconciliation Act of 1987 (OBRA) requires health care facilities to hire nursing assistants
   a. who hold certificates.
   b. who study hard.
   c. who hold certificates or licenses from state-approved training programs and have completed the Nursing Assistant Competency Evaluation examination.
   d. who hold up well under stress.

2. Candidates for the competency examination must have completed a state-approved training course consisting of
   a. a maximum of 75 hours of hard labor.
   b. a minimum of 25 hours of classroom time.
   c. a minimum laboratory experience of 45 hours.
   d. a minimum of 75 hours of theory, lab practice, and supervised patient care.

3. The Clinical Skills Examination requires the involvement of
   a. an actor.
   b. a director.
   c. a producer.
   d. an agent.

4. Some of the tasks you may be asked to demonstrate are
   a. cooking, cleaning, and shopping.
   b. fishing, hunting, and gathering.
   c. toileting, applying a safety device, and personal care.
   d. occupying a made bed.

5. During the clinical skills examination, you should
   a. ask questions of the actor.
   b. draw conclusions about patient diagnoses.
   c. offer examples of how excellent you are.
   d. demonstrate competencies you have acquired during training.

6. After the clinical skills examination, you will be asked to take a written (oral in some situations) examination consisting of
   a. 100 true or false questions.
   b. 50 or more multiple-choice questions.
   c. 75 hours of written testimony.
   d. 50 open-book questions.

7. An important part of the multiple-choice examination includes the use of
   a. oral responses of the patient.
   b. medical terms and abbreviations.
   c. multiplication tables.
   d. study groups.

8. Upon completing your training course, you have a ____________ within which you must complete the testing process and register with the Nurse Aide Registry.
   a. "doorway to disaster"
   b. "hallway to success"
   c. "window of opportunity"
   d. "house of cards"

9. The Nurse Aide Registry keeps an official list of
   a. registered nursing assistants.
   b. missed "windows of opportunity."
   c. examination appointments.
   d. examination fees.

10. The best contacts for possible employment are
   a. local health care facilities.
   b. family and friends.
   c. help wanted classified advertisements in the newspaper.
   d. all of the above.

11. Most prospective employers require that you
   a. fill out an application.
   b. work the first pay period for free.
   c. pay for an application.
   d. bring a friend to be with you during the interview.

12. You should be sure to include your ____________ skills on your résumé.
   a. animal
   b. dancing
   c. singing
   d. people

13. Be sure that your stated objective on the résumé
   a. relates to the job for which you are applying.
   b. is clearly written.
   c. relates to the training you have received.
   d. all of the above.

14. It is important to ____________ and shake the interviewer's hand when the interview is over.
   a. smile
   b. look very serious

c. frown
d. avoid eye contact during the interview

15. It is preferred that you accept in writing because this gives you a chance to
a. write a thank-you note.
b. restate the salary, hours, or shifts you will work and the date you will start the job.
c. give a verbal reply.
d. change the agreement to better suit your expectations.

16. After you have been hired, you can expect
a. to relax and quit learning.
b. an orientation to the new job provided by the employer.
c. to take a vacation immediately.
d. to know everything about how to do your new job.

17. To make the most of your years of work in the future, you should
a. consult a psychic.
b. create a career path to use as a guide.
c. avoid further training.
d. avoid change whenever possible.

18. Education or career counselors at local colleges can provide you with free information on
a. how to advance your training.
b. how to get funding for school.
c. how to develop a career path.
d. all of the above.

19. Guidelines for keeping a job include ___________ and _____________.
a. tardiness; not coming to work
b. using alcohol; drugs before coming to work
c. violating confidentiality rules; abusing patients
d. none of the above

20. The most appropriate person to ask to write a reference letter about your work ethic and skill set would be
a. your spiritual counselor.
b. your neighbor.
c. an instructor who mentored you.
d. your mother.

21. For women, an appropriate outfit to wear to an interview would be
a. a scrub top and bottom.
b. a dark skirt, modest blouse, hose, and practical dress shoes.
c. brightly colored dress with dangling earrings and necklace to match.
d. a white starched lab coat over a bright-colored top with dress pants.

22. For men, an appropriate outfit to wear to an interview would be
a. a striped, short-sleeve shirt with a collar and colored jeans.
b. a white button-down shirt with a tie, dark pants, and dress shoes.
c. any clean and ironed scrub outfit.
d. earth-tone pants with a brightly colored shirt.

23. A course usually offered as a mandatory yearly in-service is
a. training about a new pain management pump.
b. information about a new procedure to dress a wound.
c. CPR renewal.
d. budget reconciliation.

24. A good reason for a nursing assistant to want to seek new employment at a different facility is because
a. she is genuinely satisfied with her position and pay.
b. her commute is too short to her current job.
c. her coworkers are volatile and harassing.
d. she is praised for her competency and skill.

25. A nursing assistant should give her current employer a(n) ________ after she has secured a new job in another facility and will leave her current position.
a. résumé
b. letter of reference
c. evaluation
d. resignation letter

TRUE OR FALSE QUESTIONS

Determine whether each question is true or false. In the space provided, write "T" for true and "F" for false. If the statement is false, rewrite it on the line provided to make it a true statement.

_____ **1.** In health care, the ability to be flexible with the hours you are willing and able to work is important to getting hired.

____

_____ **2.** If a job is offered to you, get a written statement concerning the conditions of employment.

____

_____ **3.** Gaining experience as a nursing assistant offers many opportunities for employment if you decide to change your career in the future.

____

_____ **4.** It is important to practice your interviewing skills with a friend, especially if you have never been in an interview before.

____

_____ **5.** You should arrive exactly at the time your interview is scheduled.

____

_____ **6.** Being bilingual in the health care field has no benefits whatsoever.

____

_____ **7.** Employers never reimburse you for any training courses you take to learn new skills.

____

_____ **8.** It is important to have many disciplinary referrals as possible in your employee file so when it comes time to change jobs or ask for a promotion, your employer can have record of your work ethic.

____

_____ **9.** Tardiness or being late for work is one of the most common reasons people get fired from their job.

____

_____ **10.** Being positive, simply stating why you are leaving a job, and thanking your current employer for the experience to work are important components to include in a letter of resignation.

____

FILL-IN-THE-BLANK QUESTIONS

Provide the meaning of the following abbreviations.

1. OBRA _____________________________
2. CSE _____________________________
3. ac _____________________________
4. hs _____________________________
5. PCA _____________________________
6. NA _____________________________
7. CPR _____________________________
8. CNA _____________________________

EXERCISE 36-1

Objective: To demonstrate the use of a career plan for a nursing assistant.

Directions: Label the career path shown in Figure 36-1 with the careers in the following word list. Next, starting with the year you will begin working as a nursing assistant, label each new job with an additional 5 years until you have completed the career path.

Word List

Food Service Worker
Laboratory Director/Manager
Advanced Nursing Assistant
Medical Assistant
Laboratory Aide
Radiologist, MD
Registered Nurse
Patient Care Technician
EKG Technician

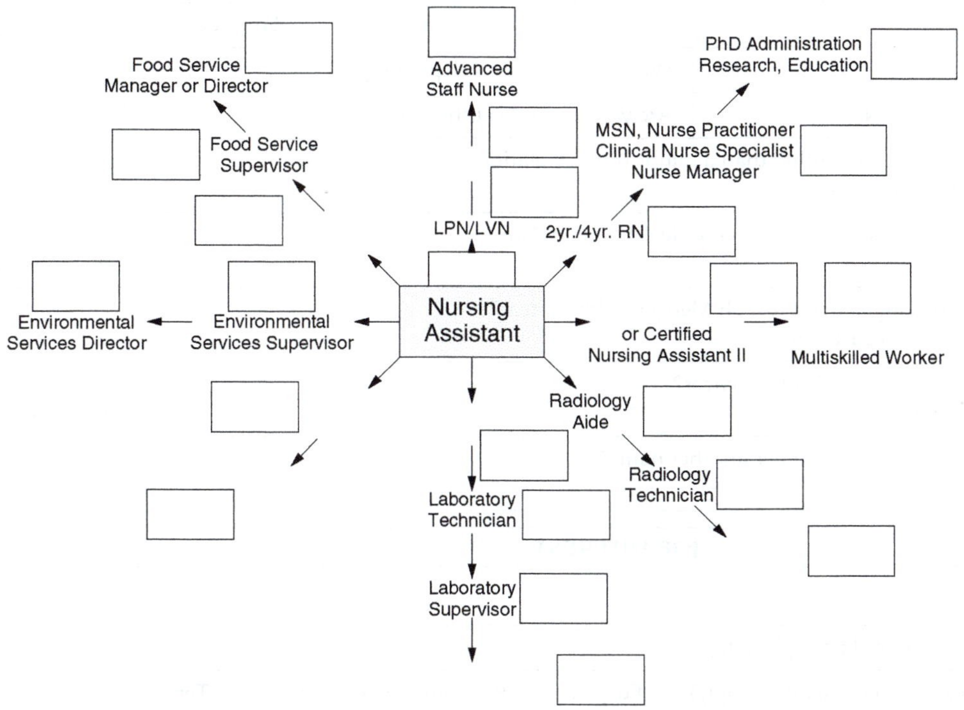

FIGURE 36-1

EXERCISE 36-2

Directions: Using Figure 36-2, fill in the blanks with your own information. Should you not be able to answer a question, place a "NA" for *not applicable* in that box. Use black or blue ink and print all information as neatly as you can. Place this in a file you created with your résumé and interviewing information. Because many applications ask for the same information, having this basic information with you to recall information quickly from one job to the next becomes easy.

SAINT JOSEPH MERCY HEALTH SYSTEM
A Member of Mercy Health Services

APPLICATION FOR EMPLOYMENT

Please indicate Unit desired:
☐ St. Joseph Mercy Hospital, Ann Arbor
☐ McPherson Hospital, Howell
☐ Saline Community Hospital, Saline
☐ Other______________________
please specify

We are an equal opportunity employer. Qualified applicants are considered for employment without regard to race, color, religion, sex, height, weight, national origin, age, marital or veteran status, or the presence of a non-job-related medical condition or disability. It is the applicant's responsibility to notify Saint Joseph Mercy Health System of any reasonable accommodation necessary to perform the essential duties of the position for which the applicant has applied.

Important - Please Type or Print Clearly in Ink

PERSONAL DATA

Date	Social Security Number
Last Name First Middle	
Address City State Zip Code	
Home Telephone ( )	Work or Alternate Telephone ( )
Are you age 18 or older? ☐ Yes ☐ No	Are you currently authorized to work in the U.S.? ☐ Yes ☐ No

Have you ever been convicted of a crime other than a minor traffic violation?
If yes, give circumstances, place, and date: ☐ Yes ☐ No

Have you ever been employed at a Saint Joseph Mercy Health System Unit?
If yes, give date(s) and location(s): ☐ Yes ☐ No

Do you have any relative(s) working at Saint Joseph Mercy Health System?
List Name(s)/Relationship/Unit/Department ☐ Yes ☐ No

Have you ever been employed by Mercy Health Services?
If yes, give date(s) and location(s): ☐ Yes ☐ No

Have you ever worked or attended school under another name?
If yes, what name(s): ☐ Yes ☐ No

JOB INTEREST

Position Desired:

Department or Clinical Area Preferred (if applicable)

Indicate your availability to work (check all that apply) ☐ Full-time ☐ Part-time ☐ Contingent ☐ Temporary
☐ Days ☐ Afternoons ☐ Midnights ☐ Weekends ☐ Holidays ☐ Shift Rotations

If Part-time, specify days and hours available:

Earliest Date Available__________________ Minimum Pay Required $ ____________ Per Hour

How did you hear of this position? ☐ Newspaper/Journal* ☐ School* ☐ Recruitment visit/job fair*
☐ Employee ☐ Relative ☐ Friend ☐ Other*
*Please Specify______________________________

Are you currently employed? ☐ Yes ☐ No

May we contact your present employer? ☐ Yes ☐ No *Contact must be made before an employment offer is finalized

01030R 8/97 (PC)D

FIGURE 36-2 Application for Employment (Courtesy of Saint Joseph Mercy Health System, Ann Arbor, MI).

EDUCATION AND TRAINING

	Date Started	Date Finished	School Name and Location	Major	Graduated	Degree/ Diploma	GPA
High School					☐ Yes ☐ No Yrs. Completed____		
College/ University					☐ Yes ☐ No Yrs. Completed____		
College/ University					☐ Yes ☐ No Yrs. Completed____		
Technical/ Vocational					☐ Yes ☐ No Yrs. Completed____		
Other					☐ Yes ☐ No Yrs. Completed____		

Student Clinical Rotations, Internship Programs	Date Started	Date Finished	Name of Facility	Type of Clinical

Describe work related skills, qualifications, achievements and contributions that you would bring to Saint Joseph Mercy Health System: ____________________

____

____

PROFESSIONAL CERTIFICATION REGISTRATION DATA

What profession(s) are you licensed, certified or registered to practice?

____

____

By examination in: State Number Expiration date

By endorsement in (reciprocity): State Number Expiration date

Are there restrictions on your license? ☐ Yes ☐ No If yes, please explain:

Are you eligible for licensure, certification or registry? ☐ Yes ☐ No

Profession Anticipated Date of Exam

List any current memberships in professional or technical associations. (Those which indicate race, color, religion, sex, or national origin may be excluded.)

____

____

____

____

____

FIGURE 36-2 (*cont.*)

EMPLOYMENT HISTORY

Beginning with your CURRENT or most RECENT employer, list the last four positions held including Military Service in date order. (Should you choose to list volunteer activities, those which indicate race, color, religion, sex, national origin may be excluded.)

Name of Employer	Position Held	From (Month/Year) To (Month/Year)
Address	Name and Title of Supervisor	Hours Per Week
City State Zip	Telephone # ( )	Base Hourly Rate/Salary
Type of Business	Reason for Leaving	
Duties		

Name of Employer	Position Held	From (Month/Year) To (Month/Year)
Address	Name and Title of Supervisor	Hours Per Week
City State Zip	Telephone # ( )	Base Hourly Rate/Salary
Type of Business	Reason for Leaving	
Duties		

Name of Employer	Position Held	From (Month/Year) To (Month/Year)
Address	Name and Title of Supervisor	Hours Per Week
City State Zip	Telephone # ( )	Base Hourly Rate/Salary
Type of Business	Reason for Leaving	
Duties		

Name of Employer	Position Held	From (Month/Year) To (Month/Year)
Address	Name and Title of Supervisor	Hours Per Week
City State Zip	Telephone # ( )	Base Hourly Rate/Salary
Type of Business	Reason for Leaving	
Duties		

Please Read The Following Carefully And Sign Where Indicated Below:

I have read all the questions and answers, and certify that the information given by me in this application is correct to the best of my knowledge. I understand that any false statements or answers or omissions may be grounds for dismissal. I further understand that my employment is contingent upon the satisfactory completion of a physical examination, including a drug screen, to be conducted by Saint Joseph Mercy Health System. I specifically authorize Saint Joseph Mercy Health System and Mercy Health Services to release all records or other information pertaining to any disciplinary action taken against me during my employment. I hereby release Saint Joseph Mercy Health System and Mercy Health Services, and their agents and employees from any liability whatsoever resulting from the release of such records or information. I hereby waive my right to written notice from my present and/or former employers whenever a disciplinary report, letter or reprimand, or other disciplinary action regarding me is divulged by my present or former employers, including but not limited to reports of disciplinary action which by law must be disclosed pursuant to M.C.L. 333.20175(5).

Signature of Applicant ______________________________ Date ______________

FIGURE 36-2 (*cont.*)

TO BE COMPLETED BY HIRING DEPARTMENT

Position Title	Base Hourly Rate of Pay
Department Name	Position Code Pay Grade
Department/Cost Center Number	Hours/pay period
Employment Status ☐ New Hire ☐ Rehire Starting Date and Time ______________	Shift Hours _____ AM / PM to _____ AM / PM Days _____ AM / PM to _____ AM / PM Afternoons _____ AM / PM to _____ AM / PM Midnights (Work hours and/or work days may change according to department needs.)
☐ Full-time ☐ Non-Exempt ☐ Hourly ☐ Part-time ☐ Exempt ☐ Salaried I ☐ Contingent ☐ Salaried II ☐ Term Expires ___/___/___ ☐ Temporary Expires ___/___/___	**Special Conditions of Employment, If Any** (Weekends, holidays, shift rotation, etc.)

☐ Offer reviewed by Human Resources ______________ (Specialist initials)

Authorized Management Signature ______________________ Date ____________

I accept the above offer and in consideration of my employment I agree to conform to the rules, regulations and policies of Saint Joseph Mercy Health System. I understand the first 180 days of employment are designated as an orientation period.

New Employee Signature ______________________ Date ____________

FIGURE 36-2 (*cont.*)

EXERCISE 36-3

Directions: Using the following template, create your own résumé and save it to a computer hard drive or a USB. Even though you may think you do not have a lot of work experience, be sure to include any job in which someone left you in a decision-making role, you have taken care of people as a volunteer or for pay, or organized events. It is important for a potential employer to see that you are responsible and can solve problems. Tailor the résumé to include only those areas in which you have experience, and delete those subheadings for areas that you may not have experience, like community or volunteer work. Be sure to include things like CPR certification and your CNA certification, if you already have received this training.

The last line of your résumé should include a line that states, "References upon request." On a separate piece of paper, title it with your name, address, phone number(s), and e-mail account. List three references who have agreed to be a reference for you and who can speak positively about your work ethic and morals. Consider placing a previous employer; someone affiliated with your spiritual practice; and a counselor, teacher, or coworker on this reference sheet. Refer to Figure 36-3 as an example.

Cathy Sands
3899 Pine St
Durham NC 12345
(555) 490-5555

OBJECTIVE

- Dedicated, service-focused individual seeking nursing assistant entry position
- Highly motivated to begin nursing career and continuing education to earn a RN license

PERSONAL TRAITS

- Reliable worker with demonstrated ability to learn new concepts and skills
- Solid work history, reputation as a team player and passion for helping others
- Background includes experience caring for terminally ill grandparent
- Healthy and energetic; current on all immunizations (including tuberculosis and hepatitis B)

WORK EXPERIENCE

Waitress
6/2008-6/2010 Chili's, Oak Creek location, part-time hostess and waitress

- Received "exemplary" and "exceeds expectations" ratings on all performance reviews Cited for excellence in interpersonal communications, teamwork, customer service, flexibility and reliability
- Demonstrated ability to interact with customers from diverse cultures and backgrounds
- Transformed "difficult" customers into loyal, repeat guests by finding win-win resolutions to problems

FIGURE 36-3 Sample résumé

Primary Care Provider
10/2008-3/2010

- Shared joint responsibility (along with mother) for the care of terminally ill grandparent in our home
- Learned the basics of taking patient vital signs and providing care from a home healthcare nurse and nursing assistant training program
- Assisted home nurse and hospice staff with all aspects of daily care, including bathing, feeding and dressing
- Helped to ensure grandparent's last year was comfortable and dignified

AFFILIATIONS

Orange Country Animal Shelter, Volunteer
Good Sheppard Church, assist with Sunday school class

EDUCATION

6/2009, Riverside High Durham NC 27710 Graduated with 30 average; played on soccer team
6/2010 Vance Granville Successfully completed nurse assistant training course; registered with NC Nursing Board

SKILLS

Skill Name	Skill Level	Last Used/Experience
Customer Service	Expert	Currently used/3 years
Interpersonal Communications	Expert	Currently used/3 years
MS Outlook	Intermediate	Currently used/3 years
MS Word	Intermediate	Currently used/3 years

ADDITIONAL INFORMATION

Available for all shifts, extended hours and weekend assignments.

References Available upon request

FIGURE 36-3 ***(cont.)***

THE NURSING ASSISTANT IN ACTION

1. You are driving to an interview when you get stuck in commuter traffic. You do not have a cell phone with you, and you know you will be late for the interview. What should you do?

2. The nurse you are assigned to work with is demeaning and frequently makes you feel incompetent. She never has anything nice to say to you or about the patients for whom you care. You dread going to work when you know she will work the same day as you. Her negativity has influenced many of your coworkers as well, and you find it increasingly difficult to stay positive. What should you do?

3. You enjoy your job, but you feel like you need to be more challenged intellectually. You heard there is a job opening on the unit two floors up, where the type of patient care is more complex. You love what you do, and the people with whom you work are great. Your boss has been really kind and supportive of you in the last three years you have worked for her. You are not sure how to go about looking into this new opportunity and the advances it might offer. What should you do?

4. A coworker just received notice that she got the job that you both applied for in the same facility you currently work. You know that she had some disciplinary referrals and had a previous track record of being tardy to work. Your work ethic is stronger and your employee record is stellar. You are left to wonder why you were not chosen for the job for which you applied, and are hurt by the fact that you were not recognized for your hard work. What should you do?

____

____

____

____

____

5. You have applied for and been offered a job a few miles from your home. The pay is better, the shift better suits your caregiving needs, and the job is more challenging. However, you have just received your 10-Year Pin and the "Employee of the Year Award" at your current job. You are grateful to your current employer for supporting you all these years and know that writing a resignation letter is the professional thing to do. What should your letter of resignation say?

____

____

____

____

____

LEARNING ACTIVITIES

1. Find someone in your life who manages a business or even a trusted friend. For approximately 15 minutes, have them pretend to interview you for a nursing assistant job. Practice answering basic questions, including questions that allow you to speak about your work ethic and about some of your weaknesses when working with others. Be sure to consider how you made attempts to overcome and change these weaknesses into a positive experience, or add what you learned about yourself and how you have grown professionally. Keep your answers succinct and short. Once finished, ask the person for constructive feedback about your body language, the words you used, length of time it took you to answer, and the quality of the answers you gave.

Before a real interview occurs, practice by asking yourself some common interview questions a potential employer may ask. Watch yourself in the mirror, and assess your body language and facial expressions. Record and replay your answers to hear yourself. Critique your own answers, voice modulation, and enthusiasm when responding.

Interviewing is an art form and a way to market yourself. Only practice and critiquing helps you overcome your initial nervousness and affords you the opportunity to "sell" yourself in a professional manner.

2. A few days before an interview occurs, go through your clothes closet and pick out an outfit that is appropriate for an interview. Check to make sure it is clean and free of stains and odors. Try it on to make sure it fits.

For women, try adding simple accessories like stud earrings, one ring, a pin, or modest necklace. Any makeup should be sensible and minimal to accent your natural beauty. For men, a tie tack, watch, and a ring is appropriate, but leave necklaces home, or place them inside dress shirts and take off any earrings. Body piercings and tattoos should be covered. For both men and women, make sure you have hose/socks and shoes that are practical and are in good condition. If your hair is long, try tying it back or grooming it away from your face. Nails should be ½" above the top of the fleshy tip of each finger and filed. A clear or light-colored polish can be worn.

If something is not quite right with your outfit, then you have time to buy something more suitable or fix what is wrong. Do not wait until the night before the interview to do this. The more you prepare, the less stress you will encounter when it is time to interview.